Manual Therapy Masterclasses

The Vertebral Column

For Churchill Livingstone:

Commissioning Editor: Mary Law
Development Editor: Kim Benson
Project Manager: Lucy Thorburn
Production Manager: Marina Maher
Layout and Cover Design: Marie Prime

Manual Therapy Masterclasses
The Vertebral Column

Edited by

Karen S. Beeton

Principal Lecturer, Department of Allied Health Professions — Physiotherapy
University of Hertfordshire, Hatfield, United Kingdom

Foreword by

Gwendolen A Jull and **Ann P Moore**

CHURCHILL
LIVINGSTONE

EDINBURGH LONDON NEW YORK OXFORD PHILADELPHIA ST LOUIS SYDNEY TORONTO 2003

Churchill Livingstone
An imprint of Elsevier Limited.

ISBN 0 443 07403 8

British Library Cataloguing in Publication Data
A catalogue record for this book is available from the British
Library.

Library of Congress Cataloging in Publication Data
A catalog record for this book is available from the Library of
Congress.

Note
Medical knowledge is constantly changing. As new
information becomes available, changes in treatment,
procedures, equipment and the use of drugs become
necessary. The author/contributors and the publishers have
taken great care to ensure that the information given in this
text is accurate and up to date. However, readers are strongly
advised to confirm that the information, especially with
regard to drug usage, complies with the latest legislation and
standards of practice.

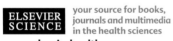
your source for books,
journals and multimedia
in the health sciences
www.elsevierhealth.com

The
Publisher's
policy is to use
**paper manufactured
from sustainable forests**

Printed by Grafos S.A. Arte sobre papel, Spain.

Contents

Contributors

Kim Bennell
Associate Professor, School of Physiotherapy,
The University of Melbourne, Melbourne, Victoria,
Australia

Geert Crombez
Professor, Department of Experimental Clinical and
Health Psychology, University of Ghent, Ghent,
Belgium

Mark J Comerford
Senior Director, Kinetic Control, Southampton,
United Kingdom

Lawrence DeMann Jr
Director, Manhattan Chiropractic Center,
New York, USA

Robert Elvey
Senior Lecturer, School of Physiotherapy,
Curtin University of Technology, Bentley, Perth,
Australia

Linda Exelby
Clinical Specialist, Pinehill Hospital, Hitchin,
North Herts, United Kingdom

Peter Gibbons
Head, School of Health Sciences, Faculty of Human
Development, Victoria University, Melbourne, Australia

Toby Hall
Adjunct Senior Fellow — Teaching, School of
Physiotherapy, Curtin University of Technology,
Bentley, Perth, Australia

Julie Hides
Clinical Supervisor, The University of Queensland,
Mater Hospital Back Stability Clinic, Mater
Misericordiae Health Sciences, South Brisbane,
Queensland, Australia

Gwendolen A Jull
Associate Professor, Department of Physiotherapy,
The University of Queensland, St. Lucia, Brisbane,
Queensland, Australia

Karim Khan
Sports Physician, Department of Family Practice and
Orthopaedics, University of British Columbia,
Vancouver, BC, Canada

Diane G Lee
Clinical Director, Delta Orthopaedic Physiotherapy
Clinic, Delta, BC, Canada

Christopher McCarthy
Research Physiotherapist, The Centre for
Rehabilitation Science, University of Manchester
and Manchester Royal Infirmary, Manchester,
United Kingdom

Jenny McConnell
McConnell and Clements Physiotherapy, Mosman,
Sydney, New South Wales, Australia

Heather McKay
Associate Professor, Department of Family Practice
and Orthopaedics, University of British Columbia,
Vancouver, BC, Canada

Sarah Mottram
Director, Kinetic Control, Southampton, United
Kingdom

Peter B O'Sullivan,
Senior Lecturer, School of Physiotherapy,
Curtin University of Technology, Bentley, Perth,
Australia

Carolyn Richardson
Associate Professor, Department of Physiotherapy,
The University of Queensland, St. Lucia, Brisbane,
Queensland, Australia

Stephen E Sandler
Senior Lecturer, The British School of Osteopathy,
Founder and Director of The Expectant Mothers
Clinic, London, United Kingdom

Philip Tehan
School of Health Sciences, Faculty of Human
Development, Victoria University, Melbourne, Australia

Johan W S Vlaeyen
Department of Medical, Clinical & Experimental
Psychology, Clinical and Experimental Psychology,
Maastricht University, Maastricht, The Netherlands

Foreword

In developing the objectives for the *Manual Therapy* journal, it was considered important to produce a journal for the publication of scientific works in the field and, at the same time, have a special feature which focused on the clinical management of patients. Hence a Masterclass section was instituted where leading clinicians and researchers are invited to contribute work on aspects of contemporary clinical practice.

Spinal pain is the most common musculoskeletal disorder of modern day society and accordingly, is the most common disorder managed by practitioners of manual therapy. Not surprisingly, several of the Masterclass features published in *Manual Therapy* have focused on aspects of disorders of the vertebral column. The series of Masterclasses brought together in this volume present some of the many circumstances that confront the practitioner in their daily clinical practice. Collectively, they reflect the biopsychosocial model of spinal pain, which is the basis of current treatment approaches. Chapters deal with the entire spectrum of issues, ranging from the physical or 'mechanism-based' clinical reasoning and diagnostic process used by manual therapy clinicians to understand patients' presenting pain and functional problems, to psychosocial issues which need to be considered in the holistic management of the spinal pain patient.

This collection of papers also reflects contemporary manual therapy practice, and contributors have taken the opportunity to add a postscript to their original work. Manual therapy is no longer focused almost exclusively on manipulative therapy. Presentations deal with examination and management of all systems, including the articular, muscle and neural systems and, accordingly, the management approaches are inclusive of manipulative therapy and other pain relieving techniques, therapeutic exercise and education in a multi-modal management regime. This is in accord with conclusions of the latest systematic reviews for evidence-based clinical practices. Notably, this Masterclass collection includes the key changes that have occurred in therapeutic exercise in recent times with the increasing understanding of the nature of motor control problems associated with spinal pain syndromes. Of importance, the manual therapist's concerns with preventative health and healthy lifestyle are beginning to emerge and are an important area for future manual therapy practice.

This collection of Masterclasses also reflects the multi-disciplinary nature of modern manual therapy. Manual therapy is not discipline specific; rather, all disciplines have taken up the challenge of evidence based practice and this is reflected in this series of papers. We have not solved the problem of spinal pain, and clinicians can push the boundaries with their experiences and ideas. The international exchange of knowledge and practice between disciplines can only further the research in the field and the practice of the clinician to the ultimate benefit of the patient.

As co-editors of *Manual Therapy*, we trust that clinicians will enjoy this series of papers on contemporary manual therapy practice for the vertebral column. We extend our congratulations to Karen Beeton, the Editorial Committee member responsible for this section of the journal, for compiling this series. We look forward to her continuing work with *Manual Therapy* in the production of the Masterclass section.

Gwendolen A. Jull
Ann P. Moore
Manual Therapy Editors

Preface

Manual Therapy is an international peer-reviewed journal that presents current research on all aspects of manual and manipulative therapy of relevance to clinicians, educators, researchers and students with an interest in this field. The journal, which is now in its 8th year of publication, includes review articles, original research papers, case reports, abstracts, book reviews and a bibliography. Such is the quality of the papers published, it is one of the few allied health journals to be indexed in Index Medicus and Medline.

One of the core components of the *Manual Therapy* journal is the Masterclass. The purpose of the Masterclass section is to describe in detail clinical aspects of patient management within a theoretical, evidence-based framework. This may relate to specific treatment techniques, a particular management strategy or the management of a specific clinical entity. Illustrations are a key aspect of the Masterclass in order to facilitate the integration of the clinical concepts by the readers. The authors are all leading clinicians and researchers in the manual therapy field. The Masterclass section of *Manual Therapy* provides an opportunity for these authors to present their approach to a wider audience. These Masterclasses therefore represent the cutting edge of clinical practice today.

Elsevier Science, the publishers of *Manual Therapy*, have decided to republish selected Masterclasses in two books. This book features a compilation of previously published Masterclasses on the subject of the vertebral column. The other book is a compilation of previous Masterclasses focusing on the peripheral joints. The purpose of this initiative was to draw together topics of related interest and to facilitate accessibility of these articles for the readers. The Masterclass authors were invited to write a short postscript if they wished, reflecting on any developments in the evidence base and/or new developments in clinical practice since the original publication of their paper.

Manual Therapy Masterclasses — The Vertebral Column consists of 15 Masterclasses on all aspects of assessment and management of the spine. The Masterclasses have been classified according to the regional areas of the spine and cervical, thoracic, lumbar and sacroiliac joints depending on the main focus of the article. There is also a section on general spinal issues and an index is included.

The postscripts which accompany the articles raise three issues. First, they demonstrate the breadth of research currently being carried out in the various fields and secondly, they draw on new evidence to support the use of the clinical concept or management strategy. Thirdly, they highlight the progression in the clinical reasoning and decision-making processes underpinning the concepts and the developments in clinical practice as a result of the increased knowledge base. In summary this collection of Masterclasses emphasize that manual therapy practice today is not static but a vibrant, expanding and innovative area of practice that is moving forward and is underpinned with a greater evidence base than ever before. This is so crucial in view of the drive today for all therapists to demonstrate evidence-based, efficient, effective practice.

It is hoped that, by bringing these clinically focused articles together in a book, it will become a valuable resource for clinicians when working in their practice or stimulate therapists when developing their own research interests. It is envisaged that it will be an additional resource for undergraduate and post-graduate students who wish to explore this field, as well as for educators. Manual therapists, whatever their professional background and area of work, are faced with challenges every day. It is hoped that these articles will enable them to draw on research based, current practice so facilitating the achievement of the best possible outcome of care for patients.

The articles demonstrate the breadth of clinical practice available to therapists today. With the increasing emphasis placed on supporting clinical findings with research evidence this compilation of Masterclasses aims to fulfil that need.

Karen Beeton
Editorial Committee Manual Therapy

Cervical Spine

SECTION CONTENTS

1

Management of cervical headache

G. A. Jull

Department of Physiotherapy, The University of
Queensland, Brisbane, Australia

The success of physical therapies in the management of headache relies in the first instance on an
accurate differential diagnosis of a cervical musculoskeletal origin to the headache. Examination
should identify a symptomatic pattern of headache
characteristic of neck dysfunction and these symptoms must be associated with relevant physical
impairments in the cervical articular and muscle
systems. Dysfunction in the upper three cervical
joints, poor activation levels and endurance capacity of the deep and postural supporting muscles of
the neck, shoulder girdle region and deficits in
kinaesthesia have been identified in the cervical
headache patient. Treatment needs to be precise
and comprehensive to address each aspect of this
interrelated dysfunction if long-term success of
treatment is to be achieved. *Manual Therapy* (1997)
2(4), 182–190

INTRODUCTION

The International Headache Society's publication
'The Classification of Headache' (IHS 1988) is tes-
timony to the many different headache forms.
Cervical headaches are those that arise from musculoskeletal impairment in the neck and physical
therapies such as manipulative therapy, therapeutic exercise and electrophysical agents have
traditionally been the treatments of choice. It is
estimated that cervical headaches account for
15–20% of all chronic and recurrent headaches
(Pfaffenrath & Kaube 1990; Nilsson 1995) and they
are the most common persistent symptom following neck trauma such as whiplash injury (Balla
& Iansek 1988).

   The success of any treatment depends on the
patient having the condition for which treatment

is applicable. The first step to successful management is to perform an accurate differential diagnosis. The diagnosis of cervical headache requires the presence of a pattern of symptoms and cervical musculoskeletal signs that distinguishes it from headaches that may have accompanying neck tension or pain but whose cause is elsewhere (Henry et al 1987). In some cases this is not a difficult task. In others, especially the chronic benign headache forms inclusive of migraine without aura, tension headache and cervical headache, the task can be more difficult because of the considerable symptomatic overlap. Additionally, cervical musculoskeletal impairments have also been found in persons with tension headache and migraine (Vernon et al 1992; Kidd & Nelson 1993). Patients can suffer a mixed headache form or two types of headache concurrently (Lance 1993), indicating that physical treatments may offer partial relief, but are not the whole solution to the patient's headache syndrome. This highlights the need for well-defined physical criteria and a pattern of relevant physical impairment in the cervical articular, muscular and nervous systems to make a diagnosis of cervical headache. Such physical impairment would not be present when the cervical spine has no major role in the aetiology of a headache form.

Treatment must address the specific impairments and successful outcomes rely on skilled delivery of treatment. Consistent with the international mood of demanding evidence-based practices and proof of effectiveness of treatment, it is now mandatory that clinicians adopt or develop suitable symptomatic, physical and functional outcome measures and these should be utilized in their daily clinical practice.

DETERMINING A CERVICAL MUSCULOSKELETAL ORIGIN TO HEADACHE SYMPTOMS

HISTORY AND SYMPTOMATIC FEATURES OF CERVICAL HEADACHE

In the process of establishing the diagnosis of cervical headache, the clinician seeks a pattern and behaviour of symptoms suggestive of a role of cervical dysfunction in the pathogenesis of headache. Over the past two decades in particular, there has been considerable research into the characterization of cervical headache and a symptom complex is emerging. Some features appear to be quite discriminatory while others do not have such high sensitivity or specificity. This probably reflects the shared access to the trigeminocervical nucleus by all headache forms (Lance 1993).

Cervical headache is classically described as an unilateral headache (Sjaastad et al 1983) but it can be bilateral with often one side predominant (Jull 1986a; Watson & Trott 1993). The description of a band-like, bilateral or whole head headache is more typical of a tension headache (Lance 1993). Cervical headache has side consistency (Sjaastad et al 1989a; D'Amico et al 1994). It should not change sides within or between attacks as can occur quite readily in migraine headaches. A patient reporting headaches that switch sides should alert clinicians to a negative feature in the problem-solving process of cervical headache diagnosis. Cervical headache is typically associated with pain in the neck or suboccipital region (Bogduk & Marsland 1986) but the presence of this pain alone is not diagnostic. What is more indicative of a neck-related cause is that the onset of pain is in the neck with subsequent spread of pain to other areas of the head. In contrast, the onset of classical migraine has been shown to be more typically in the head with neck pain arising later (Sjaastad et al 1989b). The area of head pain has few distinguishing features. It is commonly reported in the occipital and suboccipital area, radiating to frontal, retro-orbital or temporal areas. This distribution reflects the greater representation of the ophthalmic division in the trigeminocervical nucleus (Bogduk 1994).

Furthermore, there is little relationship between area of pain and segmental source of dysfunction (Jull 1986a). In considering other musculoskeletal causes of headache, head or face pain more in the distribution of the mandibular or maxillary divisions of the trigeminal nerve should alert the clinician to a differential examination of the craniomandibular complex. The intensity of cervical headache can be mild, moderate or severe. It is most commonly moderate. It can fluctuate in intensity between and even within a headache period, which is different from migraine, which, if uncontrolled, inevitably builds up to a severe intensity with each episode. Other symptoms may accompany cervical headache such as nausea, lightheadedness or dizziness, or visual disturbances but they are not dominant features that characterize headaches such as migraine with aura or cluster headaches (Sjaastad & Bovim 1991).

The temporal pattern or the frequency and duration of headache can be a key feature in differential diagnosis (Lance 1993) and many recurrent headaches such as migraine, cluster and even tension headache have a characteristic pattern. In contrast, cervical headaches often lack a regular pattern (Sjaastad 1992). They are typically precipitated by sustained neck postures or movements but patients often have difficulty in recognizing aggravating factors (Sjaastad et al 1983; Pfaffenrath et al 1987). Stress may be a provocative factor but this is common to many headaches and is not necessarily of differential diagnostic assistance even though its management may be a vital aspect of a patient's treatment. Cervical headache patients often report difficulties in identifying factors that ease their headaches. Lying down and resting may help as do simple analgesics for some patients. Interestingly, it can be the lack of response to medications successful for other headache forms that may add to the picture of a cervical headache (Bovim & Sjaastad 1993; Sjaastad et al 1993).

Onset of cervical headache can occur at any age and commonly relates to trauma, degenerative joint disease or, with the increasingly sedentary nature of modern day work, to postural strains. Not all patients can identify a specific incident related to headache onset and attempting to link headaches to some traumatic incident in a patient's past can be a misleading exercise. The length of history of headache is variable and often prolonged. As occurs in most headache forms, the incidence of cervical headache is more prevalent in females and, unlike migraine, there appears to be no particular familial tendency.

Outcome measures suitable for research can sometimes be difficult to employ in a clinical setting, often because of time and convenience for both the patient and clinician. Rather than abandon all formal outcome measures, simple outcome measures can be used in the clinical setting. Records of frequency, intensity (VAS scale) and duration of headache can be kept by the patient on a daily or at least a weekly basis. The Neck Disability Index (Vernon & Moir 1991) or the Northwick Park Neck Pain Questionnaire (Leak et al 1994) are reliable and sensitive scales easily employed in the clinical setting to monitor change in functional status.

PHYSICAL IMPAIRMENT IN THE MUSCULOSKELETAL SYSTEM IN CERVICAL HEADACHE

A musculoskeletal condition usually manifests in pain associated with physical impairments in the articular, neuromuscular and nervous systems. The musculoskeletal condition of cervical headache is no exception. The confirmation of a musculoskeletal origin of headache as opposed to another cause requires that a pattern of relevant physical impairment is present. As in many headache forms, there are no reliable laboratory or radiological tests suitable for diagnostic use on a widespread basis. This means that the clinical physical examination is of primary importance. Lack of clear evidence of musculoskeletal dysfunction would suggest that the headache is not of cervical origin.

The physical examination encompasses assessment of the function of three systems: the articular system, the muscle system and neuromotor control and the nervous system. These systems are assessed collectively through analyses of postural form and active movement tests that consider the range, pattern, control and pain responses to movements in each plane. This is followed by more specific tests that aim to detect the precise impairments in each system. The importance of striving to have measures of relevant physical impairment cannot be overemphasized and currently they are lacking in many areas.

The physical impairments in the cervical spine will be discussed as pertaining to the articular, muscle and neural systems although it is recognized that this is an artificial division as the systems are highly interlinked in both normal function as well as in a pain state.

ARTICULAR SYSTEM

The joint impairment that is pathognomonic of cervical headache is painful joint dysfunction within the upper three segments (C0–3). These are the segments that have access to the head via the trigeminocervical nucleus (Bogduk 1994). There may be associated joint dysfunction in other regions of the cervical or thoracic spines. In the physical examination, tests of active movement and manual examination of the cervical segments are used to elicit this joint dysfunction and techniques are well described in manipulative therapy texts.

Active movement examination can be very informative in some patients with respect to pain responses and the demonstration of abnormal range or poor control of movement. However, in the context of a population whose cause of headache may or may not reside in cervical musculoskeletal dysfunction, examination of active movements has been shown to have poor sensitivity to differentiate subjects with and without a neck complaint (Treleaven et al 1994; Sandmark & Nisell 1995). Thus a negative response in this examination is not helpful in differential diagnosis.

The clinical method of manual examination has been used to detect symptomatic cervical joint dysfunction in a number of studies of cervical headache (Jaeger 1989; Jensen et al 1990; Watson & Trott 1993; Beeton & Jull 1994; Dreyfuss et al 1994; Treleaven et al 1994; Whittingham et al 1994; Schoensee et al 1995). Furthermore, initial studies have shown that it has high sensitivity and specificity, enabling the detection of the presence of cervical joint dysfunction in neck pain and headache patients (Jull et al 1988; Sandmark & Nisell 1995; Jull et al 1997). This evidence would suggest that at the present time, manual examination is the most appropriate clinical test to determine the presence of painful joint dysfunction in the differential diagnosis of cervical headache.

As a clinical comment, there are three elements in the assessment method of manual examination. One is the perception of motion, another is the perceived nature of tissue compliance and the

reaction of the tissues to the applied manual stress and thirdly the provocation of pain (Jull et al 1988, 1994). The presence of some joint hypomobility or hypermobility alone is not diagnostic, this being found in asymptomatic populations (Jull 1986b). The provocation of pain and the perception of the segmental muscle reaction adding to the altered segmental tissue compliance is probably a significant cue to the examining clinician (Jull et al 1994). If this is the case, it reinforces the need for a skilled manual examination and one that does not provoke pain or discomfort due to poor handling skills. The latter would result in a high probability of false positive results.

In respect of outcome measures for manual examination, it would be reasonable to suggest that the clinician formally document a qualitative motion rating for the symptomatic joints accompanied by a patient self-rating pain score. Even though studies have not shown strong intertherapist agreement in motion rating, that for intratherapist reliability appears to be acceptable (Schoensee et al 1995).

MUSCLE SYSTEM

The head, neck and shoulder girdle muscle system is necessarily complex, to enable the fulfilment of its functions of generating appropriate head movements and maintaining stability of the head–neck system in any orientation for work, vision and hearing as well as distributing the forces inherent in upper limb function (Winters & Peles 1990). The neck muscles are rich in proprioceptors and make important contribution to balance and general postural control. The muscle system and its neuromotor control have always been of interest to physiotherapists. It is known that with cervical joint injury and pain, there will be reactions in the neuromuscular system as occur with injury to any other joint in the body. The challenge is to develop measures to identify and detect the relevant dysfunctions in the neuromuscular system. Work in this area is still in its infancy but neck pain patients still require management.

Recent work in the area of muscle dysfunction in low back pain has identified impairments in the muscle system that are linked to back pain. These impairments have not been in muscle strength but in motor control (Hodges & Richardson 1996, 1997). Specific muscles within a muscle group have been found to be dysfunctional (Hides et al 1994, 1996; Hodges & Richardson 1996, 1997). They are the deep muscles with direct vertebral attachments that span the vertebrae and have more influence on joint control rather than torque production (Cholewicki & McGill 1996). The anatomy and function of the neck region is quite different to the lumbar spine and a direct extrapolation from one to the other is not possible. Yet the discoveries in the back have given some credence to several clinical theories in the neck and, combined with existing clinical, anatomical and biomechanical knowledge, have given direction to the development of some new measures of muscle function in the neck and scapular region, particularly in relation to deep and postural muscle that provides a supporting or tonic function.

All muscles in the head and neck region contribute to postural control and movement in a highly integrated and coordinated way (Vitti et al 1973; Keshner et al 1989; Keshner & Peterson 1995; Mayoux-Benhamou et al 1997). Directed by findings in the back, we have had a special clinical interest in the role of the deep muscles of the neck for joint control and support. There is a growing realization of the importance of these deep muscles. Winters & Peles (1990), in studying the interaction of several neck muscles by computer modelling, noted that if only the large muscles of the neck were simulated to produce movement, this resulted in regions of local segmental instability, particularly in near upright or neutral postures. Deep muscle activity was required to stiffen or stabilize the segments in functional midranges. Furthermore, because of the presence of the normal lordotic cervical curve, they found that contraction of the larger posterior muscles that span the curve created a tendency towards buckling of the spine. This highlights the importance of the cervical flexors in postural and segmental control. Several authors have identified the greater role of the deep neck flexors in this function of support. Conley et al (1995) studied the function of individual neck muscles using contrast shifts T2 weighted magnetic resonance imaging during exercise. They confirmed that the more superficial flexors, such as sternocleidomastoid, had a major function in torque production. The deeper muscles, including longus capitis and longus colli, demonstrated lesser but continued (or tonic) activity concomitant with a postural, supporting role. This supporting role of these deep muscles has also been confirmed by Vitti et al (1973) and Mayoux-Benhamou et al (1994).

Of relevance to the patient with cervical headache and the need to identify physical impairments linked to this problem, there is clinical evidence that the upper and deep cervical flexors, which are important muscles for cervical segmental and postural control, lose their endurance capacity in patients with neck pain (Watson & Trott 1993; Beeton & Jull 1994). The increased understanding of the tonic supporting role of the deep neck flexors and their functional differentiation from the superficial flexors, such as sternocleidomastoid, realized the need to develop a test that would target these muscles in relative isolation from their superficial counterparts (Jull 1994). The test is conducted in supine lying with the head neck region supported in a neutral position (Fig. 1.1). This test emphasizes low load to reflect the muscles' tonic function and to assess a patient's ability to hold an upper cervical flexion position. The action is reasoned to recruit all the deep neck flexors to hold the head and the cervical region in a static position. As the muscles are deep and unable to be palpated directly, an indirect quantification of their ability to hold the cervical spine position is gained by monitoring the steady position of the neck with an inflatable air filled pressure sensor (Stabilizer, Chattanooga South Pacific) that is positioned suboccipitally behind the neck. Lack of a contribution of the superficial neck flexors to the action can be monitored through surface electromyography (EMG) (Fig. 1.1). Work is currently proceeding to establish the validity of this test, although initial clinical data suggest that it can depict a deficit in function in patients with neck pain. This dysfunction improves with retraining and parallels a reduction in symptoms (Beeton & Jull 1994; Grant et al 1998).

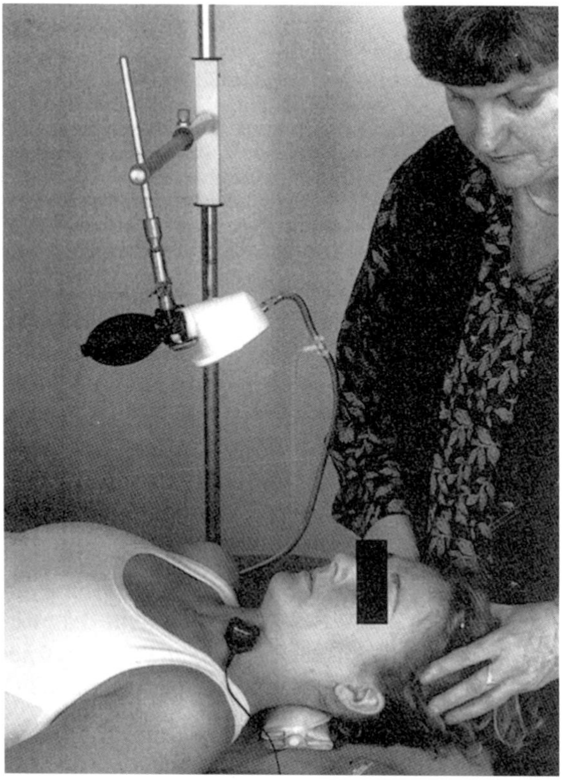

Figure 1.1 The test of holding capacity of the deep neck flexors. The head is in a neutral position and the pressure sensor is placed suboccipitally behind the neck and inflated to 20 mmHg. The patient is instructed to very slowly flex the upper cervical spine with a gentle nodding action and hold the position steady for 10 seconds. This should occur with minimal activity in the superficial muscles. An ideal response is that the patient can increase pressure by 10 mmHg. Most neck pain patients' initial performance is an increase of 2–4 mmHg and they demonstrate an inability to hold the position steady.

It is also known that the small posterior suboccipital muscles are vital for control of the head and upper cervical joints especially in midrange control (Winters & Peles 1990). Conley et al (1995) noted the more continuous activity of the deep posterior muscles semispinalis cervicus and multifidus in their studies, thus suggesting a supporting role. Furthermore, Hallgren et al (1994) and McPartland et al (1997) noted atrophy in the deep suboccipital extensors in patients with chronic neck pain. As yet measures that can be clinically used to detect deficits in these specific muscles have not been developed but knowledge

of their functional role and the likely presence of impairment indicate that they should also receive specific attention in the rehabilitation of the cervical headache patient.

Postures of the shoulder girdle are closely linked to head and neck postures and control of the region. Loss of postural function in the scapular girdle muscles, such as lower trapezius and serratus anterior, is a frequent clinical finding (Janda 1994; Jull 1994; White & Sahrmann 1994), although research evidence of their dysfunction is sparse (Beeton & Jull 1994; Grant et al 1998). This probably reflects difficulty in measurement rather than an absence of interest. At the present time, the holding capacity of these muscles is tested through a modified grade 3 classic muscle test for the lower trapezius (Fig. 1.2).

It is held that other axioscapular muscles, such as the levator scapulae, often, inappropriately, take on the postural supporting role and may become overactive (Janda 1994). This could be in response to either pain or poor motor control. Increased activity of the levator scapulae muscles may aggravate or cause pain by increasing compressive forces on cervical joints (Behrsin & Maguire 1986). Although it has been observed clinically that the impairment in the deep neck flexors, lower trapezius and serratus anterior is almost an inevitable accompaniment of neck pain, it appears that overactivity or tightness of muscles as assessed by clinical muscle length tests is not a regular feature (Treleaven et al 1994; Jull et al 1999). More work is needed in this area to understand the impairments underlying the presence of muscle tightness and why it is present in some muscles and some individuals but not others. At present, in respect to neck pain patients, it seems that it can be in response to poor patterns of motor control (Janda 1994) and less extensible or mechanosensitive neural tissues of the upper quadrant (Edgar et al 1994; Balster & Jull 1997). Assessments of neck muscle tightness at the present time are the clinical tests (Janda 1994) that can be qualitatively rated on a 0–3 scale of normal, slight, moderate to very tight.

The role and description of the cervical muscles, and particularly the deep upper cervical muscles

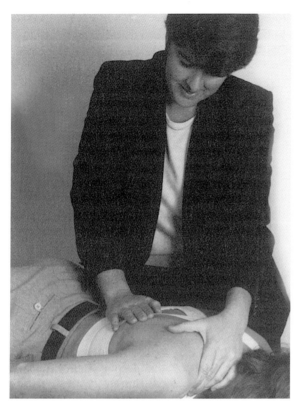

Figure 1.2 The lower trapezius is assessed by testing the patient's ability to hold the scapula adducted and depressed. To restrict the action to the lower trapezius as much as possible, load is removed from the test by leaving the arm by the side. The clinician places the scapula in position and then asks the patient to hold the position. Any substitution with muscles, such as latissimus dorsi, levator scapulae or upper trapezius, should be monitored.

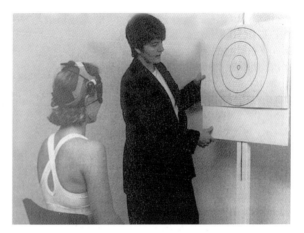

Figure 1.3 Tests of cervical kinaesthesia after Revel et al (1991). The patient's ability to relocate a relaxed starting position following excursions into sagittal, horizontal or frontal plane motion can be tested.

THE NERVOUS SYSTEM

The neurophysiological function of the nervous system is primary but this can also become a pain source when nerves are irritated mechanically or are inflamed. Compression of the C2 and C3 nerve roots has been documented as a relatively rare cause of cervical headache (Jansen et al 1989). The dura mater of the upper cervical cord and posterior cranial fossa is supplied by the ventral rami of the upper three cervical nerves (Bogduk 1994) and, therefore, can be a possible pain source in cervical headache. If inflamed, neural tissues can become sensitive to movement and elicit responses in the muscle system. This relationship of irritation of the nervous system to muscle tightness or hyperactivity and muscle inhibition is often observed clinically. Hu et al (1993, 1995) showed in animal experiments that the application of a small fibre irritant to cervical and cranial meningeal tissues resulted in an increased EMG activity in the upper trapezius and jaw muscles. The axioscapular muscles are closely related to the cervical spinal nerves and the brachial plexus. Edgar et al (1994) found, even in asymptomatic subjects, that less natural extensibility of the upper quadrant neural structures was associated with less measured length of the upper trapezius muscle. Balster & Jull (1997) confirmed an association between lesser neural extensibility and

as dynamic proprioceptors, are well known. It is likely that there is a close relationship between the joint stability role of the deep local muscle system and its role in neck kinaesthesia. There is ample evidence that kinaesthetic deficits accompany cervical joint pain, injury and disease (Revel et al 1991; Heikkila & Anstrom 1996; McPartland et al 1997; Loudon et al 1997). Of relevance is that sensitive tests of cervical kinaesthesia can be applied in the clinical setting (Fig. 1.3). Furthermore, Revel et al (1994) were able to demonstrate that improvement in kinaesthesia paralleled a decrease in neck pain, giving direction and a basis for therapeutic strategies.

heightened upper trapezius activity in an EMG study of the upper limb neural tissue provocation test (Elvey 1979). Such evidence of heightened muscle activity in muscles antagonistic to those that are important in postural control of the shoulder girdle could further compound the problem of poor active stabilization in patients with neck pain and pathology.

There are fascial connections between the upper cervical dura and the deep suboccipital extensors (Hack et al 1995) and the dura attaches to the cranial fossa and the back of the body of the C2 vertebra. Upper cervical flexion, therefore, becomes a key movement in upper quadrant neural tissue provocation tests for the cervical headache. The test can be sensitized from a neural tissue point of view by preplacing the upper or lower limb in a neural test position. While positive results of clinical tests of neural structures can be observed in the clinic in some cervical headache patients, there have been no known attempts to date to develop some quantifiable test of neural tissue sensitivity for headache patients and no investigation of the frequency of positive responses to current clinical tests in cervical headache populations.

PHYSICAL IMPAIRMENT TO DIAGNOSE A CERVICAL HEADACHE

As in painful musculoskeletal conditions in other regions of the body, it is apparent from the knowledge base to date, that the diagnosis of cervical headache or a cervical component to headache is dependent on the presence of both articular and muscle impairments accompanied by acute or long-term manifestations of poor neuromotor control. At a local measurable level, painful upper cervical joint dysfunction accompanied by impairments in the deep cervical flexors, scapular postural muscles and cervical kinaesthesia should be present. Their absence would indicate that headache has another cause. Other signs of physical impairments may be, and often are, present in the cervical headache sufferer, including postural abnormalities, muscle tightness and neural tissue mechanosensitivity, but their absence does not reject a cervical headache diagnosis.

TREATMENT STRATEGIES FOR THE CERVICAL HEADACHE PATIENT

Treatment aims to reverse the physical impairments linked to the patient's neck pain and headache, as well as preventing future episodes. Treatment should be pragmatic and dysfunction-based. It must be precise and comprehensive to cope with the often complex dysfunction that may present in the cervical headache patient. Intervention in one system alone does not guarantee resolution of impairments in other systems (Hides et al 1996) and relief of headache as an immediate response to treatment is unlikely to be translated into long-term relief. Clinicians must use outcome measures of subjective and physical impairment to monitor effects of interventions both within and between treatments.

It is probable, in light of the studies that show pain and headache relief with direct joint or nerve blocks of the upper cervical articulations (Bogduk & Marsland 1986; Drefuss et al 1994; Lord et al 1994), that joint dysfunction is a primary source of pain in many cervical headache sufferers. Yet for effective management the clinician must design treatment programmes that reflect a knowledge and understanding of the interdependence of the articular and muscle systems and their neuromotor control in normal function and their interrelationship in dysfunction.

Joint impairment is managed by a combination of therapies. Manipulative therapy can be employed to utilize both the manipulation-induced analgesic and biomechanical effects to relieve joint pain and restore motion (Vernon 1989; Herzog et al 1993; Lee et al 1993; Vicenzino et al 1994; Wright 1995). Active movement designed to influence the segment as locally as possible should be practised by the patient, not only to encourage as normal joint afferentation as possible but to more permanently establish any beneficial effects achieved by manipulative therapy techniques. It has been shown that movement gained by a specific manipulative technique performed in isolation can be lost within 48 hours (Nansel et al 1990). A joint without adequate muscle support and control will be vulnerable to further strain and pain. Additionally, achievement of muscle control is frequently commensurate with pain control (Derrick & Chesworth 1992; Beeton & Jull 1994; Richardson & Jull 1995). With the knowledge that the important cervical supporting muscles, the deep neck flexors, as well as the scapular postural supporting muscles, are dysfunctional, activation and re-education of their tonic supporting capacity becomes an essential component of treatment from the outset to both relieve and control joint pain.

It should be appreciated that the effect of lack of support by key deep and postural muscles, together with the adverse stresses likely to be imposed by overactive axioscapular muscles, has considerable impact on articular tissues. Some estimate of the contribution of this muscle dysfunction to the production of joint pain and motion abnormality can be made in the initial clinical examination by conducting a pre- and post-muscle test assessment of the painful vertebral joints notably through the pain provocative posteroanterior glide technique. It is not uncommon to find clinically that joint pain is reduced and motion improved following the reciprocal relaxation of muscles produced as a by-product of testing the activation and holding capacities of the deep cervical and lower scapular stabilizers. This is potent feedback to patients and enhances compliance with exercise when it is realized that retraining these muscles can relieve and control their neck pain and headache.

The retraining of muscle support and control is a key element of management. Initially, the tonic holding capacity of the deep supporting and postural muscles is trained and these muscles are targeted in as much isolation as possible from other muscles in the region in the first instance to ensure their accurate activation. The deep neck flexors are retrained in the supine test position with the use of feedback from the pressure sensor. A common fault is that the exercise is performed too quickly or too strongly. The upper cervical flexion action must be performed slowly and precisely with the patient training their holding capacity at a level of pressure increase that they can control. This exercise can also be used to assist in retraining kinaesthetic sense with the patient carefully targeting different pressures between 20 and 30 mmHg when these are

thought to be achievable. Care must be taken not to work into fatigue as this will encourage substitution by other muscles. The lower trapezius and serratus anterior are retrained using the same principles of improving tonic holding capacity and formal retraining is often undertaken in the prone test position. From the outset, the patient must be taught how to assume a correct neutral upright spinal postural position that they practise repeatedly during the day as part of a motor skill retraining programme. They can incorporate training of their postural muscles into this routine. The only word of caution is that the upper cervical flexors and the lower trapezius are antagonistic to muscles with could be hypertonic in response to sensitive neural tissues. If this is the case, exercise may either proceed with considerable caution or be delayed until neural tissues are sufficiently settled.

In concert with active postural retraining, ergonomic and lifestyle advice should be given to the patient to cover their work or domestic environments. Perpetuation of strains from these sources can hinder the progress of treatment.

Muscle retraining and re-education of motor control should proceed through several stages. Co-contraction exercises can be introduced to incorporate the deep cervical flexors and extensors. Rotation is an optimal resistance direction for this purpose and resistance should be aimed at a 20–30% effort in line with retraining tonic supporting function. Exercise can be performed in the lying or the correct upright sitting posture. Retraining movement patterns using the correct synergistic action between the deep and superficial neck flexors as well as re-education of the pattern of axioscapular muscle sequencing during arm movements (Janda 1994) is often necessary. Kinaesthesia may be further trained by the patient moving their head and neck accurately and repeatedly to visual targets.

It is wise to reflect on the fact that the physical changes that have developed with a prolonged history of chronic cervical headache are unlikely to resolve in a week or two. The patient and clinician must appreciate that time and dedicated work by the patient is required if a successful outcome is to be achieved in the long term. Efficacy of treatment and progress through all stages should be evaluated by the retesting of the relevant outcome measures. It is only by changing the physical impairments that there is a prospect of long-term relief.

CONCLUSION

The first step towards successful management of the cervical headache patient is the possession of a clear differential diagnosis. It is necessary to have clear outcome measures relevant to the history of headache and physical impairments associated with the condition of the cervical musculoskeletal system. Treatment must address all impairments with the aim of relieving headaches in the long term. A comprehensive treatment approach has been outlined and its efficacy is currently being evaluated in a formal clinical trial.

REFERENCES

Balla J, Iansek R 1988 Headaches arising from disorders of the cervical spine. In: Hopkins A (ed) Headache. Problems in Diagnosis and Management. Saunders, London, pp 241–267

Balster S, Jull G 1997 Upper trapezius muscle activity in the brachial plexus tension test in asymptomatic individuals. Manual Therapy 2: 144–149

Beeton K, Jull G 1994 Effectiveness of manipulative physiotherapy in the management of cervicogenic headache: a single case study. Physiotherapy 80: 417–423

Behrsin JF, Maguire K 1986 Levator scapulae action during shoulder movement. A possible mechanism of shoulder pain of cervical origin. Australian Journal of Physiotherapy 32: 101–106

Bogduk N 1994 Cervical causes of headache and dizziness. In: Boyling J, Palastanga N (eds) Grieve's Modern Manual Therapy of the Vertebral Column. Churchill Livingstone, Edinburgh, pp 317–332

Bogduk N, Marsland A 1986 On the concept of third occipital headache. Journal of Neurology. Neurosurgery and Psychiatry 49: 775–780

Bovim G, Sjaastad O 1993 Cervicogenic headache: responses to nitroglycerin, oxygen, ergotomine and morphine. Headache 33: 249–252

Cholewicki J, McGill S 1996 Mechanical stability of the in vivo lumbar spine: implications for injury and chronic low back pain. Clinical Biomechanics 11: 1–15

Conley MS, Meyer RA, Bloomberg JJ, Feeback DL, Dudley GA 1995 Noninvasive analysis of human neck muscle function. Spine 20: 2505–2512

D'Amico D, Leone M, Bussone G 1994 Side-locked unilaterality and pain localization in long-lasting headaches: migraine, tension-type headache, and cervicogenic headache. Headache 34: 526–530

Derrick L, Chesworth B 1992 Post-motor vehicle accident alar ligament instability. Journal of Orthopaedic and Sports Physical Therapy 16: 6–10

Dreyfuss P, Rogers J, Dreyer S, Fletcher D 1994 Atlanto-occipital joint pain. A report of three cases and description of an intraarticular joint block. Regional Anesthesia 19: 344–351

Edgar D, Jull GA, Sutton S 1994 Relationship between upper trapezius muscle length and upper quadrant neural tissue extensibility. Australian Journal of Physiotherapy 40: 99–103

Elvey RL 1979 Brachial plexus tension test and the pathoanatomical origin of arm pain. In: Glasgow EF,

Twomey LT (eds) Aspects of Manipulative Therapy, 1st Edition. Lincoln Institute of Health Sciences, Melbourne, pp 105–110

Grant R, Jull G, Spencer T 1998 Active stabilisation training for screen based keyboard operators — a single case study. Australian Journal of Physiotherapy 43: 235–242

Hack GD, Koritzer RT, Robinson WL, Hallgren RC, Greenman PE 1995 Anatomic relation between the rectus capitis posterior minor muscle and the dura mater. Spine 20: 2484–2486

Hallgren R, Greenman P, Rechtien J 1994 Atrophy of suboccipital muscles in patients with chronic pain: a pilot study. Journal of the American Osteopathic Association 94: 1032–1038

Heikkila H, Anstrom P 1996 Cervicocephalic kinesthetic sensibility in patients with whiplash injury. Scandinavian Journal of Rehabilitation Medicine 28: 133–138

Henry P, Dartigues JF, Puymirat E, Peytour TL, Lucas J 1987 The association of cervicalgia-headaches: an epidemiologic study. Cephalalgia 7 (Suppl 6): 189–190

Herzog W, Zhang Y, Conway P, Kawchuk G 1993 Cavitation sounds during spinal manipulative treatments. Journal of Manipulative and Physiological Therapeutics 16: 523–526

Hides J, Stokes M, Saide M, Jull G, Cooper D 1994 Evidence of lumbar multifidus wasting ipsilateral to symptoms in patients with acute/subacute low back pain. Spine 19: 165–177

Hides J, Richardson C, Jull G 1996 Multifidus muscle recovery is not automatic following acute first episode low back pain. Spine 21(23): 2763–2769

Hodges PW, Richardson CA 1996 Inefficient muscular stabilisation of the lumbar spine associated with low back pain: a motor control evaluation of transversus abdominis. Spine 21: 2640–2650

Hodges PW, Richardson CA 1997 Contraction of the abdominal muscles associated with movement of the lower limb. Physical Therapy 77: 132–144

Hu JW, Yu XM, Vernon H, Sessle BJ. 1993 Excitatory effects on neck and jaw muscle activity of inflammatory irritant applied to cervical paraspinal tissues. Pain 55: 243–250

Hu JW, Vernon H, Tatourian I 1995 Changes in neck electromyography associated with meningeal noxious stimulation. Journal of Manipulative and Physiological Therapeutics 18: 577–581

International Headache Society 1988 Classification of headache. Cephalalgia 8 (Suppl 7): 1–96

Jaeger B 1989 Are cervicogenic headaches due to myofascial pain and cervical spine dysfunction? Cephalaegia 9: 157–164

Janda V 1994 Muscles and motor control in cervicogenic disorders: Assessment and management. In: Grant R (ed) Physical Therapy of the Cervical and Thoracic Spine, 2nd Edition. Churchill Livingstone, New York, pp 195–216

Jansen J, Markakis E, Rama B, Hildebrandt J 1989 Hemicranial attacks or permanent hemicrania — a sequel of upper cervical root compression. Cephalalgia 9: 123–130

Jensen OK, Nielsen FF, Vosmar L 1990 An open study comparing manual therapy with the use of cold packs in the treatment of post concussional headache. Cephalalgia 10: 241–249

Jull GA 1986a Headaches associated with the cervical spine — a clinical review. In: Grieve GP (ed) Modern Manual Therapy of the Vertebral Column. Churchill Livingstone, Edinburgh, pp 322–329

Jull GA 1986b Clinical observations of upper cervical mobility. In: Grieve GP (ed) Modern Manual Therapy of the Vertebral Column. Churchill Livingstone, Edinburgh, pp 315–321

Jull G 1994 Headaches of cervical origin. In: Grant R (ed) Physical Therapy of the Cervical and Thoracic Spine, 2nd Edition. Churchill Livingstone, New York, pp 261–285

Jull GA, Bogduk N, Marsland A 1988 The accuracy of manual diagnosis for cervical zygapophysial joint pain syndromes. Medical Journal of Australia 148: 233–236

Jull G, Treleaven J, Versace G 1994 Manual examination: is pain provocation a major cue for spinal dysfunction? Australian Journal of Physiotherapy 40: 159–165

Jull G, Zito G, Trott P, Potter H, Shirley D, Richardson C 1997 Interexaminer reliability to detect painful upper cervical joint dysfunction. Australian Journal of Physiotherapy 43: 125–129

Jull G, Barrett C, Magee R, Ho P 1999 Further characterisation of muscle dysfunction in cervical headache. Cephalalgia 19: 179–185

Keshner E, Campbell D, Katz R, Peterson B 1989 Neck muscle activation patterns in humans during isometric head stabilization. Experimental Brain Research 75: 335–344

Keshner E, Peterson B 1995 Mechanisms controlling human stabilization. 1. Head-neck dynamics during random rotations in the horizontal plane. Journal of Neurophysiology 73: 2293–2301

Kidd RF, Nelson CM 1993 Musculoskeletal dysfunction of the neck in migraine and tension headache. Headache 33: 566–569

Lance J 1993 Mechanisms and Management of Headache, 5th Edition. Butterworth–Heinemann, Oxford

Leak AM, Cooper J, Dyer S, Williams KA, Turner-Stokes L, Frank AO 1994 The Northwick Park neck pain questionnaire, devised to measure neck pain and disability. British Journal of Rheumatology 33: 469–474

Lee M, Latimer J, Maher C 1993 Manipulation: investigation of a proposed mechanism. Clinical Biomechanics 8: 302–306

Lord S, Barnsley L, Wallis B, Bodguk N 1994 Third occipital headache; a prevalence study. Journal of Neurology, Neurosurgery and Psychiatry 57: 1187–1190

Loudon J, Ruhl M, Field E 1997 Ability to reproduce head position after whiplash injury. Spine 22: 865–868

McPartland J, Brodeur R, Hallgren R 1997 Chronic neck pain, standing balance and suboccipital muscle atrophy — a pilot study. Journal of Manipulative and Physiological Therapeutics 20: 24–29

Mayoux-Benhamou MA, Revel M, Vallee C, Roudier JP, Bargy F 1994: Longus Colli has a postural function on cervical curvature. Surgical and Radiologic Anatomy 16: 367–371

Mayoux-Benhamou MA, Revel M, Vallee C 1997 Selective electromyography of dorsal neck muscles in humans. Experimental Brain Research 113: 353–360

Nansel D, Peneff A, Cremata E, Carlson J 1990 Time course considerations for the effects of unilateral lower cervical adjustments with respect to the amelioration of cervical lateral-flexion passive end-range asymmetry. Journal of Manipulative and Physiological Therapeutics 13: 297–304

Nilsson N 1995 The prevalence of cervicogenic headache in a random population sample of 20–59 year olds. Spine 20: 1884–1888

Pfaffenrath V, Kaube H 1990 Diagnostics of cervical headache. Functional Neurology 5: 157–164

Pfaffenrath V, Dandekar R, Pollmann W 1987 Cervicogenic headache – the clinical picture, radiological findings and hypothesis on its pathophysiology. Headache 27: 495–499

Revel M, Andre-Deshays C, Minguet M 1991 Cervicocephalic kinesthetic sensibility in patients with cervical pain. Archives of Physical Medicine and Rehabilitation 72: 288–291

Revel M, Minguet M, Gergoy P, Vaillant J, Manuel J 1994 Changes in cervicocephalic kinesthesia after a proprioceptive rehabilitation program in patients with neck pain: a randomised controlled study. Archives of Physical Medicine and Rehabilitation 75: 895–899

Richardson CA, Jull GA 1995 Muscle control — pain control. What exercises would you prescribe? Manual Therapy 1: 2–10

Sandmark H, Nisell R 1995 Validity of five common manual neck pain provocating tests. Scandinavian Journal of Rehabilitation Medicine 27: 131–136

Schoensee H, Jensen G, Nicholson G, Gossman M, Katholi C 1995 The effect of mobilisation on cervical headaches. Journal of Orthopaedic and Sports Physical Therapy 21: 183–196

Sjaastad O 1992 Laterality of pain and other migraine criteria in common migraine. A comparison with cervicogenic headache. Functional Neurology 7: 289–294

Sjaastad O, Bovim G 1991 Cervicogenic headache. The differentiation from common migraine. An overview. Functional Neurology 6: 93–100

Sjaastad O, Saunte C, Hovdahl H Breivik H, Gronbaek E 1983 Cervicogenic headache. A hypothesis. Cephalalgia 3: 249–256

Sjaastad O, Fredriksen TA, Sandt Antonaci F 1989a Unilaterality of headache in classic migraine. Cephalalgia 9: 71–77

Sjaastad O, Fredriksen TA, Sandt 1989b The localisation of the initial pain of attack: a comparison between classic migraine and cervicogenic headache. Functional Neurology 6: 93–100

Sjaastad O, Joubert J, Elas T, Bovim G, Vincent M 1993 Hemicrania continua and cervicogenic headache. Separate headache or two faces of the same headache? Functional Neurology 8: 79–83

Treleaven J, Jull G, Atkinson L 1994 Cervical musculoskeletal dysfunction in post-concussional headache. Cephalalgia 14: 273–279

Vernon H 1989 Exploring the effect of a spinal manipulation on plasma beta-endorphin levels in normal men. Spine 14: 1272–1273

Vernon H, Moir SA 1991 The Neck Disability Index: a study of reliability and validity. Journal of Manipulative and Physiological Therapeutics 14: 409–415

Vernon H, Steiman I, Hagino C 1992 Cervicogenic dysfunction in muscle contraction headache and migraine: a descriptive study. Journal of Manipulative and Physiological Therapeutics 15: 418–429

Vicenzino B, Collins D, Wright A 1994 Sudomotor changes induced by neural mobilisation techniques in asymptomatic subjects. Journal of Manipulative and Physiological Therapeutics 17: 66–74

Vitti M, Fujiwara M, Basmajain J, Iida M 1973 The integrated roles of longus coli and sternocleidomastoid muscles: an electromyographic study. Anatomical Record 177: 471–484

Watson DH, Trott PH 1993 Cervical headache. An investigation of natural head posture and upper cervical flexor muscle performance. Cephalalgia 13: 272–284

White SG, Sahrmann SA 1994 A movement system balance approach to management of musculo-skeletal pain. In: Grant R (ed) Physical Therapy of the Cervical and Thoracic Spine, 2nd Edition. Churchill Livingstone, New York, pp 339–357

Whittingham W, Ellis WB, Molyneux TP 1994 The effect of manipulation (toggle recoil techniques) for headaches with upper cervical joint dysfunction: a pilot study. Journal of Manipulative and Physiological Therapeutics 17: 369–375

Winters JM, Peles JD 1990 Neck muscle activity and 3-D head kinematics during quasi-static and dynamic tracking movements. In: Winters JM, Woo SL-Y (eds) Multiple Muscle Systems: Biomechanics and Movement Organization. Springer-Verlag, New York, pp 461–480

Wright A 1995 Hypoalgesia post-manipulative therapy: a review of a potential neurophysiological mechanism. Manual Therapy 1: 11–16

POSTSCRIPT

The theme of this article emphasized that optimal management of cervical headache relied first on identifying the cervicogenic headache patient from those with the other common frequent intermittent headaches, such as migraine and tension-type headache, as well as the need to characterize musculoskeletal dysfunction in cervicogenic headache for appropriate treatment. A multimodal physical therapy treatment regime for patients with cervicogenic headache was presented based on the knowledge from research into the nature of the physical impairment associated with this form of headache. However, evidence of the efficacy of the programme had not been established.

Research has continued to enhance the understanding of the syndrome of cervicogenic headache both for diagnosis and treatment. Sjaastad et al (1998) have refined the criteria for cervicogenic headache and studies have now been conducted to investigate their reliability. Vincent (1998) and Vincent and Luna (1999) used these criteria and those for migraine and tension-type headache published by the International Headache Society (1988) to determine how well they could differentiate patients with cervicogenic, episodic tension-type headache and migraine without aura. They found that cervicogenic headache could be differentiated from migraine with 100% sensitivity and specificity if at least seven of the 18 individual criteria were present. Seven or more criteria were required to differentiate cervicogenic headache from tension-type headache with a sensitivity of 100% and a specificity of 86.2%. In a similar study Bono et al (1998) estimated that between 70% and 80% of cervicogenic headache patients could be identified if five or more of the individual criteria for cervicogenic headache were present. In these studies, the features that most distinguished cervicogenic headache were unilateral, side-locked headache and headache association with neck postures or movements, in agreement with Sjaastad et al's (1998) major criteria. Van Suijlekom et al (2000) investigated inter-observer reliability in the use of the criteria for the three headache forms and found that agreement was highest and virtually the same for migraine and cervicogenic headache (77% and 76% respectively), although identifying tension-type headache was more problematic with inter-observer agreement of 48%. The results of these studies encourage manual therapy clinicians to use the criteria as the basis for their clinical reasoning process in the examination of the chronic headache patient to enhance their diagnostic accuracy. However, the poorer agreement in the recognition of tension-type headache underlies the need for an accurate physical examination to determine the presence of comparable musculoskeletal dysfunction to distinguish cervicogenic headache from tension-type headache and migraine without aura.

Further research has now strengthened knowledge of the presence, nature and identification of physical impairment in the cervical region of the cervicogenic headache patient. Zwart (1997) was able to demonstrate that a reduction in cervical range of motion distinguished subjects with chronic cervicogenic headache from those with chronic tension-type and migraine headaches. Aligned with this measure of dysfunction, Gijsberts et al (1999) conducted an inter-therapist reliability study using three pairs of manual therapists to detect the presence or absence of painful joint dysfunction in a cohort of 105 headache subjects. They demonstrated fair to good agreement (ICCs 0.67–0.88) and, importantly, showed that the pain provoked in the cervical joints by the manual examination also accurately identified the cervicogenic headache group from those subjects with other types of headache. Zito et al (unpublished data, in preparation) also found that the presence of upper cervical dysfunction, as detected by manual examination, clearly distinguished cervicogenic headache subjects from asymptomatic subjects as well as those with migraine without aura. In a similar study (Jull et al 1997), manual examination of the upper cervical spine also distinguished cervicogenic headache subjects from asymptomatic control subjects. These studies strengthen knowledge of the association between upper cervical joint pain and dysfunction and cervicogenic headache and also support the use of manual examination in the differential assessment of patients with chronic headache.

There has also been further research into the muscle dysfunction associated with cervicogenic headache. Placzek et al (1999) determined that patients with chronic headache of likely cervical origin demonstrated less strength in cervical flexion and extension. The notion that problems in muscle control were present in the cervicogenic headache patient was also introduced in this chapter. Further research has confirmed the presence of a dysfunction in the neck flexor synergy in cervicogenic headache subjects, with these subjects having poorer performance in the craniocervical flexion test, indicative of dysfunction in the deep neck flexors (Jull et al 1999, 2002). A study of whiplash subjects, in whom headache is a common complaint, revealed increased activity in the superficial neck flexors (sternocleidomastoid muscles) in association with the poorer performance in the cranio-cervical flexion test (Jull 2000). Barton and Hayes (1996) also noted that some subjects with cervicogenic headache had prolonged EMG relaxation times in the sternocleidomastoid muscles following cervical flexor strength tests. Additionally, Bansevicius and Sjaastad (1996) demonstrated that cervicogenic headache subjects demonstrated increased EMG activity in the upper trapezius whilst performing a computer-based task requiring concentration. Thus the changes in muscle system function that are observed readily by the clinician are being confirmed in research.

A programme involving manipulative therapy and a specific exercise programme was advocated for the management of cervicogenic headache, based on the nature of the joint and muscle dysfunction found in these patients. The efficacy of these treatments has now been tested in a randomized clinical trial (Jull et al 2002). The profile of patients in the study revealed that they suffered chronic headache (mean history of 6.1 years) of moderate intensity with a mean frequency of 3.5 days per week. The effectiveness of manipulative therapy and the specific exercise programme used alone and in combination were tested and it was determined that the two treatments significantly and similarly reduced the headache symptoms and neck pain and the effects were maintained in the long term (12-month follow-up period). These results challenge the view of Sjaastad et al (1997) that physiotherapy is probably only useful for patients with minor symptoms and the benefits, if any, are only of a short-term nature.

While knowledge of the diagnosis and suitable treatment methods for cervicogenic headache has rapidly expanded in recent years, further challenges are present. One pressing need is the recognition of those cervicogenic headache patients likely to be responsive to physiotherapy management. The clinical trials have revealed that while manipulative therapy and the specific exercise programme were efficacious for the majority of subjects, 28% of subjects failed to achieve the benchmark of efficacy of at least a 50% reduction in headache frequency. An analysis utilizing all information about the history and nature of headache and physical and psychometric features was unable to distinguish those subjects likely and not likely to respond to treatment. Further research is required to identify other variables likely to influence outcome so that physiotherapy management may, in the future, be applied in an optimal manner.

REFERENCES

Bansevicius D, Sjaastad O 1996 Cervicogenic headache: The influence of mental load on pain level and EMG of shoulder-neck and facial muscles. Headache 36: 372–378

Barton PM, Hayes KC 1996 Neck flexor muscle strength, efficiency, and relaxation times in normal subjects and subjects with unilateral neck pain and headache. Archives of Physical and Medical Rehabilitation 77: 680–687

Bono G, Antonaci F, Ghirmai S, Sandrini G, Nappi G 1998 The clinical profile of cervicogenic headache as it emerges from a study based on the early diagnostic criteria (Sjaastad et al 1990). Functional Neurology 13: 75–77

Gijsberts TJ, Duquet W, Stoekart R, Oostendorp R 1999 Pain-provocation tests for C0-4 as a tool in the diagnosis of cervicogenic headache. Abstract. Cephalalgia 19: 436

International Headache Society Classification Committee 1988 Classification and diagnostic criteria for headache disorders, cranial neuralgias and facial pain. Cephalalgia 8: 9–96

Jull GA 2000 Deep cervical neck flexor dysfunction in whiplash. Journal of Musculoskeletal Pain 8 (1/2) 143–154

Jull G, Zito G, Trott P, Potter H, Shirley D, Richardson C 1997 Inter-examiner reliability to detect painful upper cervical joint dysfunction. Australian Journal of Physiotherapy 43: 125–129

Jull G, Barrett C, Magee R, Ho P 1999 Further characterisation of muscle dysfunction in cervical headache. Cephalalgia 19: 179–185

Jull G, Trott P, Potter H, Zito G, Niere K, Shirley D, Emberson J, Marschner I, Richardson C 2002 A randomized controlled trial of exercise and manipulative therapy for cervicogenic headache. Spine 27: 1835–1843

Placzek JD, Pagett BT, Roubal PJ, Jones BA, McMichael HG, Rozanski EA, Gianoto KL 1999 The influence of the cervical spine on chronic headache in women: A pilot study. The Journal of Manual and Manipulative Therapy; 7: 33–39.

Sjaastad O, Fredriksen TA, Pfaffenrath V 1998 Cervicogenic headache: Diagnostic criteria. Headache 38: 442–445

Sjaastad O, Fredriksen TA, Stolt-Nielsen A, Salvesen R, Jansen J, Pareja JA, Poughias LP Knuszewski P, Inan L 1997 Cervicogenic headache: A clinical review with a special emphasis on therapy. Functional Neurology 12: 305–317

Van Suijlekom H, den Vet H, van den Berg S, Weber W 2000 Interobserver reliability in physical examination of the cervical spine in patients with headache. Headache 40: 581–586

Vincent M 1998 Validation of criteria for cervicogenic headache. Functional Neurology 13: 74–75

Vincent MB, Luna RA 1999 Cervicogenic headache: a comparison with migraine and tension-type headache. Cephalalgia 19: 11–16

Zwart JA 1997 Neck mobility in different headache disorders. Headache 37: 6–11

2

Spinal manipulative thrust technique using combined movement theory

C. J. McCarthy

The Centre for Rehabilitation Science, University of Manchester, Manchester Royal Infirmary, Manchester, UK

Spinal manipulative thrust technique (SMTT) is employed by all manual therapy professions using different rationales for the selection of technique. A method of rationally selecting particular SMTTs is described with a view to integrating SMTT into the practice of manual therapists familiar with Combined movement theory (CMT), a corollary of the Maitland Concept. The similarities of CMT and SMTT methodologies are described and two examples of how CMT can be utilized for SMTT selection in the cervical spine are detailed. *Manual Therapy* (2001) **6(4)** 197–204.

INTRODUCTION

SMTT has been used by physiotherapists and other manual therapy professions for many years. Seminal work by authors in the field of musculoskeletal therapy including Cyriax (1941), Grieve (1991) and Maitland et al (2001) has described spinal manipulative thrusts and recommended their consideration in the management of spinal dysfunction. SMTT continues to be taught and practised and there appears to be no decline in the popularity of these techniques despite the scarcity of evidence to support their continued use (Bogduk & Mercer 1995).

Passive movement of the vertebral column is used commonly in the management of spinal dysfunction (Anderson et al 1992). One of the most popular paradigms of passive movement treatment in spinal dysfunction is the Maitland Concept (Maitland et al 2001) and the corollary of this — CMT (Edwards 1987, 1992). The aims of this article are to introduce the fundamental similarities in approach between SMTT and CMT and introduce a process of SMTT selection based upon CMT. It is hoped that by adopting this rationale of SMTT selection it may provide the user with a method of applying SMTT that integrates the two concepts.

SPINAL MANIPULATIVE THRUST TECHNIQUE

Whilst the similarities and differences between the particular manipulative techniques are not always clear from the literature, there seems to be agreement that SMTT involves a small-amplitude, high-velocity thrust to a spinal joint (Ottenbacher & DiFabio 1985) that extends beyond a restricted range of movement (Koes et al 1991). The effectiveness of SMTT in the treatment of spinal pain has been investigated in numerous randomized controlled trials with these, in turn, being analyzed in systematic reviews (Koes et al 1991, 1996). Whilst it is beyond the scope of this article to discuss these articles in great depth, it appears that SMTT produces short-term improvement in pain, and high patient satisfaction in certain spinal dysfunctions; however, the available evidence establishes little more than this.

FUNDAMENTALS OF SPINAL MANIPULATIVE THRUST TECHNIQUE

The fundamental elements that are required for the application of localized SMTT are listed below.

LOCALIZED PASSIVE MOVEMENT

SMTT aims to produce effects (local joint and paraspinal muscle effect) as a consequence of applying a passive movement towards one functional spinal unit, i.e. two spinal levels (Herzog 2000). It is essential, therefore, that spinal passive movement is localized to one functional spinal unit and the manipulative thrust be directed toward one zygapophyseal joint (Grieve 1991; Nyberg 1993).

COMBINATION OF MOVEMENTS

During SMTT the application of a high-velocity, low-amplitude thrust occurs at the end of range of movement for the joint. However, in order that the joint is not moved past its painless or 'normal' range of movement in any one plane, the joint is positioned in a manner that allows an end-range feel to be produced in a combination of mid-range positions. Thus the high-velocity, low-amplitude thrust is applied in a position where the joint has reached the end of its range of movement in that particular combination of plane movements but is not at the end of the available range for each of the movements if they were to be applied in isolation (Nyberg 1993).

In order to produce an end-of-combined-range position amenable to SMTT, the combinations of movement used are often complex and appear to contradict the normal coupled movements of the spine. The use of these 'irregular' coupled movements produces the 'lock' position commonly referred to in osteopathic literature (Hartman 1985).

APPRECIATION OF THE END-FEEL

An important indicator for the suitability of an SMTT is the quality of the end-feel of the combination of movements used to produce a 'lock' position. Whilst this sensation is difficult to quantify, the appreciation of the difference between the feel of a 'locked' joint and one that has not achieved a 'crisp or locked' end-feel is vital in deciding if a thrust technique is to be adopted (Grieve 1991).

LOCAL, HIGH-VELOCITY LOW-AMPLITUDE MOVEMENT

The final movement of an SMTT involves the production of a small amplitude displacement with an acceleration over this short distance that is high. Typically the duration of cervical SMTT is between 100 and 200 ms, with forces ranging from 100 to 150 Newtons (Herzog 2000).

THE EFFECTS OF SPINAL MANIPULATIVE THRUST TECHNIQUE

Various therapeutic effects of SMTT have been proposed in the literature, ranging from movement of the nucleus pulposus (Haldeman 1978) to reductions in paraspinal muscle hypertonicity (Herzog et al 1999). Unfortunately, the quality of the evidence on which some of these observations have been made has been poor, ranging from personal opinion (Fraser 1976) to poorly designed trials (Rupert et al 1985). More recent work has provided some evidence of the effects of SMTT, and whilst a considerable amount of work is still required in this area the available evidence would suggest that SMTT can cause cavitation within the synovial joint (Conway et al 1993; Herzog et al 1993), a temporary increase in the degree of displacement that is produced with force due to hysteresis effects (Herzog 2000) and an alteration in electromyographical activity in local and distant spinal muscles (Herzog et al 1999). These effects may, in turn, reduce the nociceptive afferent barrage to the dorsal horn (Zusman 1986) and evoke descending pain inhibitory systems (Wright 1995) resulting in analgesia.

INDICATIONS FOR SPINAL MANIPULATIVE THRUST TECHNIQUE

If one accepts the premise that SMTT is a modality aimed at affecting the zygapophyseal joint, then the type of clinical presentation that would suggest an amenity to SMTT would be one demonstrating signs and symptoms emanating from the zygapophyseal joint and local surrounding structures. These features would depend on the precise nature of the articular dysfunction but typically include:

- A history of onset suggestive of mechanical dysfunction
- Local nociceptive pain, with or without somatic pain referral patterns

- Pain that has clear mechanical aggravating and easing positions or movements
- Spinal movement patterns that when examined actively and passively suggest a movement restriction that is local to one or two functional spinal units (Grieve 1991).

CONTRAINDICATIONS FOR SPINAL MANIPULATIVE THRUST TECHNIQUE

The contraindications to cervical manipulation have been described in detail elsewhere (Grieve 1991; Barker et al 2000) and whilst it is beyond the scope of this article to discuss each of these contraindications two factors are of special note.

IRRITABILITY

The 'irritability' of a condition is a conceptual characterization that imparts information regarding the degree of provocation required to exacerbate the condition, the degree to which it is exacerbated, and the time it takes the condition to return to previous pain levels (Maitland et al 2001). Subjects demonstrating an irritable spinal pain syndrome rarely have spinal dysfunction amenable to SMTT (Grieve 1991). However, the presence of severe pain does not indicate an irritable condition and therefore does not preclude the use of appropriate SMTT.

INAPPROPRIATE END-FEEL

The practicality of producing an SMTT means that the last decision made, with regard to the suitability of performing an SMTT, is undertaken whilst assessing the quality of the end-feel (Davis 1999) or 'lock' immediately prior to applying the thrust. If this assessment reveals a quality of end-feel that does not match the manual therapist's expectations of an end-feel that would lead to a successful SMTT then the SMTT is contraindicated. In other words, if when adopting the pre-manipulative starting position, the joint does not feel as if it will 'go' then the manipulative thrust should not be performed (Hartman 1985).

SUMMARY OF SPINAL MANIPULATIVE THRUST TECHNIQUE

SMTT is a passive movement treatment modality that has some evidence for its efficacy in the treatment of certain spinal dysfunctions (Anderson et al 1992). The evidence for the exact mechanisms of effect is not fully known. The application of SMTT requires a skilled assessment of the active and passive movement dysfunction and the application of high-velocity, low-amplitude forces that are directed specifically at one spinal joint (Grieve 1991). In order to position the joint in a range where the movement restriction may be treated without producing excessive movement around the joint, passive movements are combined in order to produce a 'locked position' (Nyberg 1993). Thus, combined movements are an integral part of SMTT.

COMBINED MOVEMENT THEORY

This method of examination and treatment of spinal pain was developed by Brian Edwards (Edwards 1987) and is an important corollary of the Maitland Concept. Edwards (1987, 1992) has described the fundamentals of CMT as:

- The use of the analytical assessment principles described by Maitland et al (2001).
- An expansion of the subjective examination to encourage the manual therapist to recognize patterns of presentation suggestive of specific 'articular' movement dysfunctions and to test these hypotheses prior to planning the physical examination.
- An expansion of the active and passive movement examination of spinal regions in order to provide more comprehensive information regarding the movement pattern of dysfunction with classification of 'prime movements' and 'prime combinations'.
- An appreciation of which anatomical regions are likely to be placed on and off tension with combinations of physiological and accessory movements.

- An appreciation of regular and irregular patterns or combinations of spinal motion.
- The use of passive movements during treatment that move the joint within the range of movement in which resistance to movement is detected (typically towards the end of available passive range).
- A system of treatment progression that involves change in starting position rather than increase in the grade (Maitland et al 2001) of the passive movement undertaken.

These fundamental elements are identical to some of the key components required for the application of SMTT. Both methodologies require skilled interpretation of signs and symptoms with a view to recognition of movement dysfunction patterns suggestive of joint dysfunction. Both methodologies require an in-depth knowledge of the effects of movement combinations on the spinal zygapophyseal joint and the structures immediately adjacent to it. Both use passive movements that are conducted towards the end of range, during which resistance to movement can be detected and both methods involve the selection and progression of treatment based on starting position rather than an increase in the grade of the passive movement applied (Table 2.1). With these considerable similarities in approach it seems reasonable that CMT and SMTT could form concordant methodologies.

COMBINED MOVEMENT THEORY ASSESSMENT PROCESS

It is beyond the scope of this article to describe in detail the assessment process. What follows represents an overview of the process.

SUBJECTIVE EXAMINATION

This part of the examination follows the principles described by Maitland et al (2001) and follows a broadly hypothetico-deductive reasoning approach (Jones 1992). The use of pattern recognition (King & Bithell 1998) is encouraged and patterns of dysfunction that could represent

Table 2.1 Fundamentals of CMT and SMTT.

Combined movement theory	Spinal manipulative thrust technique
Passive movement treatment	Passive movement treatment
Movement induced in a range where resistance is detected	*Movement localized to one functional spinal unit*
Movement localized to one or two functional spinal units	Combining up to three physiological movements to place the joint in a starting position in which further movement can be applied
Combining up to three physiological movements to place the joint in a starting position in which further movement can be applied	Combining passive physiological and accessory movements
Combining passive physiological and accessory movements	Positioning of joints based on an interpretation of symptomatology and of which joint structures are likely to be tensioned in combined positions
Positioning of joints based on an interpretation of symptomatology and of which joint structures are likely to be tensioned in combined positions	*Use of irregular combinations of movement*
Use of normal/regular coupled movements and irregular combinations of movement	Progression of treatment by alteration of starting position rather than by alteration of grade of movement
Progression of treatment by alteration of starting position rather than by alteration of grade of movement	*Use of high-velocity, high-acceleration movement with low amplitude*
Use of low-velocity movement with low to high amplitude	

Differences in methodologies are italicized.

articular dysfunction are identified if present. The concepts of severity and irritability of the condition are established and used to structure the examination in terms of the extent of symptom provocation that is to be produced during the physical examination.

PHYSICAL EXAMINATION

After observation of static posture, observation of active movement is made. This is particularly relevant when observing the combination of movements that the patient can perform in order to most significantly change their symptoms, i.e. to reduce their pain in the case of severe pain presentation and reproduce their pain in the non-severe pain presentation. This movement combination forms an important re-assessment marker and has been termed the patient's 'functional demonstration' (Maitland et al 2001).

Single-plane active movements of the spinal region are then examined. The movements requiring particular attention should be evident from the information gained from the subjective examination and the functional demonstration. Active movements are ranked in order of importance to

establish the movement and combination of two movements that change symptomatology most significantly. These movements are termed the 'prime movement' and 'prime combination' respectively and represent the movements that are most significant in the mechanical presentation of the condition (Fig. 2.1).

The prime movement and prime combination are then examined passively using both physiological and accessory movements (Edwards 1992; Maitland et al 2001). It is during this process that the zygapophyseal joint demonstrating greatest movement dysfunction is established, quality of movement restriction felt and the relationship between range of passive movement and symptom provocation established. It is during combined passive physiological examination that the examiner will feel if the joint dysfunction has an end-feel quality that suggests an SMTT may be of use.

CMT INTERPRETATION PRINCIPLES

During and following the subjective and physical examination, interpretation of data should lead the examiner to form hypotheses regarding:

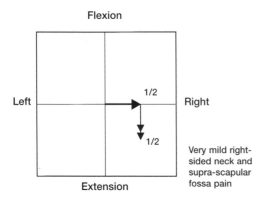

Flexion

Left — Right

1/2

1/2

Very mild right-sided neck and supra-scapular fossa pain

Extension

→ Prime movement (Right-lateral flexion).

→↓ Prime combination (Right-lateral flexion followed by extension).

Figure 2.1 Box diagram showing a graphical method of displaying the prime movement and combination of two movements forming the prime combination. These movements are established by examining the active physiological movements of the spinal region and ranking the movements to establish the two most significant movements in symptom reproduction. In this case, the prime movement is right-lateral flexion, limited to half range, and the prime combination is right-lateral flexion followed by extension, again limited to half expected range.

- The severity and irritability of the condition (Maitland et al 2001).
- The dysfunctional movement pattern associated with the condition (Edwards 1992).
- The spinal joint that is most implicated in symptomatology (Edwards 1992).
- The combination of movements/positions that most influence symptomatology (Edwards 1992).
- The position of structures that are likely sources of symptomatology, i.e. anterior or posterior joint structures (Edwards 1992).
- The regularity or irregularity of the combinations of movement producing the prime combination (Edwards 1992).
- The quality of the passive end-feel of the implicated joint's prime movement and more importantly its prime combination.
- The suitability of the implicated joint for SMTT based on the end-feel of the joint when placed in its prime combination position (Davis 1999).

SELECTION OF SMTT USING CMT

Following an interpretation of the examination, a treatment plan can be formulated. Particular SMTTs can be selected as treatment techniques using CMT. This selection process has the advantage of providing the manual therapist with a rational reasoning process that aids the integration of SMTT into practice and enables SMTT to become a technique that may be considered earlier in the resolution of the condition rather than as a technique only used after a period of mobilization. The choice of starting position for treatment depends primarily on the willingness of the examiner to reproduce symptomatology. In the first worked example, detailed below, the rationale for the starting position and progression of treatment is detailed for a situation where symptom reproduction is deemed to be acceptable.

SYMPTOM REPRODUCTION DEEMED ACCEPTABLE

In a clinical presentation where the manual therapist feels it is acceptable to reproduce symptomatology the dysfunctional joint is placed in a starting position from which symptoms can be reproduced with passive movements applied in this position.

PATIENT PRESENTATION

The patient presents with very mild right-sided neck and supra-scapular fossa pain characteristic of nociceptive and somatic referred pain. The pain is provoked with a prime movement of half-range, right-lateral flexion and a prime combination of right-lateral flexion followed by extension of the right C4/5. Passive movement examination reveals that extension performed in right-lateral flexion reproduces symptoms most significantly. Combined movement theory suggests that the structures anterior to the joint would be tensioned in this combined position. Thus, in right-lateral flexion and extension the passive movements that could be applied that would further encourage an increase in the tension of the anterior structures would be:

- Extension
- Right-lateral flexion
- Right rotation
- Anterior glide of C5 on C4
- Posterior glide of C4 on C5
- Right-lateral flexion SMTT in extension
- Right rotation SMTT in extension
- Transverse SMTT to the left in right-lateral flexion and extension.

SMTT POSITIONING

When combining the three plane movements required to produce the starting position for right-lateral flexion SMTT in right-lateral flexion and extension, the order in which the individual plane movements are combined will influence the range of movement produced and the degree to which symptomatology is reproduced. As plane movements are combined passively the range of movement that can be produced is reduced as the tension in particular structures is increased. For example, the range of extension that can be produced at C4/5 in neutral is greater than when it is performed in right-lateral flexion. Thus, when producing the starting position for the right-lateral flexion SMTT, the application of the prime movement (right-lateral flexion) as the last movement to be combined reduces the range of movement required and consequently the reproduction of symptoms.

In order that an adequate 'crisp' locked end-feel is produced whilst in mid-range for each plane movement, the combination of movements will involve the application of an irregular pattern of movements. Thus, in this example the regular combination of movements, i.e. matching the normal coupled movements of the mid-cervical spine, are extension, right-lateral flexion and right-rotation, a locked position requires an irregular movement pattern involving right-lateral flexion, extension and left rotation. As the prime movement for this example is right-lateral flexion, the starting position for the application of an SMTT could be achieved by combining right-lateral flexion, extension and left rotation in that order. (Figs 2.2 & 2.3). Right-lateral flexion followed by exten-

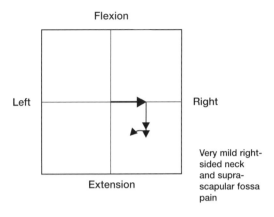

SMTT starting position (right-lateral flexion followed by extension followed by left rotation).

Figure 2.2 Box diagram showing the starting position for a right-lateral flexion SMTT with this non-severe presentation. C4–5 is placed in right-lateral flexion, extension and left rotation enabling a joint 'lock' in a mid-range combined position. This starting position utilizes the primary combination, as symptom reproduction is deemed acceptable.

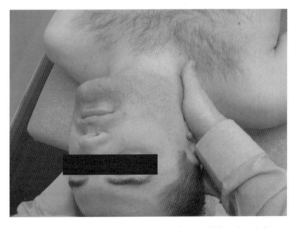

Figure 2.3 Positioning for the starting position for right-lateral flexion SMTT at C4–5 in right-lateral flexion, extension and left rotation. In this starting position the right C4–5 joint has reached 'end range' for this combination of movements but is not at end range for each movement if applied in isolation.

sion is applied first, as this is the prime movement and prime combination and symptom reproduction is acceptable in this example.

SYMPTOM REPRODUCTION DEEMED UNACCEPTABLE

In a clinical presentation when the manual therapist feels it is unacceptable to reproduce symptomatology, the dysfunctional joint is placed in a starting position from which symptoms are unlikely to be reproduced with passive movements applied in this position.

PATIENT PRESENTATION

Very severe right-sided 'nociceptive' neck and somatic supra-scapular fossa-referred pain provoked with a prime movement of half-range, right-lateral flexion and a prime combination of right-lateral flexion followed by extension of the right C4/5. CMT suggests that the structures anterior to the joint would be tensioned in this position. Thus, in left-lateral flexion and flexion the following passive movements could be applied in a position where the anterior structures are not tensioned, allowing the following therapeutic passive movements to be produced whilst avoiding symptom reproduction:

- Flexion
- Left-lateral flexion
- Left rotation
- Posterior glide of C5 on C4
- Anterior glide of C4 on C5
- Left-lateral flexion SMTT in flexion
- Left rotation SMTT in flexion
- Transverse SMTT to the right in left-lateral flexion and flexion.

SMTT POSITIONING

In order to place the joint in a position where an SMTT can be applied without reproduction of symptoms the joint must be placed in a starting position that maximally reduces the tension on the anterior joint structures whilst using an irregular movement pattern to enable a midrange lock position to be produced.

Thus, in order to produce the starting position for a left-lateral flexion thrust in flexion the movements of left-lateral flexion, flexion and

right rotation could be combined in that order. This order uses a combination of movements that is directionally opposite to the prime combination and ensures that (right rotation) the irregular pattern component (that moves the joint in a direction that may potentially reproduce symptoms) is combined in a position where only a small range of movement is available (Figs 2.4 & 2.5).

SMTT SELECTION USING CMT

SMTT selection can be based on CMT and provides the manual therapist with a method of clinical reasoning that enables SMTT to be considered as a treatment option when using combined-movement treatments. Having decided that the patient's spinal dysfunction is suitable for treatment using CMT the selection of particular SMTT can be made using information already obtained from the CMT examination. The starting position for SMTT is reasoned by

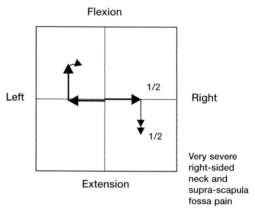

→ Prime combination (Right-lateral flexion followed by extension).

↱ SMTT starting position (left-lateral flexion followed by flexion followed by right rotation).

Figure 2.4 Box diagram showing the starting position for a left-lateral flexion SMTT with this severe presentation. C4–5 is placed in left-lateral flexion, flexion and right rotation enabling a joint 'lock' in a mid-range combined position. This position is directionally opposite to the prime combination and thus avoids symptom reproduction.

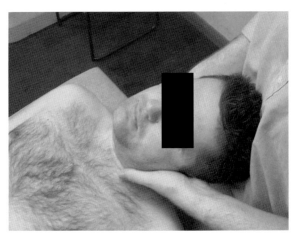

Figure 2.5 An illustration of the positioning of C4–5 in left-lateral flexion, flexion and right rotation. In this starting position the right C4–5 joint has reached 'end range' for this combination of movements but is not at end-range for each movement if applied in isolation.

analysing the combination of movements that reproduce symptomatology and placing the joint into that combined position or in its directional opposite depending on the suitability of symptom reproduction.

In order that a suitable combined end-of-range 'lock' is produced irregular patterns of movement (not matching normal coupled movement for the spinal region) are used. The order in which movements are combined to produce starting positions for SMTT is determined by the prime movement and prime combination of the dysfunction. When symptom reproduction is deemed appropriate the prime movement can be applied first. When symptoms are not to be reproduced the direction opposite of the prime movement can be applied first. The choice of irregular pattern used to form the 'lock' and the direction of SMTT will be based on the desire of the manual therapist to move the joint in a direction that will further increase the tension on, or reduce the tension on, the joint structures thought to be the source of symptoms. Two examples of the positioning for cervical SMTT

using CMT have been illustrated above; however, the principles are identical for the thoracic and lumbar spines (see Postscript).

CONCLUSION

Both CMT and SMTT provide the manual therapist with methodologies for the therapeutic passive movement of spinal dysfunctions. There is considerable overlap in the fundamental components of CMT and SMTT with both methodologies using combined movements to position the dysfunctional joint and deliver movement at the end-of-range for a combination of three plane movements. This parity of methodology enables the use of CMT as a rationale for the selection of SMTTs and it is hoped that by adopting a 'familiar' methodology in the selection of SMTT, manual therapists will find the selection of SMTTs clinically relevant.

SUMMARY POINTS

- Spinal dysfunction amenable to treatment with CMT is amenable to treatment with SMTT.
- CMT assessment provides adequate information for the selection of particular SMTTs.
- Severe pain can be treated with SMTT by adopting a starting position for techniques that is directionally opposite to the prime combination of the dysfunction.

Acknowledgements

I would like to thank Dr Brian Edwards for first showing me that CMT could be used to apply SMTT whilst attending an intermediate combined movement course at the Royal Free Hospital, London, UK in 1991 and Nikolaos Strimpakos and Dr Michael Callaghan for modelling.

REFERENCES

Anderson R, Meeker W, Wirick B, Mootz R, Kirk D, Adams A 1992 A meta-analysis of clinical trials of spinal manipulation. Journal of Manipulative and Physiological Therapeutics 14: 181–194

Barker S, Kesson M, Ashmore J, Turner G, Conway J, Stevens D 2000 Guidance for pre-manipulative testing of the cervical spine. Manual Therapy 5: 37–40

Bogduk N, Mercer S 1995 Musculoskeletal Physiotherapy: Clinical Science and Practice. In: Refshauge K, Gass E (eds) Butterworth–Heineman, Oxford

Conway PJW, Herzog W, Zhang Y, Hasler EM, Ladly K 1993 Forces required to cause cavitation during spinal manipulation of the thoracic spine. Clinical Biomechanics 8: 210–214

Cyriax J 1941 Massage, Manipulation and Local Anaesthesia, 1st edn. Hamish Hamilton Medical Books, London

Davis DG 1999 Manipulation. In: Subotnick SI (ed) Sports Medicine of the Lower Extremity, 2nd edn. Churchill Livingstone, New York, 433–454

Edwards B 1987 Clinical Assessment: The use of combined movements in assessment and treatment. In: Twomey LT, Taylor JR (eds) Physical Therapy of the Low Back Churchill Livingstone, New York, 175–224

Edwards BC 1992 Manual of Combined Movements, 1st edn. Churchill Livingstone, Edinburgh

Fraser DM 1976 Post-partum backache: a preventable condition? Canadian Family Physician 22: 1434–1439

Grieve GP 1991 Mobilization of the Spine: A Primary Handbook of Clinical Method, 5th edn. Edinburgh, Churchill Livingstone

Haldeman S 1978 The clinical basis for discussion of the mechanics of manipulation. In: Korr I (Ed) The Neurobiologic Mechanisms in Manipulative Therapy. Plenum Press, London, p.53

Hartman LS 1985 Handbook of Osteopathic Technique, 2nd edn. Unwin Hyman, London

Herzog W 2000 Clinical Biomechanics of Spinal Manipulation. Churchill Livingstone, New York

Herzog W, Conway PJW, Kawchuk GN, Zhang Y, Hasler EM1993 Forces exerted during spinal manipulation. Spine 18: 1206–1212

Herzog W, Scheele D, Conway PJ 1999 Electromyographic responses of back and limb muscles associated with spinal manipulative therapy. Spine 24: 146–153

Jones M 1992 Clinical reasoning in manual therapy. Physical Therapy 72: 875–884

King CA, Bithell C 1998 Expertise in diagnostic reasoning: a comparative study. British Journal of Therapy and Rehabilitation 5: 78–87

Koes BW, Assendelft WJ, Van der Heijden GJMG, Bouter LM, Knipschild PG 1991 Spinal manipulation and mobilization for back and neck pain: a blinded review. BMJ 303: 1298–1303

Koes B, Assendelft W, Van der Heijden G, Bouter L 1996 Spinal manipulation for low back pain. An updated systematic review of randomized clinical trials. Spine 21: 2860–2873

Maitland GD, Hengeveld E, Banks K, English K 2001 Maitland's Vertebral Manipulation, 6th edn. Churchill Livingstone, New York

Nyberg R 1993 Manipulation: definition, types, application. In: Basmajian JV, Nyberg R (Eds) Rational Manual Therapies. Williams and Wilkins, Baltimore, 21–47

Ottenbacher K, DiFabio RP 1985 Efficacy of spinal manipulation/mobilisation therapy: a meta-analysis. Spine 10: 833–837

Rupert RL, Wagnon R, Thompson P, Ezzeldin MT 1985 Chiropractic adjustments: Results of a controlled clinical trial in Egypt. International Review of Chiropractic. Winter 58–60

Wright A 1995 Hypoalgesia post-manipulative therapy: a review of a potential neurophysiological mechanism. Manual Therapy 1: 16

Zusman M 1986 Spinal manipulative therapy: Review of some proposed mechanisms and a new hypothesis. Australian Journal of Physiotherapy 32: 89–99

POSTSCRIPT

A further example of the application of combined movement in the application of SMTT is included here. Lumbar spine manipulation is detailed below, primarily to address an issue over nomenclature regarding intersegmental motion during lumbar SMTT positioning.

LUMBAR SPINE SMTT USING CMT SELECTION

In this example the patient presents with non-severe, nociceptive right-sided lumbar pain with a segmental source of L5/S1. The prime combination is extension, right-side flexion and the therapist feels it is acceptable to reproduce this pain during treatment. Theoretically, in the prime combination position, the superior part of the right L5/S1 zygapophyseal joint capsule would be placed under tension. Maximal tension would be placed on this part of the capsule with the 'regu-

lar pattern' position of extension, right-lateral flexion and right rotation. Thus, the irregular pattern position used for SMTT would be extension, *left*-lateral flexion and right rotation (Fig. 2.6)

It is apparent from Figure 2.7 that inducing right rotation of L5 on S1, whilst in left sidelying, results in associated left-side flexion, thus producing an irregular pattern of movement at this segment or 'lock'. This method of describing the direction of movement of the spinal levels uses a description of the superior level's movement in relation to the

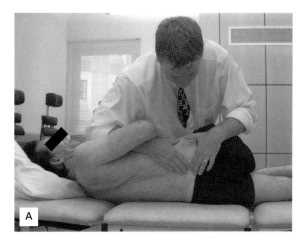

A

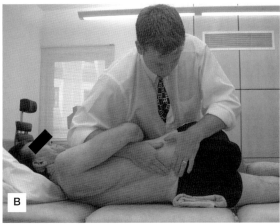

B

Figure 2.7 The starting position for a right-rotation SMTT, of L5 on S1, in extension left sideflexion. (A) illustrates the left-lateral flexion that occurs in conjunction with right rotation, when performed in left sidelying. (B) illustrates how the degree of left-lateral flexion can be accentuated by raising the pelvis up on the plinth with a towel.

Flexion

Left ———————— Right

Extension

Non-severe,
nociceptive,
right-sided
low back pain

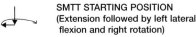

SMTT STARTING POSITION
(Extension followed by left lateral
flexion and right rotation)

Figure 2.6 The starting position for a right rotation SMTT of L5 on S1 in left sidelying. As it is deemed acceptable to reproduce mild symptoms, the SMTT can be performed in a starting position that is similar to the primary combination. If symptom reproduction was deemed to be unacceptable the starting position would involve combining flexion with left-lateral flexion and right rotation, with more emphasis on the left-lateral flexion component and less on right rotation.

inferior level. Thus, if the method of describing intersegmental movement, which is used to describe cervical and thoracic movement, is applied to the lumbar spine it effectively means that when performing a typical rotation technique in left side-lying, right rotation is actually being induced — a procedure that has conventionally been labelled as a left rotation technique by some clinicians.

Thoracic Spine

SECTION CONTENTS

3

Rotational instability of the midthoracic spine: assessment and management

D. G. Lee

Orthopaedic Division of the Canadian Physiotherapy Association, Delta Orthopaedic Physiotherapy Clinic, Delta, British Columbia, Canada

Recent research has enhanced the understanding of instability of the spine. The principles of this research have been incorporated into the evaluation and treatment of the unstable thorax. Rotational instability of the midthorax is commonly seen following trauma to the chest. Specific mobility and stability tests have been developed to detect this instability. The tests are derived from a biomechanical model of evaluation. Treatment is based on sound stabilization principles and although the segment will remain unstable on passive testing, the patient can be trained to control the biomechanics of the thorax and return to a high level of function. *Manual Therapy* (1996) **1(5)**, 234–244

INTRODUCTION

In the literature pertaining to back pain, the musculoskeletal components of the thorax have received little attention. Research is sparse in all areas including developmental anatomy, normal biomechanics, pathomechanical processes, evaluation and treatment. And yet, midback pain is not uncommon. A biomechanical approach to assessment and treatment of the thorax requires an understanding of its normal behaviour. A working model has been proposed (Lee 1993; 1994a, b), part of which is based on scientific research (Panjabi et al 1976) and the remainder on clinical observation. This model requires validation through further research studies.

The understanding of instability of the spine has been enhanced by recent research (Hides et al

1994, 1995; Hodges & Richardson 1995a, b; Panjabi 1992a, b; Richardson & Jull 1995; Vleeming et al 1995). The principles of this research have been incorporated into the evaluation and treatment of the unstable thorax. Rotational instability of the midthorax involves both the spinal and costal components of the segment. Specific tests have been developed (Lee 1993, 1994a, b; Lowcock 1990) to detect this instability and the management is based on sound stabilization principles (Richardson & Jull 1994).

ANATOMY

The thorax can be divided into four regions according to anatomical and biomechanical differences. The midthorax is the topic of this paper and includes the T3 to T7 vertebrae, the third to seventh ribs and the sternum. Rotational instability of the thorax is most common in this region. A brief anatomical review is relevant in order to understand the normal mechanics and pathomechanics of rotation in the midthorax.

The facets on both the superior and inferior articular processes of the thoracic vertebra are curved in both the transverse and sagittal planes (Davis 1959). This orientation permits multidirectional movement and does not restrain, nor direct, any coupling of motion when the thorax rotates. Neither do they limit the amount of lateral translation that occurs in conjunction with rotation (Panjabi et al 1976). The ventral aspect of the transverse process contains a deep, concave facet for articulation with the rib of the same number (Fig. 3.1). This curvature influences the conjunct rotation that occurs when the rib glides in a superoinferior direction. A superior glide is associated with anterior rotation of the rib; an inferior glide is associated with posterior rotation.

The posterolateral corners of both the superior and inferior aspects of the vertebral body contain an ovoid demifacet for articulation with the head of the rib. Development of the superior costovertebral joint is delayed until early adolescence (Penning & Wilmink 1987; Williams et al

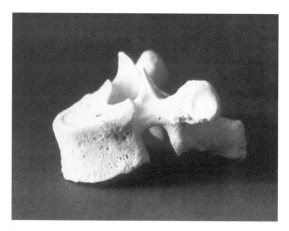

Figure 3.1 Anterolateral view of the fourth thoracic vertebra. Note the concave facet on the transverse process for articulation with the fourth rib as well as the two demi-facets on the lateral aspect of the vertebral body for articulation with the heads of the fourth and fifth ribs. Reproduced with kind permission from Diane G. Lee Physiotherapist Corporation from Lee (1994b).

1989). In the skeletally mature, the costovertebral joint is divided into two synovial cavities separated by an intra-articular ligament. Several ligaments support the costovertebral complex, including the radiate, costotransverse or interosseous ligament, lateral costotransverse ligament and the superior costotransverse ligament. Attenuation of some of these ligaments occurs when the midthorax is unstable.

The anatomy and age-related changes of the intervertebral disc in the thorax have received recent study. Crawford (1995) investigated a series of 51 cadavers aged from 19 to 91 years and tabulated the incidence and location of degeneration, Schmorl's nodes and posterior intervertebral disc prolapse. The midthoracic region was found to have the highest incidence of degenerated discs and intervertebral prolapses. Wood et al (1995) found that 73% of 90 asymptomatic individuals had positive anatomical findings at one or more levels of the thoracic spine on magnetic resonance imaging. These findings included herniation, bulging, annular tears, deformation of the spinal cord and Scheuermann end-plate irregularities. While structural changes are common, their clinical consequences are unknown. It is hypothesized (Lee 1993, 1994a, b) that some changes must take place in the intervertebral disc for the thoracic segment to become unstable in rotation. These changes may occur prior to the onset of symptoms and predispose the patient to the development of instability.

BIOMECHANICS OF ROTATION

In the cadaver, Panjabi et al (1976) found that rotation around a vertical axis was coupled with contralateral sideflexion and contralateral horizontal translation. Clinically, it appears that in the midthorax, midrange rotation can couple with either contralateral or ipsilateral sideflexion. At the limit of rotation, however, the direction of sideflexion has consistently been found to be ipsilateral (Fig. 3.2). In other words, at the limit of axial rotation, rotation and sideflexion occur to the same side. It may be that the thorax must be intact and stable both anteriorly and posteriorly for this *in vivo* coupling of motion to occur. The anterior elements of the thorax were removed 3 cm lateral to the costotransverse joints in the study by Panjabi et al (1976).

During right rotation of the trunk, the following biomechanics are proposed (Lee 1993, 1994a, b). The superior vertebra rotates to the right and translates to the left (Fig. 3.3). Right rotation of the superior vertebral body 'pulls' the superior aspect of the head of the left rib forward at the costovertebral joint, inducing anterior rotation of the neck of the left rib (superior glide at the left costotransverse joint), and 'pushes' the superior aspect of the head of the right rib backward, inducing posterior rotation of the neck of the right rib (inferior glide at the right costotransverse joint). The left lateral translation of the superior vertebral body 'pushes' the left rib posterolaterally along the line of the neck of the rib and causes a posterolateral translation of the rib at the left costotransverse joint. Simultaneously, the left lateral translation 'pulls' the right rib anteromedially along the line of the neck of the rib and causes an anteromedial translation of the rib at the right costotransverse joint. An anteromedial/posterolateral slide of the ribs *relative to the transverse processes to which they attach* is thought to occur during axial rotation.

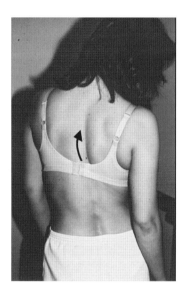

Figure 3.2 Clinically, the midthorax appears to sideflex (arrow) and rotate to the same side at the limit of rotation of the trunk. Reproduced with kind permission from Diane G. Lee Physiotherapist Corporation from Lee (1994b).

When the limit of this horizontal translation is reached, both the costovertebral and the costotransverse ligaments are tensed. Stability of the ribs both anteriorly and posteriorly is required for the following motion to occur. Further right rotation of the superior vertebra occurs as the superior vertebral body tilts to the right (glides superiorly along the left superior costovertebral joint and inferiorly along the right superior costovertebral joint). This tilt causes right sideflexion of the superior vertebra *at the limit* of right rotation of the midthoracic segment (Fig. 3.4)

DEFINITION OF INSTABILITY

Instability can be defined as a loss of the functional integrity of a system that provides stability. In the thorax, there are two systems which contribute to stability: the osteoarticularligamentous and the myofascial. Snijders and Vleeming (Snijders et al 1992; Vleeming et al 1990a, b, 1995) refer to these two systems as form and force closure. Together they provide a self-locking mechanism that is useful in rehabilitation.

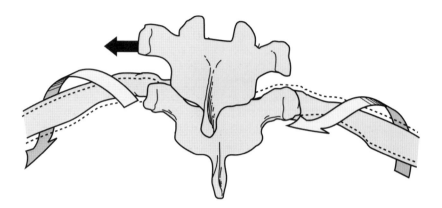

Figure 3.3 The biomechanics proposed to occur in the midthorax during right rotation of the trunk. Reproduced by permission from Lee 2003.

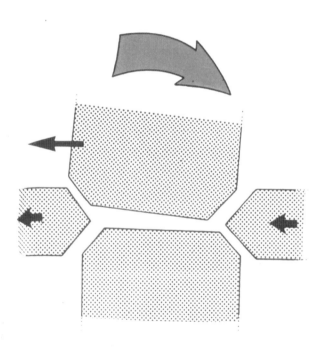

Figure 3.4 At the limit of left lateral translation, the superior vertebra sideflexes to the right along the plane of the pseudo 'U' joint formed by the intervertebral disc and the superior costovertebral joints. Reproduced by kind permission of The Journal of Manual and Manipulative Therapy from Lee (1993).

'Form closure refers to a stable situation with closely fitting joint surfaces, where no extra forces are needed to maintain the state of the system' (Snijders et al 1992; Vleeming et al 1995). The degree of inherent form closure of any joint depends on its anatomy. There are three factors that contribute to form closure: the shape of the joint surface, the friction coefficient of the articular cartilage and the integrity of the ligaments that approximate the joint. The costal components of the midthorax have considerable form closure given the shape of the costovertebral joints and the structure of the ligaments.

'In the case of force closure, extra forces are needed to keep the object in place. Here friction must be present' (Snijders et al 1992). Joints with predominantly flat surfaces are well suited to transfer large moments of force but are vulnerable to shear. Factors that increase intra-articular compression will increase the friction coefficient and the ability of the joint to resist translation. The relatively flat zygapophyseal joints provide little resistance to lateral translation and rely on the form closure of the costal components and the myofascial force closure for stability. The muscles that contribute to force closure of the midthoracic region include the transversospinalis and erector spinae groups. These muscles will be addressed in rehabilitation of the unstable thorax.

Panjabi has proposed a conceptual model that describes the interaction between the components of the spinal stabilizing system (Panjabi 1992a, b). In this model he describes the neutral zone, which is a small range of displacement near the joint's neutral position where minimal resistance is given by the osteoligamentous structures. Specific clinical tests aim to palpate the motion within the neutral zone. The range of the neutral zone may increase with injury, articular degeneration (loss of form closure) and/or weakness of the stabilizing musculature (loss of force closure). When the thorax is unstable, the neutral zone is increased.

Rotational instability of the thorax causes an increase in the neutral zone that is palpated during segmental lateral translation. The unstable segment has a softer end feel of motion, an increased quantity of translation and a variable symptom response. If the joint is irritable, the test may provoke pain. If the instability is long standing and asymptomatic, the tests are often not provocative.

CLINICAL TESTS FOR LATERAL TRANSLATION STABILITY (ROTATION)

To evaluate the stability of a midthoracic segment, it is necessary to first determine the available mobility in lateral translation. Left rotation/left sideflexion/right translation requires the left sixth rib to glide anteromedially relative to the left transverse process of T6 and the right sixth rib to glide posterolaterally relative to the right transverse process of T6 and the T5 vertebra to laterally translate to the right relative to T6. This motion is tested in the following manner. The patient is sitting with the arms crossed to opposite shoulders (Fig. 3.5). With the right hand/arm, the thorax is palpated such that the fifth finger of the right hand lies along the *sixth* rib. With the left hand, the transverse processes of T6 are fixed. With the right hand/arm the T5 vertebra and the sixth ribs are translated *purely* to the right in the transverse plane. The quantity, and in particular the end feel of motion, is noted and compared to the levels above and below.

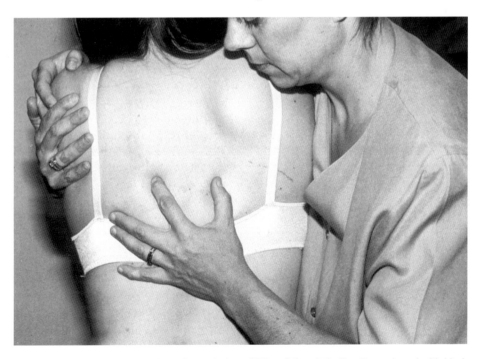

Figure 3.5 Passive mobility test for right lateral translation of T5 and the sixth ribs. Reproduced with kind permission from Diane G. Lee Physiotherapist Corporation from Lee (1994b).

Next, the stability of the T5–6 spinal component can be evaluated by restricting the sixth ribs from gliding relative to their transverse processes and then applying a lateral translation force. No motion should occur when the ribs are fixed. This test stresses the anatomical structures that resist horizontal translation between two adjacent vertebrae when the ribs between them are fixed. A positive response is an increase in the quantity of motion and a decrease in the resistance at the end of the range. To test the T5–6 segment, the patient is sitting with the arms crossed to opposite shoulders (Fig. 3.6). With the right hand/arm, the thorax is palpated such that the fifth finger of the right hand lies along the fifth rib. With the left hand, T6 and the sixth ribs are fixed bilaterally by

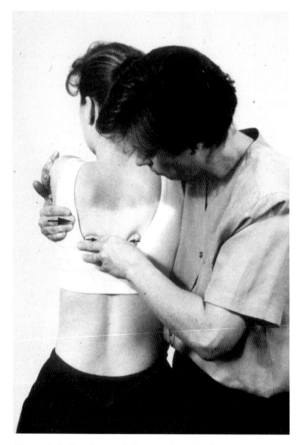

Figure 3.6 Passive stability test for right lateral translation of T5–6 with the sixth ribs fixed. Reproduced with kind permission from Diane G. Lee Physiotherapist Corporation from Lee (1994b).

compressing the ribs centrally towards their costovertebral joints (small arrows Fig. 3.6). The T5 vertebra is translated through the thorax *purely* in the transverse plane. The quantity of motion, the reproduction of any symptoms and the end feel of motion is noted and compared with the levels above and below. When the segment is stable, no motion should occur. When unstable, the same degree of motion previously noted in the mobility test can be palpated.

SUBJECTIVE AND PHYSICAL FINDINGS

Rotational instability of the midthorax can occur when excessive rotation is applied to the unrestrained thorax or when rotation of the thorax is forced against a fixed rib cage (seat belt injury). At the limit of right rotation in the midthorax, the superior vertebra has translated to the left, the left rib has translated posterolaterally and the right rib has translated anteromedially. Further right rotation results in a right lateral tilt of the superior vertebra (Fig. 3.4). Fixation of the superior vertebra occurs when the left lateral translation exceeds the physiological motion barrier and the vertebra is unable to return to its neutral position.

Initially, the patient complains of localized, central midthoracic pain that can radiate around the chest wall. The pain may be associated with numbness along the related dermatome. Sympathetic symptoms, including sensations of local coldness, sweating, burning and visceral referral, are common. If the unstable complex is fixated at the limit of rotation, very little relieves the pain. All movements, especially contralateral rotation, and sustained postures tend to aggravate the pain. If the complex is not fixed, the patient often finds that contralateral rotation and extension affords some relief.

Positionally, the following findings are noted when T5–6 is fixated in left-lateral translation and right rotation (right rotational instability). T5–T6 is right rotated in hyperflexion, neutral and extension, the right sixth rib is anteromedial posteriorly and the left sixth rib is posterolateral posteriorly. All active movements produce a 'kink' at the level of the fixation; the worst movement is often rotation (Fig. 3.7). The passive accessory mobility tests for the zygapophyseal and costotransverse joints are reduced but present. The right-lateral translation mobility test is completely blocked.

Prior to reduction of the fixation, the left-lateral translation stability test of T5–6 is normal because the joint is stuck at the limit of left-lateral translation. After the fixation is reduced, the stability test reveals the underlying excessive left-lateral translation. The reduction restores the complex to a neutral position from which the amplitude of left-lateral translation can be more effectively measured.

If the segment is not fixated at the limit of lateral translation, then both the mobility and stability tests will reveal excessive left-lateral translation. When the sixth ribs are compressed medially into the vertebral body of T5, there should be no lateral translation of T5 relative to T6. When the segment is unstable, excessive motion during this test is noted.

Segmental atrophy of multifidus can be palpated bilaterally. In the lumbar spine, Hides et al (1994) found wasting and local inhibition at a segmental level of the lumbar multifidus muscle in all patients with a first episode of acute/subacute low back pain. In a follow-up study Hides et al (1995) found that without therapeutic intervention, multifidus did not regain its original size or function and the recurrence rate of low back pain over an 8-month period was very high. They also found that the deficit could be reversed with an appropriate exercise programme. This research is consistent with clinical observation of instability in the midthorax.

TREATMENT

If the segment is fixated at the limit of lateral translation/rotation, a manipulative reduction is necessary prior to the initiation of a stabilization programme. When T5–6 is fixated in left-lateral translation/right rotation the following technique is used.

The patient is in left sidelying, the head supported on a pillow and the arms crossed to the opposite shoulders. With the left hand, the right seventh rib is palpated posteriorly with the thumb and the left seventh rib is palpated posteriorly with the index or long finger. T6 is fixed by compressing the two seventh ribs towards the midline. Care must be taken to avoid fixation of the sixth ribs, which must be free to glide relative to the transverse processes of T6. The other hand/arm lies across the patient's crossed arms to control the thorax. Segmental localization is achieved by flexing and extending the joint until a neutral position of the zygapophyseal joints is achieved. This localization is maintained as the patient is rolled supine *only until contact is made between the table and the dorsal hand.*

From this position, T5 and the left and right sixth ribs are translated laterally to the right

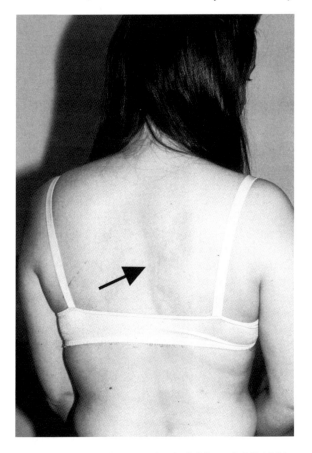

Figure 3.7 This patient sustained a left lateral shift (right rotational instability) of T5 and the sixth ribs in a motor vehicle accident. Note the 'kink' at the limit of right rotation. Reproduced with kind permission from Diane G. Lee Physiotherapist Corporation from Lee (1994b).

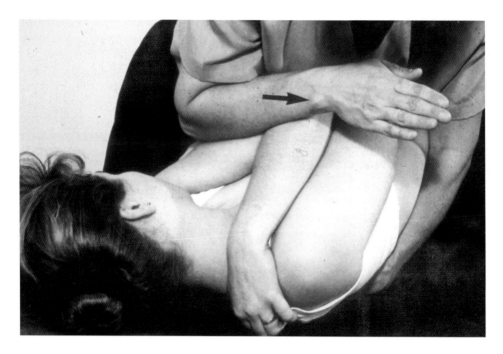

Figure 3.8 Manipulation technique for reduction of a fixated left-lateral shift of T5 and the sixth ribs relative to T6. Strong distraction must be maintained throughout the technique. Reproduced with kind permission from Diane G. Lee Physiotherapist Corporation from Lee (1994b).

through the thorax to the motion barrier. Strong longitudinal distraction is applied through the thorax prior to the application of a high-velocity, low-amplitude thrust. The thrust is in a lateral direction in the transverse plane (Fig. 3.8). The goal of the technique is to laterally translate T5 and the left and right sixth ribs relative to T6. Following reduction of the fixation, the thorax is taped (Fig. 3.9) to remind the patient to avoid end-range rotation. Stabilization is then required.

If the segment is not fixated, stabilization is begun immediately. Physiotherapy cannot restore form closure; therefore, the emphasis of treatment must be on the restoration of force closure. The goal is to reduce the dynamic neutral zone during functional activities and to avoid the end ranges of rotation, thus limiting the chances of fixation. This is accomplished through specific exercises augmented with muscle stimulation and electromyography. The first group of muscles that must be addressed are the transversospinal (multifidus) and erector spinae groups.

Essentially, the patient is taught to specifically recruit the segmental muscles isometrically and then concentrically while prone over a gym ball (Fig. 3.10). Electrical stimulation can be a useful adjunct at this time. In sidelying, specific segmental rotation can be resisted by the therapist, both concentrically and eccentrically, to facilitate the return of multifidus function. The programme is progressed by increasing the load the thorax must control. Initially, scapular motion is introduced, especially in lower trapezius work. The patient must control the neutral position of the midthorax throughout the scapular depression. The goal is to teach the patient to isolate scapular motion from spinal motion so that the scapula does not produce spinal motion during activities involving the arm. Once control is gained over the scapula, exercises involving the entire upper extremity may be added. By increasing the lever arm and then the load, the midthorax is further challenged. Gymnastic ball, proprioceptive, balance and resistive work can

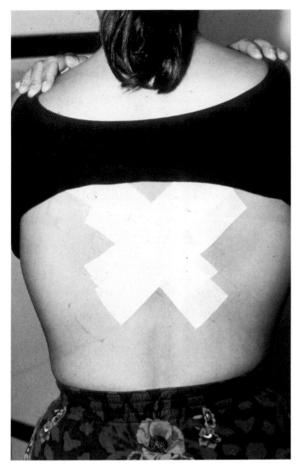

Figure 3.9 The thorax is taped for proprioceptive input to remind the patient which movements to avoid. Reproduced with kind permission from Diane G. Lee Physiotherapist Corporation from Lee (1994b).

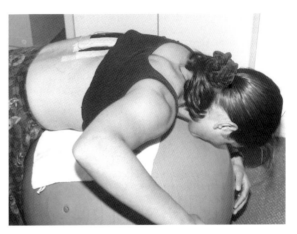

Figure 3.10 Re-education of the spinal extensors can be facilitated by electrical stimulation. Reproduced with kind permission from Diane G. Lee Physiotherapist Corporation from Lee (1994b).

be integrated into the programme as needed. The velocity of the exercises can be increased according to the patient's work and recreation demands. Initially, the load should be applied bilaterally and then progressed to unilateral work. At the completion of the programme the patient should be able to isolate specific spinal extension without scapular motion and control both bilateral and unilateral arm motion throughout midrange. They are advised to avoid any activity that places the midthorax at the limit of rotation in the direction of their instability.

CONCLUSION

Instability of the thorax can be extremely debilitating but is a treatable condition. The segment remains statically unstable and the neutral zone, on passive testing, remains increased. Through appropriate training, the region can become dynamically stable and the neutral zone controlled.

REFERENCES

Crawford RJ 1995 Normal and degenerative anatomy of thoracic intervertebral discs. Proceedings of the 9th Biennial Conference of the Manipulative Physiotherapists Association of Australia. Gold Coast, Queensland, 24–29

Davis PR 1959 The medial inclination of the human thoracic intervertebral articular facets. Journal of Anatomy 93: 68–74

Hides JA, Stokes MJ, Saide M, Jull GA, Cooper DH 1994 Evidence of lumbar multifidus muscle wasting ipsilateral to symptoms in patients with acute/subacute low back pain. Spine 19(2): 165–172

Hides JA, Richardson CA, Jull GA 1995 Multifidus inhibition in acute low back pain: recovery is not spontaneous. Proceedings of the 9th Biennial Conference of the Manipulative Physiotherapists Association of Australia. Gold Coast, Queensland, 57–60

Hodges PW, Richardson CA 1995a Neuro-motor dysfunction of the trunk musculature in low back pain Patients. Proceedings of the World Confederation of Physical Therapists Congress, Washington

Hodges PW, Richardson CA 1995b Dysfunction of transversus abdominis associated with chronic low back pain. Proceedings of the 9th Biennial Conference of the Manipulative Physiotherapists Association of Australia. Gold Coast, Queensland, 61–62

Lee DG 1993 Biomechanics of the thorax: a clinical model of in vivo function. Journal of Manual and Manipulative Therapy 1(1): 13–21

Lee DG 1994a Biomechanics of the thorax. In: Grant R (ed) Physical Therapy of the Cervical and Thoracic Spine, 2nd edn. Churchill Livingstone, New York, pp 47–64

Lee DG 1994b Manual therapy for the thorax — a biomechanical approach. Delta Orthopaedic Physiotherapy Clinic, 301 11950 80th Ave, Delta, BC V4C 1Y2

Lowcock J 1990 Thoracic joint stability and clinical stress tests. Proceedings of the Canadian Orthopaedic Manipulative Physiotherapists, Orthopaedic Division of the Canadian Physiotherapy Association Newsletter November/December 1991: 15–19

Panjabi MM 1992a The stabilizing system of the spine. Part I. Function, dysfunction, adaptation, and enhancement. Journal of Spinal Disorders 5(4): 383–389

Panjabi MM 1992b The stabilizing system of the spine. Part II. Neutral zone and instability hypothesis. Journal of Spinal Disorders 5(4): 390–397

Panjabi MM, Brand RA, White AA 1976 Mechanical properties of the human thoracic spine. Journal of Bone and Joint Surgery 58A: 642–652

Penning L, Wilmink JT 1987 Rotation of the cervical spine — A CT study in normal subjects. Spine 12(8): 732–738

Richardson CA, Jull GA 1994 Concepts of Assessment and Rehabilitation for active lumbar stability. In: Boyling JD,

Palastanga N (eds) Grieve's Modern Manual Therapy, 2nd edn. Churchill Livingstone. Edinburgh, pp 705–720

Richardson CA, Jull GA 1995 Muscle control — pain control. What exercises would you prescribe? Manual Therapy 1(1): 2–10

Snijders CJ, Vleeming A, Stoeckart R 1992 Transfer of Lumbosacral Load to Iliac Bones and Legs. Part I: Biomechanics of Self-bracing of the Sacroiliac Joints and its Significance for Treatment and Exercise. In: Vleeming A, Mooney V, Snijders CJ, Dorman T (eds) First Interdisciplinary World Congress on Low Back Pain and its Relation to the Sacroiliac Joint. San Diego, CA, Nov. 5–6, pp 233–254

Vleeming A, Stoeckart R, Volkers ACW, Snijders CJ 1990a Relation between form and function in the sacroiliac joint. Part 1: Clinical anatomical aspects. Spine 15(2): 130–132

Vleeming A, Volkers ACW, Snijders CJ, Stoeckart R 1990b Relation between form and function in the sacroiliac joint. Part 2: Biomechanical aspects. Spine 15(2): 133–135

Vleeming A, Snijders CJ, Stoeckart R, Mens JMA 1995 A New Light on Low Back Pain. In: Vleeming A, Mooney V, Dorman T, Snijders CJ (eds) Second Interdisciplinary World Congress on Low Back Pain. San Diego, CA, Nov. 9–11, 149–168

Williams P, Warwick R, Dyson M, Bannister LH 1989 Grays Anatomy. 37th edn. Churchill Livingstone, Edinburgh

Wood KB, Garvey TA, Gundry C, Heithoff KB 1995 Magnetic resonance imaging of the thoracic spine. Journal of Bone and Joint Surgery 77A(11): 1631–1637

POSTSCRIPT

Although research continues to be sparse in the area of the thorax, clinical developments have occurred since this article was first published. The original paper described tests for articular function of the thorax (form closure) with an emphasis on how to detect and manage passive rotational instability of a midthoracic segment. Since then, tests for muscle function (force closure) (Lee 2003a) and exercises using imagery for isolation and training of the local stabilizing muscles (Lee 2003b) have been developed. This postscript will introduce new tests for examining force closure and motor control of a thoracic segment as well as an exercise using imagery to facilitate the isolation of the muscles which, it is proposed, stabilize a thoracic segment.

TESTS FOR FORCE CLOSURE AND MOTOR CONTROL OF A THORACIC SEGMENT

Prone arm lift

The Prone Arm Lift test evolved (Lee 2003b) from the Active Straight Leg Raise Test (ASLR) (Mens et al 1997, 1999), which was developed to evaluate stability of the lumbopelvic region. The prone patient is asked to lift their arm off of the table (only a few degrees of lift is necessary) (Fig. 3.11) and to note any difference in the effort required to lift the left or right arm. The strategy used to stabilize the thorax during this task is observed. The arm should flex at the glenohumeral joint, the scapula should remain upwardly rotated and stable against the chest wall and the thorax should not rotate, sidebend, flex, extend or translate. If the arm is elevated to the end of its available range then the thorax will move; this is a normal biomechanical consequence. Therefore, when interpreting the findings from this test it is important to observe the thorax at the moment the arm begins to lift. The provocation of any pain is also noted. The thorax is then compressed passively (Fig. 3.12) by approximating the ribs (noted to be moving during the first part of this test) towards the midline. The Prone Arm Lift test is then repeated while this compression is maintained and any change in effort and/or pain is noted.

When a patient has a rotational instability of the midthorax and lacks dynamic control, the segment can be seen to laterally translate and rotate during the Prone Arm Lift test. The effort required to lift the arm is increased and subsequently decreases when segmental compression is applied. The patient often reports that the arm feels lighter and easier to lift when their thorax is passively stabilized (compressed) and that their pain is decreased. If the segment is fixated (see main article), this compression can result in increased effort to lift the arm and increased pain.

Force closure and the neutral zone

When the force closure mechanism is effective, it is hypothesized that contraction of the muscles of the local system (Bergmark 1989; Comerford & Mottram 2001) compresses the thoracic segment and thereby increases the stiffness and reduces the size of the neutral zone. This has been verified for the sacroiliac joint (Richardson et al 2002). To test the status of the force closure mechanism responsible for controlling lateral translation of a midthoracic segment, the patient is first instructed to recruit the local muscle system (see below). Once the patient is able to sustain a tonic contraction of the local muscles, the effect of this contraction is assessed by repeating the form closure tests for lateral translation (see main article). The stiffness should increase and no relative intersegmental or vertebrocostal motion should be felt. This means that an adequate amount of compression of the thorax has occurred and the force closure mechanism is effective. If the motion remains unchanged during activation of the local system, then the force closure mechanism is ineffective for controlling lateral translation. This is a poor prognostic sign for successful rehabilitation with exercise.

Activation/Isolation of the local stabilizers of the thorax

Coordinated action between the local and global muscle systems is required for forces to be effectively transferred through the thorax. This ensures that stability is achieved without rigidity and/or episodes of collapse. The reader is referred to Linda-Joy Lee's chapter in *The Thorax — An Integrated Approach* (Lee 2003a) for further information.

Stabilization therapy for all regions of the spine begins with activation/isolation of the local system. This can be facilitated using imagery (Franklin 1996; Lee 2001). The following exercise uses imagery to assist in the isolation of the local stabilizers of the thorax. The patient is sitting with the thorax in a neutral spine position (Lee 2003b). With one hand, the local stabilizers of the dysfunctional segment are palpated. With the other hand, a point on the midaxillary line of the rib associated with this segment (sixth rib for T6) is palpated. The patient is instructed to imagine a line or connection between these two points. They are instructed to slowly breathe in and on the outward breath to think about 'connecting' or drawing together the two points. A slow, sequential pressure can be provided from lateral to medial (ribs into spine) to provide a proprioceptive input

and thus facilitate the image of compressing the ribs into the vertebral column. A deep, slow swelling (tonic contraction) of the local stabilizers indicates a successful response. This is felt as a gradual increase in tension or firmness as opposed to a superficial, rapid bulging (phasic contraction). The latter is indicative of a superficial global muscle contraction (Moseley et al 2002).

Once the patient can isolate the local stabilizers they are instructed to maintain this contraction and breathe normally. The spine should retain its neutral position, and the scapular muscles should remain relaxed as should the global stabilizers of the thorax. Loading is then introduced to the thorax by adding controlled motions of the scapula and then the arm. With every progression introduced, it is important to ensure that the local stabilizers remain activated.

CONCLUSION

Rotational instability of the thorax remains a common clinical condition. Physiotherapy cannot alter the structural changes that have lead to the passive instability; however, we can teach the patient to dynamically control the dysfunctional segment. The tests described in this postscript can be used to determine the status of the force closure mech-

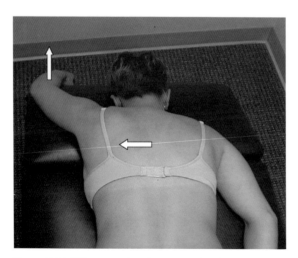

Figure 3.11 When a patient has a rotational instability of the midthorax and lacks dynamic control, the segment can be seen to laterally translate and rotate during the Prone Arm Lift test.

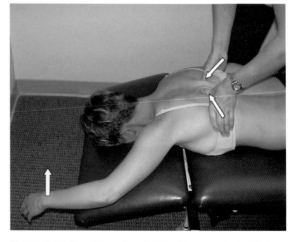

Figure 3.12 The Prone Arm Lift test is repeated whilst the therapist applies compression of the ribs towards the midline at the level of the rotational instability. Any change in effort and/or pain is noted.

anism. Once the patient is taught to isolate the local stabilizers, the tests can also be used to predict if rehabilitation is likely to be successful with appropriate motor control retraining. Although these tests appear to be effective clinically, they remain to be validated scientifically.

REFERENCES

Bergmark A 1989 Stability of the lumbar spine. A study in mechanical engineering. Acta Orthopedica Scandinavica 230 (60): 20

Comerford MJ, Mottram SL 2001 Movement and stability dysfunction — contemporary developments. Manual Therapy 6(1): 15–25

Franklin E 1996 Dynamic alignment through imagery. Human Kinetics

Lee DG 2001 Imagery for Core Stabilization — an educational video. DGL Physiotherapist Corp., www.dianelee.ca

Lee DG 2003a The Thorax — An Integrated Approach. DGL Physiotherapist Corp., www.dianelee.ca

Lee LJ 2003b Restoring force closure/motor control of the thorax. In: Lee DG (ed) The Thorax — An Integrated Approach. DGL Physiotherapist Corp., www.dianelee.ca

Mens JMA, Vleeming A, Snijders CJ, Stam HJ 1997 Active straight leg raising test: a clinical approach to the load transfer function of the pelvic girdle. In: Vleeming A, Mooney V, Dorman T, Snijders C, Stoeckart R (eds) Movement, Stability and Low Back Pain. Churchill Livingstone, Edinburgh

Mens JMA, Vleeming A, Snijders CJ, Stam HJ, Ginai AZ 1999 The active straight leg raising test and mobility of the pelvic joints. European Spine 8: 468

Moseley GL, Hodges PW, Gandevia SC 2002 Deep and superficial fibres of the lumbar multifidus muscle are differentially active during voluntary arm movements. Spine 27(2): E29

Richardson CA, Snijders CJ, Hides JA, Damen L, Pas MS, Storm J 2002 The relationship between the transversely oriented abdominal muscles, sacroiliac joint mechanics and low back pain. Spine 27(4): 399–405

Lumbar spine

SECTION CONTENTS

4

Muscle control–pain control. What exercises would you prescribe?

C. A. Richardson   G. A. Jull
Department of Physiotherapy, The University of
Queensland, Brisbane, Australia

A very specific type of exercise has been devised which is proving to provide effective pain relief for chronic and recurrent back pain sufferers. The exercise approach focuses on retraining a precise co-contraction pattern of the deep trunk muscles, the transversus abdominis and lumbar multifidus. The approach is based on the knowledge of how muscles provide stability for the spine in normal situations. It has been further developed according to research evidence that has demonstrated dysfunction in the deep trunk muscles in patients with back pain. The mechanism for pain relief with this specific exercise approach is believed to be through enhanced stability of the lumbar spine segments.
Manual Therapy (1995) **1**, 2–10

INTRODUCTION

Therapeutic exercise encompasses many well-known exercise strategies, such as rehabilitating the functional demands of the muscle system, enhancing cardiovascular fitness or improving joint and muscle flexibility. Exercise can also be used to assist in pain relief through several local or general physiological effects (McArdle et al 1991). Our particular interest has been in the use of exercise for pain control in spinal pain patients. It is our hypothesis that control of back pain and prevention of its recurrence can be assisted by enhancing muscle control of the spinal segment. The aim is to improve active segmental stabilization thereby protecting the joints from painful strains and reinjury.

In recent times, several different exercise programmes have been proposed to promote lumbar stabilization (Robison 1992; Saal & Saal 1989). The ability of such programmes to improve stabilization of the lumbar spine has been difficult to evaluate because of a lack of appropriate measurement methods. Current programmes consist of a variety of general trunk and girdle exercises and, for the most part, they seem to have had some success (Saal & Saal 1989). However, within these general programmes, it is difficult to ascertain which particular features of the exercise tasks or facilitation techniques are responsible for the more successful outcomes in some patients compared to others. Therefore, it is sometimes difficult for the clinician to know where to place the emphasis in their retraining of a back pain patient.

Our work with spinal pain patients both in the clinic and in the laboratory has led to the development of some quite specific exercise techniques for the rehabilitation of lumbar segmental control. Research is beginning to vindicate these approaches. In presenting these particular exercise techniques, it is appropriate to consider several issues. These include the mechanisms involved in providing muscle support for the lumbar motion segment and why muscle control is needed to enhance segmental stabilization in back pain patients. It is also necessary to understand which muscles are vital for segmental stabilization as well as those which demonstrate dysfunction in back pain patients. This provides a basis for identifying features to consider in exercise design for specific methods of rehabilitation of active lumbar segmental control.

MECHANISMS FOR MUSCULAR SUPPORT OF THE LUMBAR MOTION SEGMENT

The muscle system, in its function of stability, provides protection to articular structures. It can help minimize unwanted joint displacement, aid stress absorption and generally prolong the 'cartilage serving time' of the joint (Baratta et al 1988).

The development of active joint stabilization has been attributed to several muscle recruitment strategies. One strategy is the early pre-programmed recruitment of particular muscles. Specific muscles are recruited before an action is commenced to ensure that the joint is supported prior to a given movement. For example, during a jumping task, the leg extensor muscles are recruited prior to ground contact in preparation for the forces of landing (Gollhofer & Kyrolainen 1991).

The regulation of muscle stiffness is also important for the stabilization of joints (Johansson et al 1991). A mechanism for increasing joint stability through enhanced muscle stiffness is co-contraction of agonist and antagonist muscles that lie on each side of a joint (Andersson & Winters 1990). Recruiting muscles in co-contraction is considered to provide support and joint stabilization even when contractions occur at very low levels. Hoffer & Andreassen (1981) contend that contractions as low as 25% maximum voluntary contraction (MVC) are able to provide maximal joint stiffness. In addition, feedback from the joint and ligament afferents, via their effects on the gamma spindle system, may help regulate muscle stiffness (Johansson et al 1991). This occurs through the gamma system's influence on the alpha motor neurones, which control the tonic, slow twitch muscle fibres (Johansson & Sojka 1991). It appears that the tonic motor units are those most closely related to the control of joint stabilization. This is commensurate with the proposed antigravity postural supporting role attributed to these motor units.

A major advance in our understanding of how muscles contribute to lumbar stabilization came from recognizing the significant functional difference between local and global muscles. Bergmark (1989), in his dissertation on lumbar spine stability, proposed a difference between local and global muscles. Global describes the large torque-producing muscles linking the pelvis to the thoracic cage. Their role is to provide general trunk stabilization. Such muscles balance external loads and in that way help minimize the resulting forces on the spine. Local muscles refer to those attaching directly to the lumbar vertebrae. These muscles are considered to be responsible for segmental stability as well as controlling the positions of the lumbar segments.

LUMBAR SEGMENTAL STABILITY

Lumbar segmental stability is provided by osseous, ligamentous and muscle restraints. Injury and degenerative disease can affect any structure of the motion segment and can result in both abnormal segmental movement and muscle dysfunction. Panjabi (1992) considers the segment's neutral zone to be the sensitive region. This is the small range of displacement around the segment's neutral position where little resistance is offered by passive spinal restraints. The subtle movement in this region may increase with injury, disc degeneration and weakness of the muscles (Panjabi 1992).

Logically it is the muscles of the local system, which have direct attachments to the lumbar vertebrae, that have the greatest capacity to affect segmental stiffness through control of the neutral zone (Crisco & Panjabi 1990). The contributions of several of the back muscles to active segmental stabilization have been investigated in *in vitro* studies (Panjabi et al 1989; Goel et al 1993; Steffen et al 1994; Wilke et al 1995). The lumbar multifidus, in particular, has been shown to contribute to the control of the neutral zone. In a biomechanical study Wilke et al (1995) demonstrated that the multifidus provided more than two thirds of the stiffness increase at the L4–5 segment. This stabilizing role of multifidus has been recently verified *in vivo* in animal research (Kaigle et al 1995).

The abdominal muscles are often ascribed an important role in the treatment of back pain. A muscle that could be described as part of the local system, and which has not been studied extensively to date, is the transversus abdominis. Its possible importance in lumbar stabilization was first addressed by Cresswell et al (1992). These researchers studied the muscles of the back and abdominal wall using fine wire electromyography (EMG). They demonstrated that the transversus abdominis had direct links with the development of intra-abdominal pressure. Furthermore this muscle contracted with all trunk movements regardless of the primary direction of movement and it was recruited prior to all other abdominal muscles with sudden perturbations of the trunk.

Recently, more concrete evidence has emerged demonstrating the importance of transversus abdominis in the motor control associated with lumbar stabilization. Fine wire and surface EMG were used to study each abdominal muscle during three movements of the upper limb: flexion, abduction and extension (Hodges & Richardson 1997). The onset of EMG activity for transversus abdominis occurred prior to any limb movement. Additionally the pattern of onset was similar for each of the three directions of arm movement. This was different from the activity pattern of other abdominal muscles. The rectus abdominis and external and internal oblique muscles rarely preceded limb movement, and the onset of their activity varied with the movement direction. The authors concluded that in regard to stabilization of the lumbar spine, this study provided evidence for a functional differentiation between the abdominal muscles.

The local muscle system has a primary responsibility for segmental stability. It appears that both multifidus and transversus abdominis are important components of this system.

DYSFUNCTIONS IN THE LOCAL MUSCLE SYSTEM

The stabilization function of any antigravity trunk muscle is likely to be affected in low back pain patients. Their tonic fibres have an important antigravity, postural supportive role. These fibres can be affected by disuse (Richardson & Jull 1994) and by the reflex and pain inhibition associated with lumbar pain and injury (Baugher et al 1984). The nature of this dysfunction impacts on the type of exercise required to restore this stabilizing or supporting role.

A link has been established between dysfunction in the local muscles and back pain. Several researchers have demonstrated dysfunctions in the multifidus muscle of back pain patients. Hides et al (1994) reported a significant reduction in segmental multifidus cross-sectional area in patients with acute, first episode, unilateral back pain. It was proposed that this phenomenon was a result of pain and or reflex inhibition of the muscle. Rantanen et al (1993) demonstrated 'moth eaten' Type I muscle fibres in the multifidus muscle of patients with chronic back pain. Further evidence comes from Biederman et al (1991), who found that multifidus demonstrated greater fatiguability relative to other parts of the erector spinae in chronic back pain patients compared with a normal population.

Dysfunction of the transversus abdominis muscle has also been clearly shown in back pain patients. Hodges and Richardson (1995) demonstrated a motor control deficit in the this muscle. In their EMG experiment analyzing the onset of activity of the muscles of the abdominal wall in response to arm movements, the timing of onset of transversus abdominis activity was delayed in chronic low back pain sufferers compared with individuals who had never experienced back pain. Notably no significant change was detected between the two groups in any other muscle of the abdominal wall. The delayed action of transversus abdominis compared with its early recruitment prior to limb movement in normal individuals has made a significant contribution to knowledge of the mechanisms involved in poor lumbar stabilization associated with low back pain. The results are even more significant when one considers that the problem appears to be limited to the muscle that forms the deepest layer of the abdominal wall.

Evidence of the importance of the local muscles in stabilization of the lumbar spine, as well as their proven dysfunction in the back pain population, has led us to focus on these muscles in the rehabilitation of active stabilization of the lumbar spine. Indeed, a completely new type of therapeutic exercise has been developed aimed at reversing the dysfunction known to occur in the local muscle system.

EXERCISE DESIGN

In the process of developing a new concept in therapeutic exercise to enhance lumbar stabilization, each facet of the exercise was reasoned on a knowledge of stabilization, as well as a knowledge of the muscle dysfunction found in back pain patients. Several decisions had to be made to design the most suitable exercise. These included the type of muscle contraction (i.e. concentric, eccentric, isometric), the body position, the level of resistance or load, the number of repetitions and subsequently the methods of progression. These decisions were based on extensive work in the clinic as well as a number of EMG studies (Jull et al 1993; Richardson et al 1990, 1992, 1995).

TYPE OF MUSCLE CONTRACTION

Functional differences between the global and local muscle systems help direct which type of muscle contraction is needed in re-education of the local system. The length–tension relationships of the muscles involved differ during trunk movements. The global muscles span the lumbar area and they shorten or lengthen eccentrically as they produce the torque to move the trunk. The local muscles attach from vertebra to vertebra and are responsible for maintaining the position of the lumbar segments during functional trunk movement. McGill (1991) confirmed their primary segmental stabilization role in a study of the geometry of the multifidus muscle. He showed that the operational length of multifidus was virtually unchanged through a range of trunk postures.

These functional demands indicate that isometric exercise is most beneficial for re-educating the stabilizing role of these deep local muscles of the lumbar spine. At a later stage, isometric exercises for these deep lumbar muscles can be combined with dynamic functional exercise for other parts of the body.

Exercise involving co-contraction of the deep abdominal and back muscles is also in line with stabilization. Co-contraction of agonist and antagonist has been considered by several researchers in relation to joint stabilization strategies (Andersson & Winters 1990). This type of muscle activity is linked to increasing joint stiffness and support independent of the torque-producing role of muscles (Carter et al 1993). A simultaneous isometric co-contraction of transversus and multifidus, while maintaining the spine in a static neutral position, should help re-educate the stabilizing role of these muscles.

As argued previously, the tonic motor units are those most closely related to control of joint stabilization. In addition, both disuse and reflex inhibition are likely to affect the slow twitch or tonic fibre function within the muscle. Therefore a prolonged tonic-holding contraction at a low level of

MVC would be most effective in retraining the stability function of these muscles.

In summary, the evidence presented indicates that a programme for the transversus abdominis and multifidus is required for specific lumbar segmental stabilization training. It should include activating an isometric co-contraction of these muscles and training the patient to hold a low-level tonic contraction. There is one other factor in exercise design. There are patients in whom the more active global muscles, such as rectus abdominis, external oblique or thoracic erector spinae, predominate in general exercise techniques. In these patients it is almost impossible to detect if local muscle activation is occurring during general exercise. Therefore, specific exercises that isolate the local muscles as much as possible from contraction of the global muscles have proved to be the most beneficial way of targeting them in rehabilitation programmes and ensuring that the correct muscles are being reactivated.

BODY POSITION AND LEVEL OF RESISTANCE

The local muscles function to control segmental stiffness independent of the global muscle system, which is responsible for balancing the external loads. There is no need for high loaded exercise and it is logical to reduce external loading during initial rehabilitation of the local system. This is achieved by using exercise positions, such as four point kneeling or prone lying, where body weight is supported and no additional external resistance is applied. Such positions and exercises involving minimal external loading also reduce the chance of pain and reflex inhibition, which could be increased if high-load exercises were given early in rehabilitation.

Low loads have another benefit in therapeutic exercise aimed at restoring joint stabilization. The restoration of tonic function in the muscles only requires low levels of muscle contraction as tonic fibres operate at levels below approximately 30–40% MVC (McArdle et al 1991). Additionally it has been argued that only low levels of muscle force, approximately 25% MVC, are needed to develop the increased muscle stiffness required for

enhancing spinal stability. Therefore, the addition of high external loading, which is required for strength changes, is not suitable for the development of muscle stiffness for joint support. For these reasons, positions and exercises involving minimal external loading are ideal when rehabilitating the local muscles for lumbar spine stabilization.

NUMBER OF REPETITIONS, HOLDING ABILITY

A localized and specific isometric-setting exercise was developed to improve the stability role of the local muscles. This isometric co-contraction of transversus and multifidus involves retraining a specific motor skill. In order to gain maximum benefit, the exercise needs to be repeated as many times as possible throughout the day.

METHODS OF PROGRESSION

Progression of this new type of exercise can be taken through several stages. At first, it involves increasing the holding time of the isometric co-contraction as well as the number of repetitions. The setting exercise can then be progressed from low loads with minimal body weight to more functional body positions with gradually increasing external loads. In addition, advances need to be made from performing the exercise with a static neutral lumbar spine to other static positions at greater extremes of range. Finally, patients should be able to hold a co-contraction of the deep muscles during dynamic functional movements of the trunk.

SPECIFIC METHODS OF REHABILITATION

Teaching the isolated setting action of transversus abdominis and multifidus is not easy when patients have marked dysfunction in their local muscle system. The therapist needs to develop a high level of teaching skill for successful treatments. For this reason quite detailed descriptions of the exercise programme will be given. As with all therapeutic exercise, methods have to be used to detect if the correct muscles are contracting during the exercise.

The dysfunction occurs in the deep muscles of the abdominal wall and back and this can present some challenges, especially in patients whose more active global muscles attempt to substitute for the correct muscle action. Several strategies, including specific palpation, careful observation of changes in body shape and the use of pressure biofeedback, have been developed for this purpose.

METHODS OF TEACHING AN ISOMETRIC CO-CONTRACTION OF TRANSVERSUS ABDOMINIS AND MULTIFIDUS WITH A STATIC NEUTRAL SPINE

There are only a few methods of achieving an isometric co-contraction of the local muscles independently of the global muscles. The method we have developed from our clinical and research work involves the re-education of the co-contraction of transversus abdominis and multifidus as the basic functional unit of a movement skill. The isolated action of these local muscles is taught by asking the patient to gently draw in the abdominal wall, especially in the lower abdominal area. This is an action similar to that described by Lacote et al (1987) for the muscle test action of the transversus abdominis muscle. The patient also learns to simultaneously contract their multifidus muscle in an isometric setting action. This ensures the maintenance of a static neutral spine position.

Active persons without a history of chronic low back pain have little difficulty in performing this task (Richardson et al 1995). However, it is not easily achieved by patients with low back pain, both acute and chronic. If the patient is unable to perform the setting action, other techniques of facilitation and skill learning are employed. These include:

- Visualizing the correct muscle action. The local muscles form a corset-like structure that acts to tighten around the waist. The physiotherapist should demonstrate and describe the muscle action to the patient. Anatomical illustrations of the muscles involved are an effective teaching aid.
- Using instructions that cue the correct action.

Several different phrases such as 'draw your lower abdomen up and in' or 'pull your navel up towards your spine' can be used to cue the patient to the muscle action required.
- Focusing on precision. The patient has to concentrate and focus on the precise muscle action to be achieved. It should be stressed that the co-activation of the deep muscles is a gentle action. Other muscles of the body are to remain relaxed during this localized exercise.
- Facilitation techniques. Such techniques can help the patient to feel the muscle action required. These can include a deep but gentle manual pressure on the transversus abdominis or manual contact on multifidus. Another facilitation strategy is to combine the co-contraction with a contraction of pelvic floor muscles.

BODY POSITIONS FOR RE-EDUCATION

There are several different positions in which the isometric co-contraction exercise can be activated whilst keeping the global muscles relaxed and maintaining the spine in a static neutral position. Each position allows different opportunities for teaching, testing and retraining this technique. Re-education of the isometric co-contraction is commenced in the four point kneeling and prone positions. One of the major advantages of these positions, as is revealed when monitoring the abdominal wall with multichannel EMG, is that they seem to be inhibitory for a major global muscle, the rectus abdominis. These positions help to isolate the exercise to the deep local muscles.

Re-education in four point kneeling

The first position for the patient to learn to contract their local muscles is in four point kneeling (Figs 4.1A & B). Learning the action of drawing in the abdominal wall and holding this position is easiest in this position. This is probably due to the facilitatory stretch of the deep abdominal muscles resulting from the forward drift of the abdominal contents. The patient is taught to locate and main-

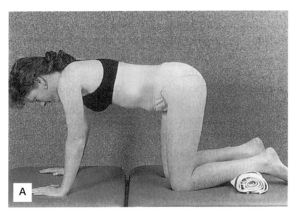
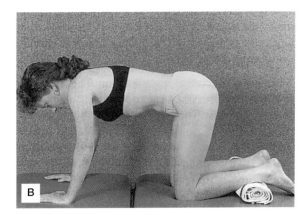

Figure 4.1 Re-education in four point kneeling. (A) The relaxed abdominal wall; (B) the abdominal drawing-in action.

tain normal thoracic and lumbar curves for the isometric exercise. The rib cage and pelvis should remain still and the patient must continue to breathe normally throughout the abdominal 'drawing in' and holding contraction.

Re-education and testing in the prone position

The prone position is a major testing and training position. It is in this position that some quantifiable evaluation of the patient's ability to co-contract the deep muscles can be made. While multichannel needle and surface EMG can be used in research to gain precise measures and descriptions of the muscle dysfunction, they cannot be readily used in the clinic. Yet some quantification of exercise performance is needed to assess the level of the patient's ability and to monitor the effectiveness of training. The pressure biofeedback unit has proved to be a useful clinical tool for assessment and to enhance training and learning in this position (Fig. 4.2). The co-contraction of the transversus abdominis and multifidus involves a drawing-in action of the abdominal wall. The pressure biofeedback unit can indirectly monitor the movement of the abdominal wall by recording a decrease in pressure as the muscles contract and support some of the weight of the abdominal contents off the sensor.

The patient is asked to lie with the pressure sensor under the lower abdomen, the lower edge in line with the anterior superior iliac spine (Fig.

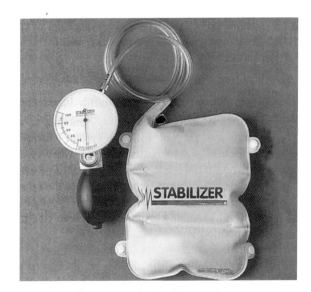

Figure 4.2 The pressure biofeedback unit.

4.3). It is inflated to 70 mmHg pressure. The instruction given to the patient is to draw the lower stomach gently off the pressure sensor and hold the position. When the correct localized contraction is performed, pressure decreases by approximately 6–8 mmHg up to a maximum of 10 mmHg in the holding position.

The simultaneous contraction of multifidus can be palpated close to the lumbar spine in the low lumbar area. Once the patient has learnt the setting action, the pressure biofeedback is invaluable in monitoring the patient's retraining of holding time of the co-contraction.

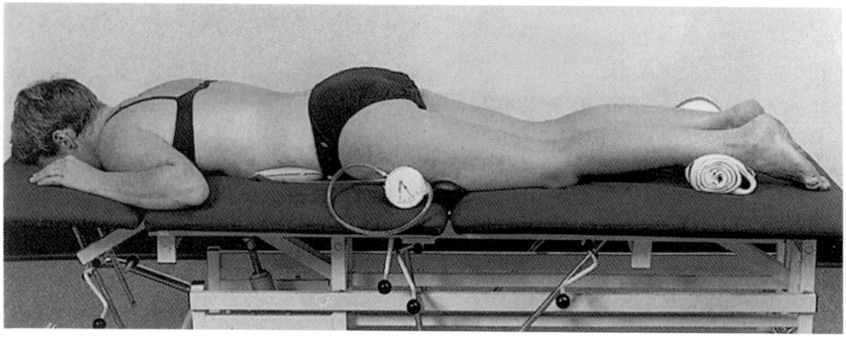

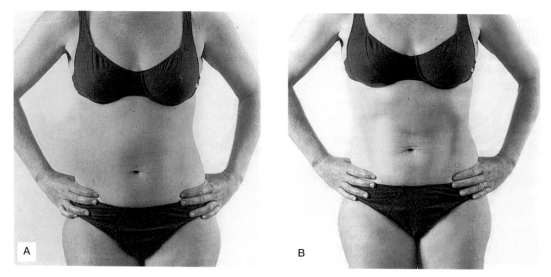

Figure 4.3 The test of the abdominal drawing-in action in prone lying. The co-contraction is monitored with the pressure biofeedback unit.

A

B

Figure 4.4 The anterior view of the co-contraction. (A) The relaxed abdominal wall; (B) the abdominal drawing in action.

Re-education in upright positions

Retraining the co-contraction in the upright standing and sitting positions is a necessary prerequisite for postural retraining and for later retraining in functional activities. The appearance of the abdominal wall when it is relaxed and when the correct action is performed is illustrated from an anterior view (Figs 4.4A & B) and from a side view (Figs 4.5A & B). The contraction of the transversus abdominis can be palpated just medial to the anterior superior iliac spines (Fig. 4.4B). Alternatively, facilitation of the co-contraction can be provided through multifidus (Figs 4.5A & B).

SUBSTITUTION STRATEGIES

The efficacy of training will relate to the accuracy with which a patient can activate and hold the deep muscle co-contraction. This setting exercise is a movement skill and patients have lesser or greater difficulty in activating the correct muscle action. When they have problems, it is not uncommon for them to use substitution strategies to mimic the correct action. The physiotherapist must be vigilant and observe or monitor substitution with the pressure biofeedback unit and correct the action.

As a basic guide the rib cage, shoulders and pelvis should remain in a constant position during

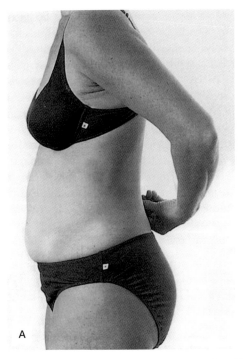
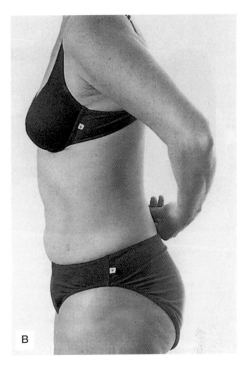

A   B

Figure 4.5 The lateral view of the co-contraction. (A) The relaxed abdominal wall; (B) the drawing-in action.

the setting action to minimize the contribution of the global muscles. Some of the substitution strategies commonly used by patients can be identified in the upright position by careful observation. One substitution manoeuvre involves sucking in the upper abdomen by taking in and holding a deep breath (Fig. 4.6). This can be done with virtually no abdominal muscle activity. If this manoeuvre is performed in the prone position using the pressure biofeedback unit, there can be a drop in pressure of 1–2 mmHg, which may be mistaken for the beginnings of a correct muscle action. Observation of the abdominal wall, asking the patient to breathe normally and palpating the contraction of either transversus abdominis or multifidus will help identify the incorrect action.

Another strategy sometimes used instead of the drawing-in action, is an abnormal bracing action involving the external obliques. In the upright position, the depression of the rib cage and the appearance of a horizontal abdominal skin crease point to the incorrect muscle action (Fig. 4.7). If performed in the prone position with pressure biofeedback, this incorrect action does not result

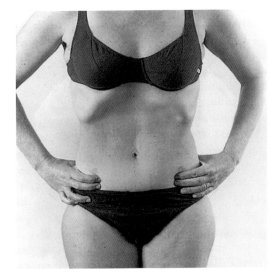

Figure 4.6 A substitution strategy utilizing breath holding and rib elevation. Note the different shape of the abdomen and rib cage compared to that with the correct action.

in a decrease in pressure. In most cases the pressure will increase by 1–2 mmHg.

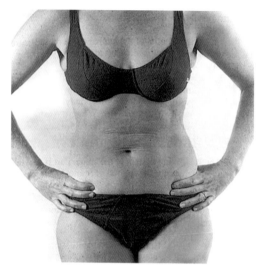

Figure 4.7 A substitution strategy of an abnormal bracing action utilizing predominantly the external oblique muscle. Note the depressed rib cage and the skin crease across the upper-middle abdomen.

PROGRESSION FROM POSITIONS OF MINIMAL EXTERNAL LOADING

Patients train in the minimally loaded prone and upright positions until they can hold an isolated contraction of the deep local muscles. An arbitrary target is the ability to perform 10 by 10 second holds in succession without fatiguing. Once this is achieved, the exercise can be progressed to slowly increase loads and functional demands.

The aim of this next stage is to integrate the local and global muscle systems. Most of the traditional stabilization programmes involving general trunk muscle co-contraction and added load are applicable at this stage (Jull & Richardson 1994). It is important that increases in load are introduced gradually with constant monitoring of the deep muscle system to ensure its continued action.

LINK BETWEEN EXERCISES AND PAIN RELIEF

The key aim of the abdominal drawing-in or setting exercise is to isolate the correct muscle action in all exercise positions and develop holding ability. Pain relief is usually concomitant with the patient mastering this task. The time taken to achieve this is variable and depends on the level of dysfunction. It may take one or two treatment sessions to help the patient master it or it may take several weeks of practice for the patient to reach this stage.

The reason for the importance of isolating the muscle action is not fully understood. Our working hypothesis is that it relates to motor control issues which are independent of the prime mover muscle action. Hodges and Richardson (1995, 1997) have demonstrated that, during limb movement, there is a separate control system for the deep abdominal muscle, transversus abdominis. This could explain the need to first train the deep muscles independently of the main torque producers, which are used to perform the functional tasks.

EVIDENCE OF EFFICACY OF THIS NEW CONCEPT IN THERAPEUTIC EXERCISE

Evidence of the link between this concept of motor control and training the deep muscles to increase segmental stability and subsequent pain relief is beginning to emerge. O'Sullivan and Twomey (1994) studied the effects of this type of exercise on patients suffering from chronic low back pain with the radiological diagnosis of spondylolysis or spondylolisthesis. On completion of the treatment period, the specific exercise group demonstrated a significant reduction in pain intensity and increase in functional mobility when compared with the control group who undertook general exercises.

The effect of this exercise on acute, first episode unilateral back pain was also studied in recent research on the multifidus muscle. Hides et al (1995) demonstrated, in a prospective controlled trial, that inhibition of the lumbar multifidus did not resolve automatically as back pain resolved. A programme of re-education of co-contraction of the deep muscles, gradually increasing the holding time, was needed to restore the segmental multifidus to its pre-injury size. Preliminary data from a 9-month follow-up suggest that the exercise group may have suffered less recurrence of back pain in this period. This is an exciting new area of clinical research which will be the focus of our future research efforts.

CONCLUSION

A very specific type of therapeutic exercise has been devised which provides effective pain relief for chronic and recurrent back pain sufferers probably through enhanced segmental stabilization. This approach was developed over several years and is based on knowledge of how muscles stabilize the spine and the dysfunction that occurs in these muscles in back pain sufferers. The success of such programmes should provide the impetus for further basic scientific research on the function of the deep muscles and the dysfunction that occurs within this system of muscles in back pain patients. As a result of increased knowledge in the area, rehabilitation exercise can be further developed and refined for more efficient and effective pain relief. In this way the scientific foundation for the practice of physiotherapy can be firmly established.

Acknowledgements

The authors wish to acknowledge the contributions of their co-researchers in the Spinal Pain Research Team at the Department of Physiotherapy, The University of Queensland: Paul Hodges, Julie Hides, Joseph Ng and Christine Hamilton.

REFERENCES

Andersson GBJ, Winters JM 1990 Role of muscle in postural tasks: spinal loading and postural stability. In: Winters JM, Woo SL-Y (eds) Multiple Muscle Systems. Springer-Verlag, New York, pp 375–395

Baratta R, Solomonow M, Zhou BH, Letson D, Chuinard R, D'Ambrosia R 1988 Muscular activation. The role of the antagonist musculature in maintaining knee stability. The American Journal of Sports Medicine 16(2): 113–122

Baugher WM, Warren RS, Marshall JL, Joseph A 1984 Quadriceps atrophy in anterior cruciate deficient knee. The American Journal of Sports Medicine 12: 192–195

Bergmark A 1989 Stability of the Lumbar Spine. A study in mechanical engineering. Acta Orthopaedica Scandinavica Supplementum 230(60): 20–24

Biederman HJ, Shanks GL, Forrest WJ, Inglis J 1991 Power spectrum analyses of electromyographic activity: discriminators in the differential assessment of patients with chronic low-back pain. Spine 16(10): 1179–1184

Carter RR, Crago PE, Gorman PH 1993 Non linear stretch reflex interaction during a contraction. Journal of Neurophysiology 69(3): 943–952

Cresswell AG, Grundstrom A, Thorstensson A 1992 Observations on intra-abdominal pressure and patterns of abdominal intramuscular activity in man. Acta Physiologica Scandinavica 144: 409–418

Crisco JJ III, Panjabi MM 1990 Postural biomechanical stability and gross muscular architecture in the spine. In: Winters JM, Woo SL-Y (eds) Multiple Muscle Systems. Springer-Verlag, New York, pp 438–450

Goel VK, Kong W, Han JS, Weinstein JN, Gilbertson LG 1993 A combined finite element and optimisation investigation of lumbar spine mechanics with and without muscles. Spine 18(11): 1531–1541

Gollhofer A, Kryolainen H 1991 Neuromuscular control of the human leg extensor muscles in jump exercises under various stretch load conditions. International Journal of Sports Medicine 12:34–40

Hides JA, Stokes MJ, Saide M, Jull GA, Cooper DH 1994 Evidence of lumbar multifidus muscle wasting ipsilateral to symptoms in patients with acute/subacute low back pain. Spine 19(2): 165–172

Hides JA, Richardson CA, Jull GA 1995 The effect of specific postural holding exercises on lumbar multifidus muscle recovery in acute low back pain patients. Proceedings of the World Confederation of Physical Therapists Congress, Washington

Hodges PW, Richardson CA 1995b Neuromotor Dysfunction of the Trunk Musculature in Low Back Pain Patients. Proceedings of the World Confederation of Physical Therapists Congress, Washington

Hodges PW, Richardson CA 1997 Feedforward contraction of transversus abdominis is not influenced by the direction of arm movement. Experimental Brain Research 114: 362–370

Hoffer J, Andreassen S 1981 Regulation of soleus muscle stiffness in premamillary cats. Journal of Neurophysiology 45: 267–285

Johansson H, Sojka P 1991 Pathophysiological mechanisms involved in genesis and spread of muscular tension in occupational muscle pain and in chronic musculoskeletal pain syndromes: a hypothesis. Medical Hypotheses 35: 196–203

Johansson H, Sjolander P, Sojka P 1991 Receptors in the knee joint ligaments and their role in the biomechanics of the joint. CRC Critical Reviews in Biomedical Engineering 18: 341–368

Jull GA, Richardson CA 1994 Rehabilitation of active stabilization of the lumbar spine. In: Twomey LT, Taylor JR (eds) Physical Therapy of the Lumbar Spine, 2nd edn. Churchill Livingstone, pp. 251–283

Jull G, Richardson C, Toppenberg R, Comerford M, Bui B 1993 Towards a measurement of active muscle control for lumbar stabilization. Australian Journal of Physiotherapy 39(3): 187–193

Kaigle AM, Holm SH, Hansson TH 1995 Experimental instability in the lumbar spine. Spine 20(24): 421–430

Lacote M, Clevalier AM, Miranda A, Bleton JP, Stevenin P 1987 Clinical Evaluation of Muscle Function. Churchill Livingstone, Edinburgh, pp 290–293

McArdle WD, Katch FI, Katch VL 1991 Exercise Physiology, Energy, Nutrition and Human Performance, 3rd edn. Lea and Febiger, Philadelphia, pp 384–417

McGill SM 1991 Kinetic potential of the lumbar trunk musculature about three orthogonal orthopaedic axes in extreme postures. Spine 16(7): 809–815

O'Sullivan PB, Twomey LT 1994 Evaluation of specific stabilising exercise in the treatment of chronic low back pain with radiological diagnosis of spondylolysis or spondylolisthesis. Thesis, Curtin University of Technology, Western Australia

Panjabi M 1992 The stabilizing system of the spine. Part II neutral zone and instability hypothesis. Journal of Spinal Disorders 5: 390–397

Panjabi M, Abumi K, Duranceau J, Oxland T 1989 Spinal stability and intersegmental muscle forces: a biomechanical model. Spine 14(2): 194–200

Rantanen J, Hurme M, Falck B, Alaranta H, Nykvist F, Lehto M, Einola S, Kalimo H 1993 The lumbar multifidus muscle five years after surgery for a lumbar disc herniation. Spine 18(5): 568–574

Richardson CA, Jull GA 1994 Concepts of Rehabilitation for spinal stability. In: Boyling JD, Palastanga N (eds) Grieve's Modern Manual Therapy of the Vertebral Column 2nd edn. Churchill Livingstone, Edinburgh, pp 705–720

Richardson C, Toppenberg R, Jull G 1990 An initial evaluation of eight abdominal exercises for their ability to provide stabilization for the lumbar spine. Australian Journal of Physiotherapy 36(1): 6–11

Richardson CA, Jull GA, Toppenberg R, Comerford M 1992 Techniques for active lumbar stabilization for spinal protection: a pilot study. Australian Journal of Physiotherapy 38(2): 105–112

Richardson CA, Jull GA, Richardson BA 1995 A Dysfunction of the Deep Abdominal Muscles Exists in Low Back Pain Patients. Proceedings of the World Confederation for Physical Therapy Congress, Washington

Robison R 1992 The new back school prescription: stabilization training part 1. Occupational Medicine 7: 17–31

Saal JA, Saal JS 1989 Non operative treatment of herniated lumbar disc with radiculopathy: An outcome study. Spine 14(4): 431–437

Steffen R, Nolte LP, Pingel TH 1994 Rehabilitation of the postoperative segmental lumbar instability — a biomechanical analysis of the rank of the back muscles. Rehabilitation 33: 164–170

Wilke HJ, Wolf S, Claes LE, Arand M, Wiesend A 1995 Stability increase of the lumbar spine with different muscle groups: a biomechanical in vitro study. Spine 20(2): 192–198

POSTSCRIPT

The main article presented a new paradigm of exercise that addressed the motor control problems in the muscles and focused on improving the mechanical support of the spinal joints through specific deep muscle contraction exercises. The new back pain exercise programme was considered to involve specific exercises that would compensate for a damaged passive system and, therefore, give spinal stability and pain control. In essence, this exercise paradigm has not changed, but research has widened its perspectives. A new insight into therapeutic exercise for both prevention and treatment of low back pain has evolved in a relatively short period of time from an increased knowledge of the neurophysiological mechanisms involved in joint protection as well as the recognition and understanding of the impairments existing in these motor control mechanisms in low back pain patients.

An important new concept has evolved, which has influenced the way deep muscle contraction is integrated into function, and hence modified our 'Muscle Control–Pain Control' model. The control of joint protection and support, through specific patterns of muscle recruitment, is strongly influenced by the presence of gravity and by the sensitivity of the sensory system within the antigravity musculature and weight-bearing joints in monitoring the weight-bearing load. There is evidence that skeletal muscle recruitment patterns change when the effects of gravity are minimized (Richardson & Bullock 1986). This area of motor control has been able to be studied through our current involvement in space (microgravity) research in which the neuromuscular system demonstrates a remodelling or neural plasticity when exposed to weightlessness in a similar pattern to that seen in low back pain patients (Richardson 2002).

Based on this new information, exercise to reverse motor problems would need to initially involve specific exercise for the deep, local muscles to develop kinaesthetic awareness to enhance the lumbopelvic support mechanisms in preparation for weight bearing (Richardson et al 2002). Real-time ultrasound enhances the efficiency of this process. This stage would be followed as quickly as possible by weight-bearing exercise for the functional integration of the deep, local muscle system into the antigravity muscle system to support and protect the joints in a gravitational environment. This integration stage would need to involve progressive (measured) increases in weight-bearing load through a gradual increase in gravitational, proprioceptive load cues. This stage would improve the ability of the antigravity muscles to be recruited in response to weight bearing to protect the joint from injury.

MEDICAL DIAGNOSIS OF MUSCLE IMPAIRMENTS — MUSCLE CONTROL–PAIN CONTROL

There are many different types of exercise programmes for the prevention and treatment of low back pain that also work on a model of muscle control–pain control. In many ways these programmes have a similar focus and all involve a combination of various types of exercise, including cognitive activation of deep muscles, emphasis on postural control and weight bearing, joint alignment exercises, muscle strengthening/lengthening, facilitation techniques to activate inhibited muscles, and increasing muscular endurance, as well as various methods of increasing proprioceptive input.

As clinical diagnosis and testing procedures for each back pain programme are quite different, to date there have been no means of comparing programmes and identifying the elements of each programme that are effective in the control and management of mechanical spinal pain and to decide which, if any, are the optimal programmes for both prevention and treatment. The main reason for this has been a deficiency, in current medical and health science practice, of a precise musculoskeletal medical diagnosis on which to base the conservative management of low back pain.

Medical diagnostic procedures of the musculoskeletal impairments involved in low back pain are currently being developed in collaboration with biomedical engineers at the University of Queensland. These measures are being tested in space-related 'bed rest' research in collaboration with the European Space Agency. It is anticipated that the results of these research studies will lead to new screening tests for the diagnosis of impairments in the joint protection mechanisms, and allow exercise prescription to be more efficient for future 'muscle control–pain control' management of low back pain.

REFERENCES

Richardson C 2002 The health of the human skeletal system for weight-bearing against gravity: The role of deloading the musculo-skeletal system in the development of musculo-skeletal injury. Gravitational Physiology 9(1): 7–10.

Richardson CA, Bullock MI 1986 Changes in muscle activity during fast, alternating flexion-extension movements of the knee. Scandinavian Journal of Rehabilitation Medicine 18: 51–58

Richardson CA, Snijders CJ, Hides JA, Damen L, Pas M. Storm J 2002 The relation between the transversus abdominis muscle, sacroiliac joint mechanics, and low back pain. Spine 27 (4): 399–405

5

Lumbar segmental 'instability': clinical presentation and specific stabilizing exercise management

P. B. O'Sullivan

School of Physiotherapy, Curtin University of Technology, Perth, Australia

Lumbar segmental instability is considered to represent a significant subgroup within the chronic low back pain population. This condition has a unique clinical presentation that displays its symptoms and movement dysfunction within the neutral zone of the motion segment. The loosening of the motion segment secondary to injury and associated dysfunction of the local muscle system renders it biomechanically vulnerable in the neutral zone. The clinical diagnosis of this chronic low back pain condition is based on the report of pain and the observation of movement dysfunction within the neutral zone and the associated finding of excessive intervertebral motion at the symptomatic level. Four different clinical patterns are described based on the directional nature of the injury and the manifestation of the patient's symptoms and motor dysfunction. A specific stabilizing exercise intervention based on a motor learning model is proposed and evidence for the efficacy of the approach provided. *Manual Therapy* (2000) **5(1)**, 2–12

INTRODUCTION

Back-related injury is a growing problem in the Western industrialized world, which is placing an increasing burden on the health budget (Indahl et al 1995). Estimates of lifetime incidence of low back pain range from 60 to 80% (Long et al 1996) and although most low back pain episodes (80–90%) subside within 2 to 3 months, recurrence is common (Hides et al 1996). Of major concern are the 5–10% of people who become disabled with a chronic back pain condition, which accounts for up to 75–90% of the cost (Indahl et al 1995). In spite of the large number of pathological conditions that can give rise to back pain, 85% of this population are classified as having 'non specific low back pain' (Dillingham 1995). More recently there has been increased focus on the identification of different subgroups within this population (Coste et al 1992; Bogduk 1995).

Lumbar segmental instability is considered to represent one of these subgroups (Friberg 1987). Traditionally, the radiological diagnosis of spondylolisthesis, in subjects with chronic low back pain attributable to this finding, has been considered to be one of the most obvious manifestations of lumbar instability (Nachemson 1991; Pope et al 1992), with reports of increased segmental motion occurring with this condition and spondylolysis (Friberg 1989; Mimura 1990; Montgomery & Fischgrund 1994; Wood et al 1994). Lumbar segmental instability, in the absence of defects of the bony architecture of the lumbar spine, has also been cited as a significant cause of chronic low back pain (Long et al 1996). A number of studies have reported increased and abnormal intersegmental motion in subjects with chronic low back pain, often in the absence of other radiological findings (Sihvonen & Partanen 1990; Gertzbein 1991; Lindgren et al 1993).

The limitation in the clinical diagnosis of lumbar segmental instability lies in the difficulty to detect accurately abnormal or excessive intersegmental motion, as conventional radiological testing is often insensitive and unreliable (Dvorak et al 1991; Pope et al 1992). Because of this, the finding of increased and abnormal intersegmental motion of a single motion segment on radiological examination is considered to be significant only if it confirms the clinical finding of lumbar segmental instability at the corresponding symptomatic level (Kirkaldy-Willis & Farfan 1982). Although the sensitivity, specificity and predictive value of physical examination findings are largely unproven (Nachemson 1991), recent research indicates that skilled manipulative physiotherapists can distinguish subjects with symptomatic spondylolysis from low back pain patients without spondylolysis, based on the finding of increased intersegmental motion at the level above the pars defects (Phillips 1994; Avery 1996).

Because of these limitations the effective management of lumbar segmental instability first relies on accurate clinical diagnosis. This article outlines the common clinical presentations of lumbar segmental instability and the specific exercise management of these conditions based on a motor learning model.

DEFINITION OF LUMBAR SEGMENTAL INSTABILITY

Panjabi (1992) redefined spinal instability in terms of a region of laxity around the neutral position of a spinal segment called the 'neutral zone'. This neutral zone is shown to be increased with intersegmental injury and intervertebral disc degeneration (Panjabi et al 1989; Mimura et al 1994; Kaigle et al 1995), and decreased with simulated muscle forces across a motion segment (Panjabi et al 1989; Kaigle et al 1995; Wilke et al 1995). The size of the neutral zone is considered to be an important measure of spinal stability. It is influenced by the interaction between what Panjabi (1992) described as the passive, active and neural control systems:

- The passive system constituting the vertebrae, intervertebral discs, zygapophyseal joints and ligaments
- The active system constituting the muscles and tendons surrounding and acting on the spinal column
- The neural system comprising the nerves and central nervous system which direct and control the active system in providing dynamic stability.

In light of this, Panjabi (1992) defined spinal instability as a significant decrease in the capacity of the stabilizing systems of the spine to maintain intervertebral neutral zones within physiological limits so there is no major deformity, neurological deficit or incapacitating pain.

DYNAMIC STABILIZATION OF THE LUMBAR SPINE

Bergmark (1989) hypothesized the presence of two muscle systems that act in the maintenance of spinal stability.

1. The 'global muscle system', which consists of large torque producing muscles that act on the trunk and spine without directly attaching to it. These muscles include rectus abdominis, obliquus abdominis externus and the thoracic part of lumbar iliocostalis and provide general trunk stabilization, but they are not capable of having a direct segmental influence on the spine.
2. The local muscle system, which consists of muscles that directly attach to the lumbar vertebrae, and are responsible for providing segmental stability and directly controlling the lumbar segments. By definition lumbar multifidus, psoas major, quadratus lumborum, the lumbar parts of the lumbar iliocostalis and longissimus, transversus abdominis, the diaphragm and the posterior fibres of obliquus abdominis internus all form part of this local muscle system.

Growing evidence is emerging that the local system muscles function differently to global system muscles, and the relationship between the two muscle systems alters depending on the loading conditions placed on the spine (O'Sullivan et al 1997a).

Cholewicke and McGill (1996) reported that the lumbar spine is more vulnerable to instability in its neutral zone and at low load when the muscle forces are low. Under these conditions lumbar stability is maintained *in vivo* by increasing the activity (stiffness) of the lumbar segmental muscles (local muscle system). The coordinated muscle recruitment between large trunk muscles (the global muscle system) and small intrinsic muscles (the local muscle system) during functional activities ensures that mechanical stability is maintained. Under such conditions they suggest that intersegmental muscle forces as low as 1–3% maximal voluntary contraction may be sufficient to ensure

segmental stability. While the global muscle system provides the bulk of stiffness for the spinal column, the activity of the local muscle system is considered necessary to maintain the segmental stability of the spine. In situations where the passive stiffness of a motion segment is reduced, the vulnerability of the spine towards instability is increased (Cholewicke & McGill 1996).

It is proposed that co-contraction of local system muscles, such as transversus abdominis, diaphragm and lumbar multifidus, results in a stabilizing effect on the motion segments of the lumbar spine, particularly within the neutral zone, providing a stable base on which the global muscles can safely act (Wilke et al 1995; Hodges & Richardson 1996; Allison et al 1997). The segmental stabilizing role of lumbar multifidus, with separate segmental innervation, acts to maintain the lumbar lordosis and ensure control of individual vertebral segments particularly within the neutral zone (Panjabi et al 1989; Goel et al 1993; Steffen et al 1994; Kaigle et al 1995; Wilke et al 1995). The deep abdominal muscles are primarily active in providing rotational and lateral stability to the spine via the thoracolumbar fascia, while maintaining levels of intra-abdominal pressure (McGill 1991; Cresswell 1993). The intra-abdominal pressure mechanism, primarily controlled by the diaphragm, transversus abdominis and pelvic diaphragm, produces a stiffening effect on the lumbar spine (McGill & Norman 1987; Aspden 1992; Cresswell 1993; Hodges et al 1997).

DYSFUNCTION OF THE NEUROMUSCULAR SYSTEM IN THE PRESENCE OF LOW BACK PAIN

The literature reports varying disruptions in the patterns of recruitment and co-contraction within and between different muscle synergies in low back pain populations (O'Sullivan et al 1997b). There is growing evidence that the deep abdominals and lumbar multifidus muscles are preferentially adversely affected in the presence of acute low back pain (Hides et al 1996), chronic low back pain (Roy et al 1989; Biedermann et al 1991;

Hodges & Richardson 1996) and lumbar instability (Sihvonen et al 1991; Lindgren et al 1993; O'Sullivan et al 1997d). There have also been reports that compensatory substitution of global system muscles occurs in the presence of local muscle system dysfunction. This appears to be the neural control system's attempt to maintain the stability demands of the spine in the presence of local muscle dysfunction (Richardson & Jull 1995; Edgerton et al 1996; O'Sullivan et al 1997d). There is also evidence to suggest that the presence of chronic low back pain often results in a general loss of function and de-conditioning as well as changes to the neural control system, affecting timing of patterns of co-contraction, balance, reflex and righting responses (O'Sullivan et al 1997b). Such disruptions to the neuromuscular system leave the lumbar spine potentially vulnerable to instability, particularly within the neutral zone (Cholewicke & McGill 1996).

CLINICAL DIAGNOSIS OF LUMBAR SEGMENTAL INSTABILITY

Questionnaire data completed by subjects diagnosed with lumbar segmental instability involved in recent clinical trials revealed that half of the subjects developed their back pain condition secondary to a single event injury while the other half developed their back pain gradually in relation to multiple minor traumatic incidents (O'Sullivan 1997). The subjects' main complaint was of chronic and recurrent low back pain and associated high levels of functional disability. Subjects commonly reported a poor outcome from general exercise and resistance training programmes as well as aggravation from spinal manipulation and mobilization. The back pain was most commonly described as recurrent (70%), constant (55%), 'catching' (45%), 'locking' (20%), 'giving way' (20%) or accompanied by a feeling of 'instability' (35%) (O'Sullivan 1997). On physical examination, active spinal movement revealed good ranges of spinal mobility, with the presence of 'through range' pain or a painful arc rather than end-of-range limitation, and the inability to return to erect standing from forward bending without the use of the hands to assist this motion. Segmental shifts or hinging were commonly observed to be associated with the painful movement. Abolition or significant reduction of pain with deep abdominal muscle activation during the provocative movement was often noted. Neurological examination and neural tissue provocation tests were generally normal (O'Sullivan 1997). These findings are consistent with those reported by other researchers (Kirkaldy-Willis & Farfan 1982; Paris 1985) and with a movement control problem within the neutral zone.

DIRECTIONAL PATTERNS OF LUMBAR SEGMENTAL 'INSTABILITY'

The directional nature of instability based upon the mechanism of injury, resultant site of tissue damage and clinical presentation is well understood in the knee and shoulder, but poorly understood in the lumbar spine. Dupuis et al (1985) reported, on the basis of experimental and radiological data, that the location of the dominant lesion in the motion segment determines the pattern of instability manifested. As the motion within the lumbar spine is three-dimensional and involves coupled movements, tissue damage is likely to result in movement dysfunction in more than one direction of movement.

The following clinical classifications have developed from clinical observation and have not been scientifically validated. They are based on the mechanism of injury to the spine, resultant tissue damage, the reported and observed aggravating activities and movement problems relating to a specific movement quadrant or quadrants. They provide a basis by which patients can be assessed and movement dysfunction analysed in a segmental and individual specific manner.

Common to all the patient presentations is the reported vulnerability and observed lack of movement control and related symptoms within the neutral zone. This is associated with the inability to initiate co-contraction of the local muscle system within this zone. It appears that these patients develop compensatory movement strategies which 'stabilize' the motion segment out of the neutral zone and towards an end-range position

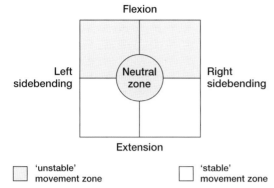

Figure 5.1 Unstable movement zone — flexion pattern. (Reproduced by kind permission of W.B. Saunders.)

(such as flexion, lateral shift or extension). This is achieved by the recruitment of global system muscles and by generating high levels of intra-abdominal pressure (bracing) during low load tasks, in what appears to be a sub-optimal attempt to preserve segmental stability.

'Flexion' pattern

The 'flexion' pattern appears to be most common. These patients primarily complain of central back pain and relate their injury to either a single flexion/rotation injury or to repetitive strains relating to flexion/rotational activities. They predominantly report the aggravation of their symptoms and 'vulnerability' during flexion/rotational movements, with an inability to sustain semi-flexed postures (Fig. 5.1). These patients present with a loss of segmental lumbar lordosis at the level of the 'unstable motion segment'. This is often noticeable in standing and is accentuated in sitting postures with a tendency for them to hold their pelvis in a degree of posterior pelvic tilt. This loss of segmental lordosis is increased in flexed postures and is usually associated with increased tone in the upper lumbar and lower thoracic erector spinae muscles with an associated increase in lordosis in this region (Fig. 5.2). Movements into forward bending are associated with the initiation of movement, and a tendency to flex more at the symptomatic level than at the adjacent levels. This movement is usually associated with an arc of pain into flexion and an inability to return from

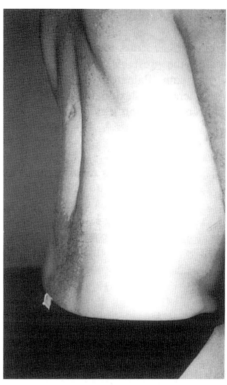

Figure 5.2 Flexion pattern: patient who sustained a flexion injury displays signs and symptoms of segmental instability at L5/S1 during flexion/rotation movements. Note, in sitting, the segmental loss of lower lumbar lordosis with upper lumbar and lower thoracic spine compensatory lordosis. (Reproduced by kind permission of W.B. Saunders.)

flexion to neutral without use of the hands to assist the movement. During backward bending, extension above the symptomatic segment with an associated loss of extension at the affected segment is often observed. Specific movement testing reveals an inability to differentiate anterior pelvic tilt and low lumbar spine extension independent of upper lumbar and thoracic spine extension. Movement tests such as squatting, sitting with knee extension or hip flexion, 'sit to stand' and forward loaded postures reveal an inability to control a neutral segmental lordosis, with a tendency to segmentally flex at the unstable motion segment, posteriorly tilt the pelvis and extend the upper lumbar and thoracic spine.

Specific muscle tests reveal an inability to activate lumbar multifidus in co-contraction with the

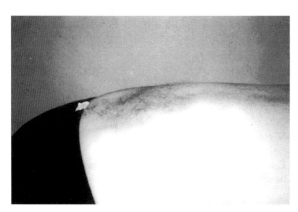

Figure 5.3 Flexion pattern: the same patient as in figure 5.2 in the neutral resting position in four point kneeling. Note the posterior tilt of the pelvis and loss of lower lumbar segmental lordosis with upper lumbar compensatory lordosis. (Reproduced by kind permission of W.B. Saunders.)

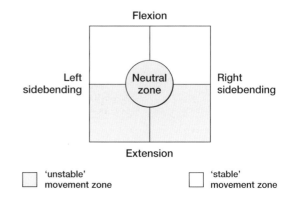

Figure 5.4 Unstable movement zone — extension pattern. (Reproduced by kind permission of W.B. Saunders.)

deep abdominal muscles at the 'unstable' motion segment within a neutral lordosis. Many patients are unable even to assume a neutral lordotic lumbar spine posture, particularly in four point kneeling and sitting (Fig. 5.3). Attempts to activate these muscles are commonly associated with bracing of the abdominal muscles with a loss of breathing control and excessive co-activation of the thoracolumbar erector spinae muscles and external oblique. This is associated with a further flattening of the segmental lordosis at the unstable motion segment, often resulting in pain. Palpatory examination reveals a segmental increase in flexion and rotation mobility at the symptomatic motion segment.

Extension pattern

Patients in a second group report central low back pain and relate their injury to an extension/rotation incident or repetitive traumas usually associated with sporting activities involving extension/rotation. They report their symptoms to be aggravated by extension and extension/rotation movements and activities such as standing, carrying out overhead activities, such as throwing, fast walking, running and swimming (Fig. 5.4). In the standing position they commonly exhibit an increase in segmental lordosis at the

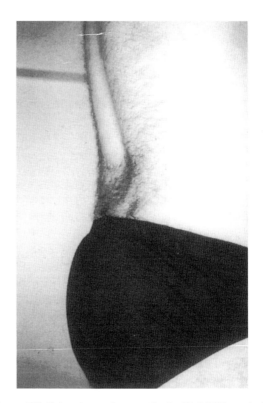

Figure 5.5 Extension pattern: patient with L5/S1 grade 1 spondylolisthesis complaining of extension-related pain presenting in standing with an anterior pelvic tilt and increased lower lumbar lordosis with associated hyperactivity of the lumbar erector spinae and superficial lumbar multifidus muscles and an inability to isolate the activation of the deep abdominal muscles without dominant activation of these muscles. (Reproduced by kind permission of W.B. Saunders.)

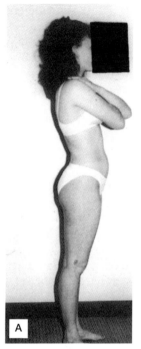
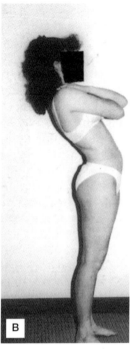

Figure 5.6 (A) Extension pattern: patient with a lumbar segmental instability at L4/5 complaining of extension-related pain. The patient's natural standing posture holds the low lumbar spine in lordosis with associated anterior tilt of the pelvis and upper lumbar and thoracic spine kyphosis. Note the increased tone of the upper compared to the lower abdominal wall. (B) Extension pattern: patient during backward bending. Note the lack of posterior pelvic rotation and upper lumbar and thoracic spine extension, resulting in segmental hinging at L4/5 and associated pain. (Reproduced by kind permission of W.B. Saunders.)

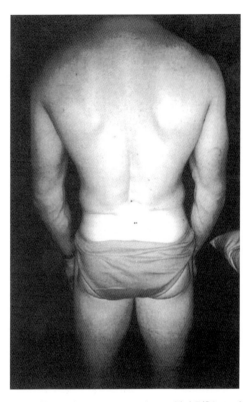

Figure 5.7 Extension pattern: patient with L5/S1 grade 1 spondylolisthesis complaining of extension-related pain and presenting with segmental hinging at the unstable segment during backward bending (note the skin crease at the level of the mobile segment). (Reproduced by kind permission of W.B. Saunders.)

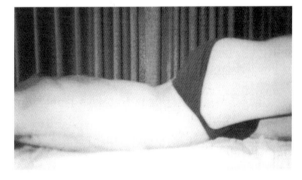

Figure 5.8 Extension pattern: patient with L4/5 grade 1 spondylolisthesis complaining of extension-related pain and presenting with segmental hinging at the unstable segment during hip extension in prone. Note the dominant activation of the back muscles and hamstrings, the lack of hip extension and associated inactivation of the deep abdominal and gluteal muscles during the manoeuvre. (Reproduced by kind permission of W.B. Saunders.)

unstable motion segment sometimes with an increased level of segmental muscle activity at this level and the pelvis is often positioned in anterior pelvic tilt (Fig. 5.5). Extension activities reveal segmental hinging at the affected segment with a loss of segmental lordosis above this level and associated postural 'sway' (Figs 5.6 & 5.7). Hip extension and knee flexion movement tests in prone reveal a loss of co-contraction of the deep abdominal muscles and dominant patterns of activation of the lumbar erector spinae, resulting in excessive segmental extension/rotation at the unstable level (Fig. 5.8). Forward bending movements commonly reveal a tendency to hold the lumbar spine in lordosis (particularly at the level of the unstable

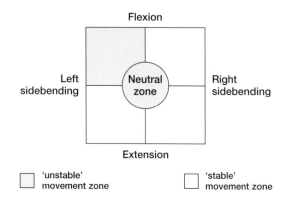

Figure 5.9 Unstable movement zone ± lateral shift pattern. (Reproduced by kind permission of W.B. Saunders.)

motion segment) with a sudden loss of lordosis at mid range flexion commonly associated with an arc of pain. Return to neutral again reveals a tendency to hyperlordose the spine segmentally before the upright posture is achieved, with pain on returning to the erect posture and the necessity to assist the movement with the use of the hands. Specific movement tests reveal an inability to initiate posterior pelvic tilt independent of hip flexion and activation of the gluteals, rectus abdominis and external obliques.

Specific muscle tests reveal an inability to co-contract segmental lumbar multifidus with the deep abdominal muscles in a neutral lumbar posture — with a tendency to 'lock' the lumbar spine into extension and brace the abdominal muscles. Attempts to isolate deep abdominal muscle activation is commonly associated with excessive activation of the lumbar erector spinae, external oblique and rectus abdominis and an inability to control diaphragmatic breathing. Palpatory examination reveals a segmental increase in extension and rotation mobility at the symptomatic motion segment.

Lateral shift pattern

A third presentation is the recurrent lateral shift. This is usually uni-directional and is associated with unilateral low back pain. These patients commonly relate a vulnerability to reaching or rotating in one direction associated with flexed postures (Fig. 5.9). This is the same movement direction that they report 'injuring' their back.

They present in standing with a loss of lumbar segmental lordosis at the affected level (similar to patient presentation one) but with an associated lateral shift at the same level. Palpation of the lumbar multifidus muscles in standing commonly reveals resting muscle tone on the side ipsilateral to the shift, and atrophy and low tone on the contralateral side. The lateral shift is accentuated when standing on the foot ipsilateral to the shift and is observed during gait as a tendency to transfer weight through the trunk and upper body rather than through the pelvis (Fig. 5.10). Sagittal spinal movements reveal a shift further laterally at midrange flexion and this is commonly associated with an arc of pain. A loss of rotary and lateral trunk control in the direction of the shift can be observed in supine postures with asymmetrical leg loading and unilateral bridging, and in four point kneeling when flexing one arm. Sitting to standing and squatting usually reveals a tendency towards lateral trunk shift during the movement with increased weight bearing on the lower limb ipsilateral to the shift.

Specific muscle testing reveals an inability to bilaterally activate segmental lumbar multifidus in co-contraction with the deep abdominal muscles, with dominance of activation of the quadratus lumborum, lumbar erector spinae and superficial lumbar multifidus on the side ipsilateral to the shift and an inability to activate the segmental lumbar multifidus on the side contralateral to the lateral shift. This is associated with bracing of the abdominal wall and loss of breathing control. Palpatory examination reveals an increase in intersegmental flexion at the symptomatic level and a uni-directional increase in rotation and sidebending in the direction of the shift.

Multi-directional pattern

This is the most serious and debilitating of the clinical presentations and is frequently associated with a traumatic injury and high levels of pain and functional disability. Patients describe their provocative movements as being multi-directional in nature (Fig. 5.11). All weight-bearing postures

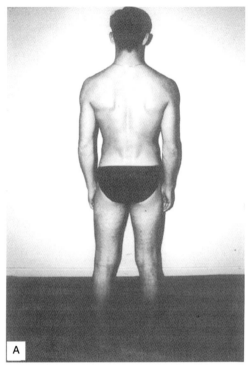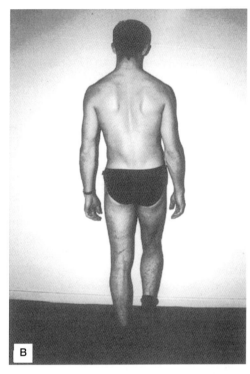

Figure 5.10 Lateral shifting pattern: patient with lumbar segmental instability at L4/5 complaining of an unstable movement zone in flexion to the left. (A) Patient presents in standing with a loss of segmental lordosis at L4/5 associated with a left-lateral segmental shift. (B) The left-lateral shift is accentuated when single leg-standing on the left with a tendency to transfer weight through the trunk rather than through the pelvis. (Reproduced by kind permission of W.B. Saunders.)

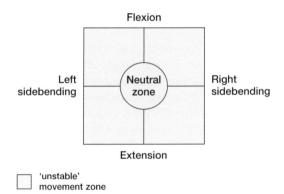

Figure 5.11 Unstable movement zone — multi-directional pattern. (Reproduced by kind permission of W.B. Saunders.)

are painful and difficulty is reported in obtaining relieving positions during weight bearing. Locking of the spine is commonly reported following sustained flexion, rotation and extension postures. These patients may assume a flexed, extended or laterally shifted spinal posture. Excessive segmental shifting and hinging patterns may be observed in all movement directions with 'jabbing' pain and associated back muscle spasm. These patients have great difficulty assuming neutral lordotic spinal positions, and attempts to facilitate lumbar multifidus and transversus abdominis co-contraction (especially while maintaining weight-bearing positions) are usually associated with a tendency to flex, extend or laterally shift the spine segmentally, with associated global muscle substitution, bracing of the abdominal wall and pain. Palpatory examination reveals multi-directional increased intersegmental motion at the symptomatic level. If these patients present with high levels of irritability and an inability to tolerate compressive loading in any position, they have a poor prognosis for conservative exercise management.

AIMS OF THE PHYSICAL EXAMINATION

1. Identify the symptomatic hypermobile motion segment and correlate this with radiological findings if present.
2. Identify direction specificity of the 'instability' problem.
3. Determine the neuromuscular strategy of dynamic stabilization; (a) observe for loss of dynamic trunk stabilization during functional movement and limb loading tests (Sahrmann 1993), (b) identify local muscle system dysfunction and faulty patterns of global muscle system substitution (Richardson & Jull 1995; Richardson et al 1999).
4. Determine the relationship between symptoms and local muscle system control.

MANAGEMENT OF LUMBAR SEGMENTAL INSTABILITY

MOTOR LEARNING MODEL

A recent focus in the physiotherapy management of chronic low back pain patients has been the specific training of muscles whose primary role is considered to be the provision of dynamic stability and segmental control to the spine, i.e. transversus abdominis, diaphragm and lumbar multifidus, based on the identification of specific motor-control deficits in these muscles (Richardson & Jull 1995; O'Sullivan et al 1997a, c). This approach is based on a motor learning model whereby the faulty movement pattern or patterns are identified and the components of the movement are isolated and retrained into functional tasks specific to the patient's individual needs (O'Sullivan et al 1997a). This model of exercise training has been shown to be effective with long-term reductions in pain and functional disability in subjects with chronic low back pain with a diagnosis of lumbar segmental instability (O'Sullivan 1997; O'Sullivan et al 1997c; 1998b). This specific exercise intervention represents, in its simplest

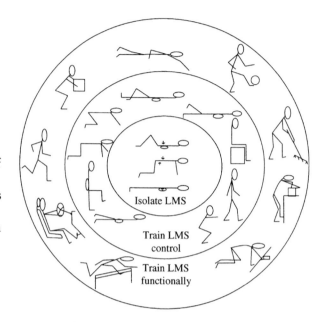

Figure 5.12 Stages of rehabilitation based on a motor learning model (LMS = local muscle system). (Reproduced by kind permission of W.B. Saunders.)

form, the process of motor learning described by Fitts and Posner (Shumway-Cook & Woollacott 1995) who reported three stages in learning a new motor skill (Fig. 5.12).

FIRST STAGE OF TRAINING

The first is the cognitive stage where, in the early training period, a high level of awareness is demanded of subjects in order that they isolate the co-contraction of the local muscle system without global muscle substitution. The aim of the first stage is to train the specific isometric co-contraction of transversus abdominis with lumbar multifidus at low levels of maximal voluntary contraction and with controlled respiration, in weight bearing within a neutral lordosis.

Progression of first stage

1. Train independence of pelvis and lower lumbar spine from thoracic spine and hips to achieve a neutral lordosis without global muscle substitution.
2. Train central and lateral costal diaphragm breathing control.

3. Maintaining neutral lordosis, facilitate the 'drawing up and in' contraction of the pelvic floor and lower and middle fibres of transversus abdominis with gentle controlled lateral costal diaphragm breathing and without global muscle substitution. This is facilitated in non-weight-bearing postures such as four point kneeling, prone or supine only if accurate co-contraction cannot be facilitated in weight-bearing postures such as sitting and standing.

4. Facilitate bilateral activation of segmental lumbar multifidus (at the unstable level) in co-contraction with transversus abdominis and controlled lateral costal diaphragm breathing while maintaining a neutral lordosis.

5. Train co-contraction in sitting and standing with postural correction.

Strategies to inhibit global muscle substitution

1. Obliquus externus abdominis and rectus abdominis:
   — focus on pelvic floor contraction
   — facilitate upper lumbar lordosis and lateral costal diaphragm breathing to open sternal angle
   — focus on optimal postural alignment in weight bearing.

2. Thoracolumbar erector spinae:
   — avoid thoracic spine extension and excessive lumbar spine lordosis
   — ensure independence of pelvis and low lumbar spine movement from thoracic spine and hips
   — facilitate lateral costal diaphragm breathing
   — use of palpatory and electromyograph biofeedback, and muscle release techniques.

In the early stages the instruction is to cease the contraction if global muscle substitution occurs, breathing control is lost, muscle fatigue occurs or there is an increase in resting pain. Training is performed a minimum of once a day (10–15 minutes) in a quiet environment. Once this pattern of muscle activation has been isolated then the contractions must be performed with postural correction in sitting and standing and the holding contraction increased from 10 to 60 seconds prior to its integration into functional tasks and aerobic activities such as talking. At this stage a degree of pain control is expected in these postures. This provides a powerful biofeedback for the patient. This stage may take 3–6 weeks to achieve.

SECOND STAGE OF TRAINING

The second phase of motor learning is the associative stage, where the focus is on refining a particular movement pattern. The aim is to identify two or three faulty and pain-provocative movement patterns based on the examination and break them down into component movements with high repetitions (i.e. 50–60). The patient is taken through these steps whilst isolating the co-contraction of the local muscle system. This is first carried out while maintaining the spine in a neutral lordotic posture and finally with normal spinal movement. At all times segmental control and pain control must be ensured. This can be performed for sit to stand, walking, lifting, bending, twisting, extending etc. The patients carry out the movement components on a daily basis with pain control and gradually increase the speed and complexity of the movement pattern until they can move in a smooth, free and controlled manner. Patients are encouraged to carry out regular aerobic exercise, such as walking, while maintaining correct postural alignment, low level local muscle system co-contraction and controlled respiration. This helps to increase the tone within the muscles and aids the automaticity of the pattern.

Patients are encouraged to perform the co-contractions in situations where they experience or anticipate pain or feel 'unstable'. This is essential, so that the patterns of co-contraction eventually occur automatically. This stage can last from between 8 weeks to 4 months depending on the performer, the degree and nature of the pathology and the intensity of practice, before the motor pattern is learned and becomes automatic. It is at this stage that patients commonly report the ability to carry out previously aggravating activities without pain and are able to cease the formal specific exercise programme. They are instructed to maintain local muscle system control functionally with postural awareness, while maintaining regular levels of general exercise.

THIRD STAGE OF TRAINING

The third stage is the autonomous stage where a low degree of attention is required for the correct performance of the motor task (Shumway-Cook & Woollacott 1995). The third stage is the aim of the specific exercise intervention, whereby subjects can dynamically stabilize their spines appropriately in an automatic manner during the functional demands of daily living. Evidence that changes to automatic patterns of muscle recruitment can be achieved by this intervention is supported by surface electromyography data and the long-term positive outcome for subjects who had undergone this treatment intervention (O'Sullivan et al 1997c; 1998a; 1998b) (Fig. 5.13).

CONCLUSION

The successful management of chronic low back pain conditions greatly depends on the accurate identification of subgroups within the population who respond to specific interventions. An individual motor learning exercise approach designed

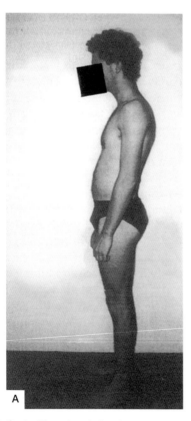
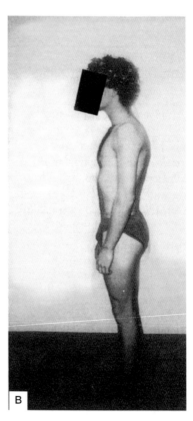

Figure 5.13 (A) Patient with a chronic low back pain condition associated with a multi-directional instability pattern associated with a spondylolisthesis at L5/S1, prior to specific exercise intervention. Note the sway posture and poor tone of the lower abdominal wall. (B) The same patient following a 10-week specific exercise intervention programme focused on training the co-contraction of the deep abdominal muscles with segmental lumbar multifidus and integrating this muscle control into functional tasks based on a motor learning model. Note the tone in the lower abdominal wall and correction of the sway posture compared to the pre-intervention photo. (Reproduced by kind permission of W.B. Saunders.)

to enhance optimal segmental spinal control for patients with lumbar segmental instability is a logical management strategy for this condition. The success of this approach depends on the skill and ability of the physiotherapist to accurately identify the clinical problem and the specific motor control dysfunction present and facilitate the correction of the faulty movement strategies. It will also be greatly influenced by the severity of the patients condition and their level of compliance. Evidence for the efficacy of this approach is growing although clinical trials comparing this to other exercise approaches is required.

Acknowledgements

All figures are reproduced by kind permission of W.B. Saunders from Twomey and Taylor (eds) 2000 Physical Therapy of the Low Back, 3rd edn. W.B. Saunders, Philadelphia.

REFERENCES

Allison G, Kendle K, Roll S, Schupelius J, Scott Q, Panizza J 1997 The role of the diaphragm during abdominal hollowing exercises. Australian Journal of Physiotherapy 44(2): 95–102

Aspden R 1992 Review of the functional anatomy of the spinal ligaments and the lumbar erector spinae muscles. Clinical Anatomy 5: 372–387

Avery A 1996 The reliability of manual physiotherapy palpation techniques in the diagnosis of bilateral pars defects in subjects with chronic low back pain. Master of Science Thesis, Curtin University of Technology, Western Australia

Bergmark A 1989 Stability of the lumbar spine. A study in mechanical engineering. Acta Orthopaedica Scandinavica 230(60)(Suppl). 20–24

Biedermann HJ, Shanks GL, Forrest WJ, Inglis J 1991 Power spectrum analysis of electromyographic activity. Spine 16(10): 1179–1184

Bogduk N 1995 The anatomical basis for spinal pain syndromes. Journal of Manipulative and Physiological Therapeutics 18(9): 603–605

Cholewicke J, McGill S 1996 Mechanical stability of the in vivo lumbar spine: implications for injury and chronic low back pain. Clinical Biomechanics 11(1): 1–15

Coste J, Paolaggi J, Spira A 1992 Classification of non-specific low back pain II. Clinical diversity of organic forms. Spine 17(9): 1038–1042

Cresswell A 1993 Responses of intra-abdominal pressure and abdominal muscle activity during dynamic loading in man. European Journal of Applied Physiology 66: 315–320

Dillingham T 1995 Evaluation and management of low back pain: and overview. State of the Art Reviews 9(3): 559–574

Dupuis P, Yong-Hing K, Cassidy D, Kirkaldy-Willis W 1985 Radiological diagnosis of degenerative spinal instability. Spine 10(3): 262–276

Dvorak J, Panjabi M, Novotny J, Chang D, Grob D 1991 Clinical validation of functional flexion-extension roentgenograms of the lumbar spine. Spine 16(8): 943–950

Edgerton V, Wolf S, Levendowski D, Roy R 1996 Theoretical basis for patterning EMG amplitudes to assess muscle dysfunction. Medicine and Science in Sports and Exercise 28(6): 744–751

Friberg O 1987 Lumbar instability: a dynamic approach by traction-compression radiography. Spine 12(2): 119–129

Friberg O 1989 Functional radiography of the lumbar spine. Annals of Medicine 21(5): 341–346

Gertzbein S 1991 Segmental instability of the lumbar spine. Seminars in Spinal Surgery 3(2): 130–135

Goel V, Kong W, Han J, Weinstein J, Gilbertson L 1993 A combined finite element and optimization investigation of lumbar spine mechanics with and without muscles. Spine 18(11): 1531–1541

Hides J, Richardson C, Jull G 1996 Multifidus recovery is not automatic following resolution of acute first episode of low back pain. Spine 21(23): 2763–2769

Hodges P, Richardson C 1996 Inefficient muscular stabilization of the lumbar spine associated with low back pain: a motor control evaluation of transversus abdominis. Spine 21(22): 2640–2650

Hodges P, Butler J, McKenzie D, Gandevia S 1997 Contraction of the human diaphragm during rapid postural adjustments. Journal of Physiology 505(2): 539–548

Indahl A, Velund L, Reikeraas O 1995 Good prognosis for low back pain when left untampered. Spine 20(4): 473–477

Kaigle A, Holm S, Hansson T 1995 Experimental instability in the lumbar spine. Spine 20(4): 421–430

Kirkaldy-Willis W, Farfan H 1982 Instability of the lumbar spine. Clinical Orthopaedics and Related Research 165: 110–123

Lindgren K, Sihvonen T, Leino E, Pitkanen M 1993 Exercise therapy effects on functional radiographic findings and segmental electromyographic activity in lumbar spine instability. Archives in Physical Medicine and Rehabilitation 74: 933–939

Long D, BenDebba M, Torgenson W 1996 Persistent back pain and sciatica in the United States: patient characteristics. Journal of Spinal Disorders 9(1): 40–58

McGill S 1991 Electromyographic activity of the abdominal and low back musculature during the generation of isometric and dynamic axial trunk torque; Implications for lumbar mechanics. Journal of Orthopaedic Research 9: 91–103

McGill S, Norman R 1987 Reassessment of the role of intra-abdominal pressure in spinal compression. Ergonomics 30(11): 1565–1688

Mimura M 1990 Rotational instability of the lumbar spine — a three dimensional motion study using bi-plane X-ray analysis system. Nippon Seikeigeka Gakkai Zasshi 64(7): 546–559

Mimura M, Panjabi M, Oxland T, Crisco J, Yamamoto I, Vasavada A 1994 Disc degeneration affects the multidirectional flexibility of the lumbar spine. Spine 19(12): 1371–1380

Montgomery D, Fischgrund J 1994 Passive reduction of spondylolisthesis on the operating room table: a prospective study. Journal of Spinal Disorders 7(2): 167–172

Nachemson A 1991 Instability of the lumbar spine. Neurosurgery Clinics of North America 2(4): 785–790

O'Sullivan P 1997 The efficacy of specific stabilizing exercise in the management of chronic low back pain with radiological diagnosis of lumbar segmental instability. PhD Thesis, Curtin University of Technology, Western Australia

O'Sullivan P, Twomey L, Allison G 1997a Dynamic stabilization of the lumbar spine. Critical Reviews of Physical and Rehabilitation Medicine 9(3&4): 315–330

O'Sullivan P, Twomey L, Allison G 1997b Dysfunction of the neuro-muscular system in the presence of low back pain — implications for physical therapy management. Journal of Manual and Manipulative Therapy 5(1): 20–26

O'Sullivan P, Twomey L, Allison G 1997c Evaluation of specific stabilising exercise in the treatment of chronic low back pain with radiological diagnosis of spondylolysis and spondylolisthesis. Spine 15(24): 2959–2967

O'Sullivan P, Twomey L, Allison G, Sinclair J, Miller K, Knox J 1997d Altered patterns of abdominal muscle activation in patients with chronic back pain. Australian Journal of Physiotherapy 43(2): 91–98

O'Sullivan P, Twomey L, Allison G 1998a Altered abdominal muscle recruitment in back pain patients following specific exercise intervention. Journal of Orthopaedic and Sports Physical Therapy 27(2): 1–11

O'Sullivan P, Twomey L, Allison G, Taylor J 1998b Specific stabilizing exercise in the treatment of chronic low back pain with clinical and radiological diagnosis of lumbar segmental 'instability'. Third Interdisciplinary World Congress on Low Back and Pelvic Pain, Vienna, Austria: 366–367

Panjabi M 1992 The stabilizing system of the spine. Part 1 and Part 2. Journal of Spinal Disorders 5(4): 383–397

Panjabi M, Abumi K, Duranceau J, Oxland T 1989 Spinal stability and intersegmental muscle forces. A biomechanical model. Spine 14(2): 194–199

Paris S 1985 Physical signs of instability. Spine 10(3): 277–279

Phillips D 1994 A comparison of manual diagnosis with a diagnosis established by a uni-level spinal block procedure. Master of Science Thesis, Curtin University of Technology, Western Australia

Pope M, Frymoyer J, Krag M 1992 Diagnosing instability. Clinical Orthopaedics and Related Research 296: 60–67

Richardson C, Jull G 1995 Muscle control — pain control. What exercises would you prescribe? Manual Therapy 1(1): 2–10

Richardson C, Jull G, Hodges P, Hides J 1999 Therapeutic exercise for the spinal segmental stabilization in low back pain: scientific basis and clinical approach. Churchill Livingstone, Edinburgh

Roy S, Deluca C, Casavant D 1989 Lumbar muscle fatigue and chronic low back pain. Spine 14: 992–1001

Sahrmann S 1993 Diagnosis and treatment of muscle imbalances associated with regional pain syndromes. Manipulative Physiotherapists Association of Australia — Eighth Biennial Conference — post conference workshop. Perth, Western Australia: 1–27

Shumway-Cook A, Woollacott M 1995 Motor control — Theory and Practical Applications. Williams & Wilkins, Baltimore

Sihvonen T, Partanen J 1990 Segmental hypermobility in lumbar spine and entrapment of dorsal rami. Electromyography and Clinical Neurophysiology 30: 175–180

Sihvonen T, Partanen J, Hanninen O, Soimakallio S 1991 Electric behaviour of low back muscles during lumbar pelvic rhythm in low back pain patients and healthy controls. Archives of Physical Medicine and Rehabilitation 72: 1080–1087

Steffen R, Nolte L, Pingel T 1994 Importance of the back muscles in rehabilitation of postoperative segmental lumbar instability — a biomechanical analysis. Rehabilitation (Stuttgart) 33(3): 164–170

Wilke H, Wolf S, Claes L, Arand M, Wiesend A 1995 Stability increase of the lumbar spine with different muscle groups. Spine 20(2): 192–198

Wood K, Popp C, Transfeldt E, Geissele A 1994 Radiographic evaluation of instability in spondylolisthesis. Spine 19(15): 1697–1703

6

Nerve trunk pain: physical diagnosis and treatment

T. M. Hall   R. L. Elvey
School of Physiotherapy, Curtin University of
Technology, Perth, Australia

The management of peripheral neuropathic pain or nerve trunk pain relies upon accurate differential diagnosis. In part neurogenic pain has been attributed to increased activity and abnormal processing of non-nociceptive input from the nervi nervorum. For neurogenic pain to be identified as the dominant feature of a painful condition there should be evidence of increased nerve trunk mechanosensitivity from all aspects of the physical examination procedure. Consistent dysfunction should be identified on key active and passive movements, neural tissue provocation tests as well as nerve trunk palpation. A local cause for the neurogenic pain disorder should also be identified if the condition is to be treated by manual therapy. A treatment approach is presented which has been shown to have efficacy in the relief of pain and restoration of function in cervicobrachial pain disorders where there is evidence according to the outlined examination protocol of nerve trunk pain. *Manual Therapy* (1999) **4(2),** 63–73

INTRODUCTION

In recent years there has been a great deal of interest in the role neural tissue may play in pain disorders. The consideration that pain may be neurogenic is not new (Marshall 1883; Madison Taylor 1909) but the more recent development of examination and treatment techniques can be attributed to Elvey (1979) and Butler (1991). Their work in formulating and describing the brachial plexus tension test and the upper limb tension test led to a rebirth of interest in neural tissue as a pain source. However, the unfortunate nomenclature, brachial plexus tension test (Elvey 1979) and upper limb tension test (Butler 1991) coupled with adverse mechanical tension of the nervous system (Butler 1989), led many physiotherapists to a pre-occupation with faulty neural tissue mechanics.

In more recent years there has been an increase in the understanding of pain physiology and there has been much interest into the area of neural tissue involvement in pain disorders (Greening & Lynn 1998; Zusman 1998), particularly from a physiotherapy perspective. This knowledge requires careful consideration in the management of neural tissue disorders and has necessitated a change in the understanding of the physical treatment of pain (Butler 1998), particularly in regard to neuropathic pain (Elvey 1998).

The purpose of this article is to present a scheme for the clinical examination to evaluate the involvement of neural tissue in a disorder of pain and dysfunction, together with a treatment approach where there is a reversible musculoskeletal cause of the neuropathic pain disorder.

PERIPHERAL NEUROPATHIC PAIN

The term 'peripheral neuropathic pain' has been suggested to embrace the combination of positive and negative symptoms in patients in whom pain is due to pathological changes or dysfunction in peripheral nerves or nerve roots (Devor & Rappaport 1990). Positive symptoms include pain, paraesthesia and spasm. In contrast, anaesthesia and weakness are negative sensory and motor symptoms, respectively.

Two types of neuropathic pain following peripheral nerve injury have been recognized: 'dysaesthetic pain' and 'nerve trunk pain' (Asbury & Fields 1984). Dysaesthetic pain results from volleys of impulses arising in damaged or regenerating nociceptive, afferent fibres. Characteristically dysaesthetic pain is felt in the peripheral sensory distribution of a sensory or mixed nerve. This pain has features that are not found in deep pain arising from either somatic or visceral tissues. These include abnormal or unfamiliar sensations, frequently having a burning or electrical quality; pain felt in the region of the sensory deficit; pain with a paroxysmal brief shooting or stabbing com-

ponent; and the presence of allodynia (Fields 1987; Devor 1991).

In contrast, nerve trunk pain has been attributed to increased activity in mechanically or chemically sensitized nociceptors within the nerve sheaths (Asbury & Fields 1984). This kind of pain is said to follow the course of the nerve trunk. It is commonly described as deep and aching, similar to a 'toothache' and made worse with movement, nerve stretch or palpation (Asbury & Fields 1984). Peripheral nerve trunks are known to be mechanosensitive, for they possess afferents within their connective tissues that are normally capable of mechanoreception (Hromada 1963; Thomas et al 1993). These afferents are known as the nervi nervorum; the majority are unmyelinated forming a sporadic plexus in all the connective tissues of a peripheral nerve and have predominantly 'free' endings (Hromada 1963). Electrophysiological studies by Bove and Light (1995) demonstrated that at least some of the nervi nervorum have a nociceptive function because they respond to noxious mechanical, chemical and thermal stimuli. Most nervi nervorum studied by Bove and Light (1997) were sensitive to excess longitudinal stretch of the entire nerve they innervated, as well as to local stretch in any direction and to focal pressure. They did not respond to stretch within normal ranges of motion. This evidence is supported by clinical studies that show under normal circumstances nerve trunks are insensitive to non-noxious mechanical deformation (Kuslich et al 1991; Hall & Quintner 1996).

Recent evidence has shown that the nervi nervorum contain neuropeptides including substance P and calcitonin gene related peptide, indicating a role in neurogenic vasodilation (Zochodne 1993; Bove & Light 1997). Bove and Light (1997) suggested that local nerve inflammation is mediated by the nervi nervorum, especially in cases with no intrafascicular axonal damage. In keeping with this, it has been postulated that the spread of mechanosensitivity along the length of the nerve trunk, distant to the local area of pathology seen in nerve trunk pain, is mediated through neurogenic inflammation via the nervi nervorum (Quintner 1998). The entire nerve trunk then behaves as a sensitized nociceptor, generating impulses in response to minor mechanical stimuli (Devor 1989).

The mechanism of neurogenic inflammation may help to explain mechanical allodynia of structurally normal nerve trunks, where the pathology is more proximal in the nerve root. An alternative explanation is that non-nociceptive input from the presumed nerve trunk mechanoreceptors is being processed abnormally within the central nervous system (Hall & Quintner 1996). This is probably the result of a sustained afferent nociceptive barrage from the site of nerve damage (Sugimoto et al 1989), a pathological process termed 'central sensitization' (Woolf 1991). In the lumbar spine the most commonly cited form of neural pathology involves nerve root compression, which usually results from intervertebral disc herniation but is also commonly caused by age-related changes (Bogduk & Twomey 1991). Slow growing osteophytes from lumbar zygapophyseal joints can compress the nerve root in the intervertebral foramen, leading to radicular symptoms and neurological signs (Epstein et al 1973).

Although pain is not a necessary feature of nerve root compression (Wiesel et al 1984), radicular pain in the absence of nerve root inflammatory changes is presumably due to chronic compression of axons within the nerve root (Bogduk & Twomey 1991). Under these circumstances there may be minimal sensitization of the nervi nervorum and little evidence of neural tissue mechanosensitivity on neural tissue provocation tests such as straight leg raise (Amundsen et al 1995). However, unless the condition is minor there should be clinical, radiological and probably electrodiagnostic evidence of compressive neurological compromise. Clinical neurological tests should include deep tendon reflexes, muscle power and skin sensation.

Alternatively, radicular pain, even when severe, may present where the axonal conduction is normal but the nerve trunk is highly mechanically sensitized. In this case clinical neurological and electrodiagnostic tests may be normal suggesting a lack of nerve root compression. What appears to be the significant factor is chemical or inflammatory (Olmarker & Rydevik 1991) sensitization of the nervi nervorum and mechanical allodynia of

peripheral nerve trunks.

In an individual patient with nerve injury it is possible that dysaesthetic pain and nerve trunk pain may exist in isolation, however, it is more common for both to be present (Asbury & Fields 1984). For this reason it might be difficult to distinguish, from the subjective description of pain, between referred pain arising from somatic tissues and referred pain arising from neural tissues (Dalton & Jull 1989; Rankine et al 1998).

The pain and paraesthesia that occur in cervical and lumbar radiculopathy may not be well localized anatomically, due to different nerve roots having a similar distribution of pain or paraesthesia. In a series of 841 subjects with cervical radiculopathy, Henderson et al (1983) found only 55% presented with pain following a typical discrete dermatomal pattern. The remainder presented with diffuse nondermatomally distributed pain. Rankine et al (1998) found that the location of pain and paraesthesia was not a good predictor of the presence of lumbar nerve root compression. As is always the case, information from the subjective examination should be interpreted with caution and within the context of the complete clinical evaluation.

CLINICAL EXAMINATION

The purpose of the clinical examination and evaluation is to diagnose the source of the patient's subjective pain complaint in order to make a diagnosis and to prescribe appropriate treatment options.

To effectively evaluate a particular disorder for manual therapy treatment, the clinician must carry out a range of physical examination tests to gain a sufficient number of consistent signs in order to make a diagnosis. For example, if a patient presents with calf pain following an injury, such as a 'pulled muscle', a number of physical examination tests correlating with each other would be required to be present before a diagnosis of muscle strain could be supported. These physical tests provide mechanical stimuli to the injured muscle tissue and so are provocative tests seeking a subjective pain response. Such tests would include a static isometric muscle contraction, calf muscle stretch and palpation of the muscle. No one test in isolation is sufficient and the physical examination findings should be consistent with the degree of trauma and subjective pain complaint ascertained from the subjective history.

In pain disorders multiple tissues are frequently involved and a very careful physical examination is required to ascertain from which tissue pain predominates. To determine whether neural tissue is involved a clinical reasoning process must be employed similar to, but more sophisticated than, the example given for calf pain and a number of very specific correlating signs must be present. For instance, it is not possible to say that a straight leg raise (SLR) test as a single test is positive or negative in the diagnosis of nerve root pathology. The mechanical stress of SLR is not isolated to the neural structures (Kleynhans & Terrett 1986). SLR induces posterior pelvic rotation within a few degrees of lifting the leg from the horizontal (Fahlgren Grampo et al 1991). Structures in the posterior thigh, pelvis and lumbar spine, including hamstring muscles, lumbar facet joints, lumbar intervertebral ligaments, muscles and the intervertebral discs as well as neural tissues, must be mechanically provoked. The findings from the SLR test must be interpreted within the clinical context of a number of other procedures before a diagnosis of nerve root pathology can be made.

The importance of accurate diagnosis or determination of the tissue of the primary source of origin of pain lies in providing accurate treatment prescription.

PHYSICAL SIGNS OF NEURAL TISSUE INVOLVEMENT

According to Elvey and Hall (1997) the physical signs of neuropathic pain should include the following:

1. Antalgic posture
2. Active movement dysfunction
3. Passive movement dysfunction, which correlates with the active movement dysfunction
4. Adverse responses to neural tissue provocation tests, which must relate specifically and anatomically to 2 and 3

5. Mechanical allodynia in response to palpation of specific nerve trunks, which relate specifically and anatomically to 2 and 4
6. Evidence from the physical examination of a local cause of the neurogenic pain, which would involve the neural tissue showing the responses in 4 and 5.

Under normal circumstances peripheral nerve trunks slide and glide with movement adapting to positional changes of the trunk and limbs (McLellan & Swash 1976; Breig 1978). When neural tissue is sensitized limb movement and positional change cause a provocative mechanical stimulus resulting in pain and therefore noncompliance. This lack of compliance will be demonstrated by painful limitation of movement caused by muscles antagonistic to the direction of movement acting to prevent further pain. Muscle contraction, as measured by electromyography, in response to painful mechanical provocation of upper and lower quarter peripheral nerve trunks, has been demonstrated in normal subjects as well as subjects who have a neuropathic pain disorder (Hall et al 1995; Hall & Quintner 1996; Balster & Jull 1997). In those subjects with a neuropathic pain disorder, due to heightened neural tissue mechanosensitivity, muscle activity occurs at the onset of pain provocation, whereas in normal subjects muscle activity occurs according to the level of the subject's pain tolerance (Hall et al 1995). It appears that muscles are recruited via central nervous system processes to prevent pain associated with the provocation of neural tissue (Hall & Quintner 1996).

POSTURE

A particular antalgic postural position that would shorten the anatomical distance over which a peripheral nerve trunk courses may be the first clinical consideration of neuropathic pain. For example, the patient who presents with severe leg pain associated with sensitization of the S1 nerve root will frequently adopt an antalgic posture of knee flexion, ankle plantar flexion and lumbar spine ipsilateral lateral flexion (Fig. 6.1).

A similar example in a patient with a brachial plexopathy would be a combination of shoulder

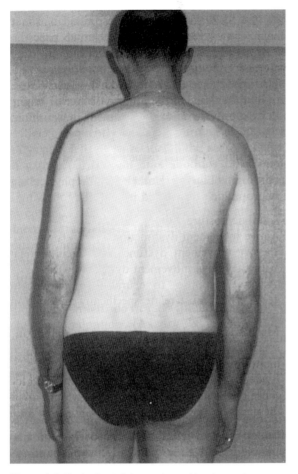

Figure 6.1 Typical antalgic posture of lumbar spine right-lateral flexion associated with right leg pain.

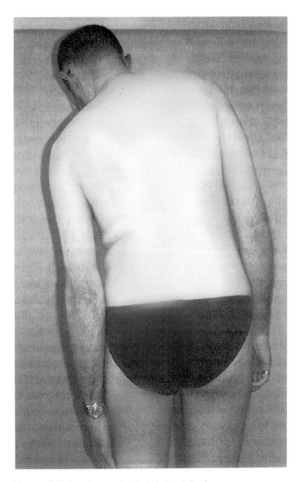

Figure 6.2 Lumbar spine left-lateral flexion.

girdle elevation, cervical spine ipsilateral lateral flexion and elbow flexion. Guarded postures to avoid movement of the sensitized nerve site have been demonstrated in an animal model (Laird & Bennett 1993). The most likely mechanism for altered posture is protective muscle contraction or spasm. The magnitude of an antalgic posture will vary with the severity of pain.

ACTIVE MOVEMENT

An analysis of an antalgic posture will indicate painful limitation of specific active movements that will provide further evidence that neural tissue is involved in a painful disorder. Depending

on which neural tissue is involved some movements will be more provocative than others.

Figures 6.2 and 6.3 demonstrate active movement limitation of lumbar lateral flexion that is consistent with the antalgic posture secondary to sensitization of right lower quarter neural tissues.

In the lower quarter, lumbar flexion, with hip flexion and knee extension, is provocative to the sciatic nerve, its terminal branches and the L4–S3 nerve roots. If pain is provoked or the range of movement is limited, it is possible to consider a process to differentiate between pathology in the lumbar somatic structures and neural tissues by positioning the ankle in dorsiflexion or the cervical spine in flexion and repeating the movement.

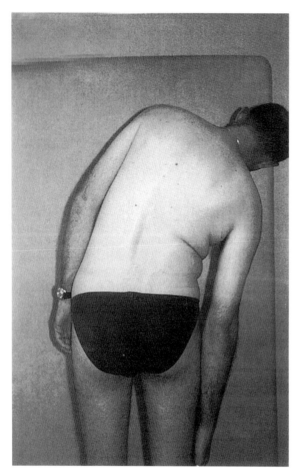

Figure 6.3 Lumbar spine right-lateral flexion.

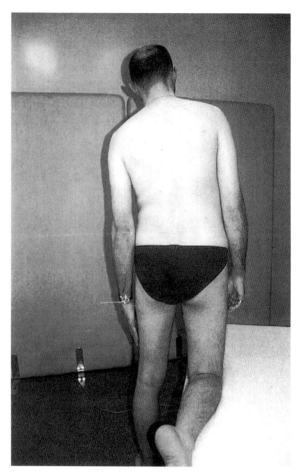

Figure 6.4 Lumbar spine left-lateral flexion with knee flexion.

Should neural tissue be involved, the response to active lumbar flexion would be more painful and the range of movement further limited by pain. Great care must be taken to prevent compensatory involuntary movement of knee flexion, which is presumably a protective hamstring muscle response.

In contrast to the sciatic nerve the femoral nerve arises from the L2 to L4 nerve roots and will be mechanically stimulated by a combination of, among other movements, lumbar contralateral lateral flexion, hip extension and knee flexion. Again differentiation of somatic and neural structure as the source of pain can be considered by using a combination of remote movements sensitizing the neural structures.

Figures 6.4–6.6 demonstrate an increasingly limited range of lumbar spine left-lateral flexion with neural sensitizing manoeuvres, utilizing the sciatic and femoral nerve trunks.

In the upper quarter various active movements will be affected depending on the particular nerve tract involved. Shoulder abduction and contralateral lateral flexion of the cervical spine will affect the brachial plexus and associated tracts of neural tissue (Elvey 1979; Reid 1987), and, as such, are the most likely movements to be affected in the presence of increased mechanosensitivity of the neural tissues forming the brachial plexus.

If active shoulder abduction or cervical spine contralateral lateral flexion is painful or limited in range, the clinician can differentiate between local

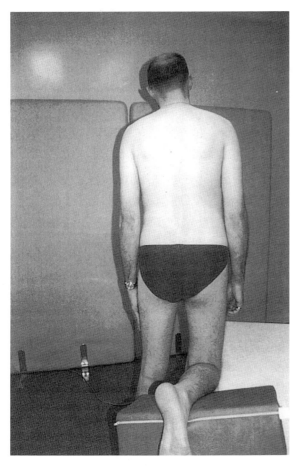

Figure 6.5 Lumbar spine left-lateral flexion with increased knee flexion.

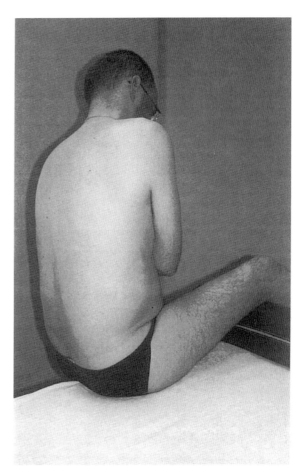

Figure 6.6 Lumbar spine left-lateral flexion with hip flexion and knee off full extension.

pathology and neural tissue by repeating the movement with neural sensitizing manoeuvres such as wrist extension. Wrist extension will place greater provocation on the upper quarter neural tissue (Kleinrensink et al 1995; Lewis et al 1998) via the median and ulnar nerve trunks. With an understanding of applied anatomy the clinician can examine active movements in various ways to support the clinical hypotheses of a neuropathic pain disorder.

PASSIVE MOVEMENT DYSFUNCTION

It is obvious that both active and passive movement have the same mechanical stimulus effect on neural tissues. Therefore in neuropathic pain

disorders there should be consistent limitation of range of passive movement by pain in the same direction as active movement limitation.

The flexion/adduction manoeuvre of the hip and the quadrant position of the shoulder (Maitland 1991) are two important passive movement tests of those joints. Not only do these movements stress the hip joint and shoulder complex but certain peripheral nerve trunks (Breig & Troup 1979; Elvey & Hall 1997). For example, the sciatic nerve lies posterior and lateral to the axis of motion of hip flexion adduction, so this movement will be provocative to the sciatic nerve and hence the L4–S3 nerve roots. A determination of possible neural tissue involvement where flexion adduction of the hip is painfully limited can be made by performing the same movement with the knee more extended. A significant increase in painful limitation of movement should be seen if neural tissue were involved in the condition.

ADVERSE RESPONSES TO NEURAL TISSUE PROVOCATION TESTS

A variety of tests have been described that have been shown to mechanically stimulate various components of the neural system, and hence can be used provocatively. The most common of these provocative manoeuvres is the SLR test (Goddard & Reid 1965). Others described include the slump test (Louis 1981), the femoral nerve stress test (Sugiura et al 1979), the passive neck flexion test (Yuan et al 1998), the median nerve stress test (Kleinrensink et al 1995) and the 'brachial plexus tension test' (Elvey 1985).

A methodological approach to neural tissue provocation tests for the upper quarter has been documented (Elvey & Hall 1997). This approach offers guidelines for examination, thus allowing the test technique to be tailored to the severity of a neuropathic pain disorder. The suggested approach incorporates provocative manoeuvres directed to the median, radial and ulnar nerve trunks from a proximal to distal direction and vice versa.

A similar flexible approach is recommended for the lower quarter. For a disorder involving the lumbar spine, provocative manoeuvres directed to the sciatic, femoral and obturator nerve trunks are required. The addition of sensitizing manoeuvres may be necessary. With the SLR test these would include, among others, ankle dorsiflexion, medial hip rotation and hip adduction, which have all been shown to increase the mechanical provocation on the sciatic nerve tract (O'Connell 1951; Breig & Troup 1979). For provocative tests to the femoral and obturator nerve lumbar spine contralateral lateral flexion may be used as a sensitizing manoeuvre. Neural tissue provocation tests are passive movement tests. The examiner must appreciate changes in muscle tone or activity in addition to a subjective pain response. Increased muscle activity is a reflection of increased mechanosensitivity of the neural tissue being tested and is indicated by an increase in

resistance to movement (Hall et al 1998). This increase in resistance should coincide with the patient's report of onset of pain (Hall et al 1995) and reproduction of pain complaint. Symptom reproduction is the second important response. Figures 6.7 and 6.8 demonstrate provocative manoeuvres to the femoral and sciatic nerve trunks as well as associated nerve roots for the patient previously illustrated.

MECHANICAL ALLODYNIA IN RESPONSE TO PALPATION OF SPECIFIC NERVE TRUNKS

An example has been given of an acute muscle tear where pain on palpation is an important aspect of diagnosis. Likewise, if the nervi nervorum is sensitized and pain is provoked by stress applied through the length of the nerve then it should also follow that focal pressure directly over the nerve trunk would also be painful. It is well known that normal peripheral nerve trunks and nerve roots are painless to non-noxious mechanical pressure (Howe et al 1977; Kuslich et al 1991; Hall & Quintner 1996). According to Dyck (1987), the entire extent of the sciatic nerve trunk is invariably tender when a lumbosacral nerve root is traumatized. Similar findings have been reported in cervical radiculopathy (Hall & Quintner 1996).

The spread of mechanosensitivity along the length of the nerve trunk following proximal nerve trauma has been reported elsewhere (Devor & Rappaport 1990) and has been interpreted as reflecting mechanosensitivity of regenerating axon sprouts freely growing, or arrested in disseminated microneuromas. An alternative construct has been put forward by Bove & Light (1997), who suggested that abnormal responses to mechanical provocation of neural tissue in radiculopathy arise from the nervi nervorum. The spread of sensitization of the nervi nervorum has been attributed to neurogenic inflammation (Quintner 1998).

In the clinical setting, palpation of neural tissue must be undertaken with great care. Mild pressure should be applied to the nerve trunks on the uninvolved side first in order to allow the patient to make a comparison. In some instances palpation

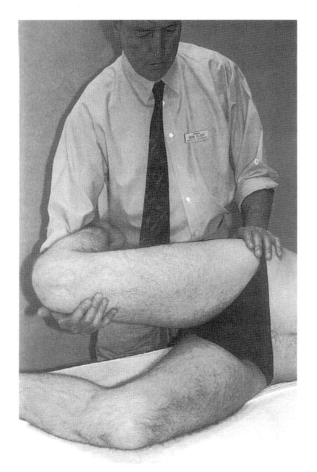

Figure 6.7 Hip extension with knee flexion, provocative to the femoral nerve and associated nerve roots.

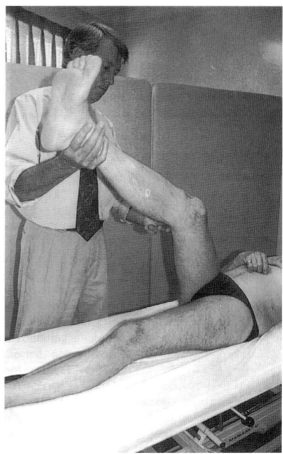

Figure 6.8 Hip flexion with knee flexion, provocative to the sciatic nerve and associated nerve roots.

can be made directly over the nerve trunk, which can be identified as a distinct structure. In other locations nerve trunks must be palpated through muscle and it is less easy to distinguish the nerve as a structure. Under these circumstances broad-based pressure is applied in the area of the nerve trunk and the response is compared to that on the uninvolved side.

Many nerves can be readily palpated but in the clinical context of upper and lower quarter pain syndromes, the most relevant and commonly palpated include the median, radial, ulnar, axillary, suprascapular and dorsal scapular nerves. In the lower quarter these include the sciatic, tibial, common peroneal and femoral nerves. Figures 6.9 and 6.10 demonstrate palpation of the femoral and common peroneal (fibular) nerves.

EVIDENCE OF A LOCAL AREA OF PATHOLOGY

Many peripheral neurogenic pain disorders present at the physical examination with all the features discussed. This does not mean that they are amenable to manual therapy treatment. It is quite possible for other conditions, such as painful diabetic neuropathy or a painful neuropathy caused by tumour infiltration, to cause all of the features discussed so far, including limitation of active and passive movement (Elvey & Hall 1997). Therefore the clinician must determine a cause for the neuropathic pain disorder.

As an example in the lower quarter, intervertebral disc pathology will often result in radicular leg pain and a specific lumbar motion segment

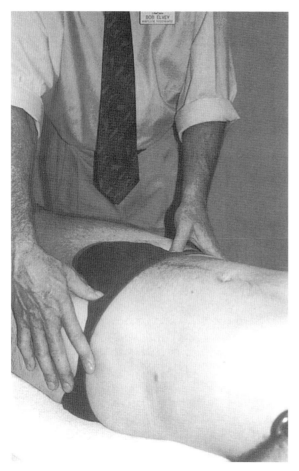

Figure 6.9 Palpation of the femoral nerve.

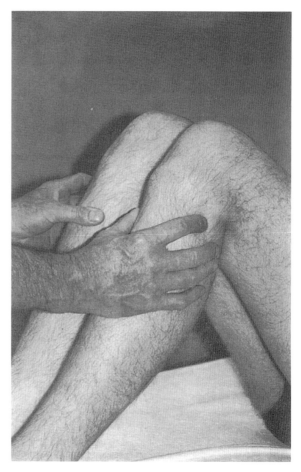

Figure 6.10 Palpation of the common peroneal (fibular) nerve.

dysfunction. Palpatory examination procedures of the lumbar spine would reveal aberrant spinal segmental mobility associated with pain. An example of this would be an L5 radiculopathy, which may have all the features previously discussed together with an L4/5 or an L5/S1 motion segment dysfunction. This would then suggest a spinal cause of the leg pain. Without the palpation findings it may not be possible to determine such a cause and further medical investigation would be necessary to exclude nonmusculoskeletal causes. Figure 6.11 shows a typical test technique in the determination of a local area of pathology. In this patient example, passive intervertebral segmental mobility tests reveal dysfunction at L4/5.

We propose that the above scheme of examination will be both sensitive and specific in determining the presence of abnormal nerve trunk mechanosensitivity and the presence of nerve trunk pain. To date, one study has used this examination protocol to determine the incidence of nerve trunk pain in a particular disorder (Hall et al 1997). In this investigation one third of subjects with chronic cervicobrachial pain syndrome were found to have neural tissue mechanosensitization as the dominant source of the subjective complaint of pain. Whilst there were no laboratory tests to confirm these physical examination findings, the findings from this study have some validity because all subjects found to have nerve trunk pain responded positively to a prescribed treat-

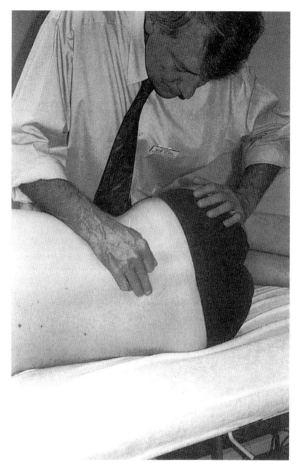

Figure 6.11 Local area of pathology at L4/5 determined by passive intervertebral segmental mobility tests.

ment programme specifically aimed at addressing nerve trunk mechanosensitivity.

TREATMENT

Diagnosis is the most important factor in the prescribed management of all pain disorders. A distinction has been made between two types of peripheral neuropathic pain disorders: dysaesthetic pain and nerve trunk pain. This distinction is important in regard to manual therapy treatment options, which should be different.

Under normal circumstances peripheral nerve trunks are protected to some degree from the effects of nerve stretch and compression (Sunderland 1990). Gross macro scale structural injury to the perineurial sheath occurs at 27% beyond the *in situ* strain of that particular nerve trunk (Kwan et al 1992). However, severe conduction loss may occur at much lower strains, even as low as 6% (Kwan et al 1992). Sunderland (1990) stated that as the fasciculi are stretched, their cross-sectional area is reduced, the intrafascicular pressure is increased, nerve fibres are compressed, and the intrafascicular microcirculation is compromised. Even slight pressure on the outside of a nerve will lead to external hyperaemia, oedema and demyelination of some axons lasting up to 28 days (Bove & Light 1997). Elsewhere it has been observed that 8% elongation of a defined nerve segment may result in impaired venular flow. At elongation of approximately 10–15%, an upper stretch limit is reached where there is complete arrest of all blood flow in the nerve (Lundborg & Rydevik 1973; Ogato & Naito 1986).

In a compression neuropathy, the nerve's microcirculation will be compromised and it is likely that minimal nerve stretch will lead to further compromise of nerve function. For these reasons it is unwise to treat a compressed nerve trunk with stretching or lengthening techniques.

The treatment of nerve trunk pain can involve the use of passive movement techniques. We believe that nerve 'lengthening' or stretching techniques are contraindicated. We advocate the use of gentle, controlled oscillatory passive movements of the anatomical structures surrounding the affected neural tissues at the site of involvement. Treatment can be progressed by using passive movement techniques in a similar manner but involving movement of the surrounding anatomic tissues or structures and the affected neural tissues together in an oscillatory movement (Elvey 1986).

A cervical lateral glide technique described by Elvey (1986) is an example of a treatment approach that has been found to be most useful. In the case of a C6 nerve root involvement the arm should be positioned in some degree of abduction, with the elbow flexed and the hand resting on the abdomen. The technique involves gently gliding the C5/6 motion segment to the contralateral side in a slow oscillating manner.

The onset of muscle activity represents the range of oscillatory movement or the treatment barrier (Elvey & Hall 1997). Should this barrier not be reached, the patient's arm is positioned in a greater range of abduction or elbow extension. Progression of the technique on subsequent days is made by performing the technique with the shoulder in a gradually increased range of abduction. At some point in the treatment a home exercise programme should be incorporated, which is an adjunct to the treatment provided by the clinician.

Evidence for the effcacy of this type of approach has been demonstrated in subjects with lateral elbow pain (Vicenzino et al 1995) and chronic cervicobrachial pain (Hall et al 1997). Hall et al (1997) showed significant improvements in pain, functional capacity, and cervical spine and shoulder girdle mobility after a 4-week treatment period utilizing this concept of management. Improvements were shown to be maintained 3 months after the end of treatment.

CONCLUSION

To successfully manage neuropathic pain disorders it is necessary to make a differential diagnosis. An outline of examination has been presented that will enable differential diagnosis and treatment prescription. A treatment approach has been briefly outlined, which has been shown to provide effective relief for chronic cervicobrachial pain sufferers (Hall et al 1997).

REFERENCES

Amundsen T, Weber H, Lilleas F, Nordal H, Abdelnoor M, Magnaes B 1995 Lumbar spinal stenosis: clinical and radiologic features. Spine 20(10): 1178–1186

Asbury AK, Fields HL 1984 Pain due to peripheral nerve damage: an hypothesis. Neurology 34: 1587–1590

Balster S, Jull G 1997 Upper trapezius muscle activity during the brachial plexus tension test in asymptomatic subjects. Manual Therapy 2(3): 144–149

Bogduk N, Twomey LT 1991 Clinical Anatomy of the Lumbar Spine, 2nd edn. Churchill Livingstone, Melbourne

Bove G, Light A 1995 Unmyelinated nociceptors of rat paraspinal tissues. Journal of Neurophysiology 73: 1752–1762

Bove G, Light A 1997 The nervi nervorum: Missing link for neuropathic pain? Pain Forum 6(3): 181–190

Breig A 1978 Adverse Mechanical Tension in the Central Nervous System: Relief by Functional Neurosurgery. Almquist and Wiksell, Stockholm

Breig A, Troup JDG 1979 Biomechanical considerations of the straight-leg-raising test. Spine 4(3): 242–250

Butler D 1989 Adverse mechanical tension in the nervous system: a model for assessment and treatment. Australian Journal of Physiotherapy 35(4): 227–238

Butler DS 1991 Mobilisation of the Nervous System. Churchill Livingstone, Melbourne

Butler D 1998 Commentary: Adverse mechanical tension in the nervous system: a model for assessment and treatment. In: Maher C (ed) Adverse Neural Tension Revisited. Australian Physiotherapy Association, Melbourne, pp 33–35

Dalton PA, Jull GA 1989 The distribution and characteristics of neck-arm pain in patients with and without a neurological deficit. Australian Journal of Physiotherapy 35: 3–8

Devor M 1989 The pathophysiology of damaged peripheral nerves. In: Wall P Melzack R (eds) Textbook of Pain. Churchill Livingstone, Edinburgh, pp 63–81

Devor M 1991 Neuropathic pain and injured nerve: peripheral mechanisms. British Medical Bulletin 47(3): 619–630

Devor M, Rappaport HZ 1990 Pain and pathophysiology of damaged nerve. In: Fields HL (ed) Pain Syndromes in Neurology. Butterworth Heinemann, Oxford, pp 47–83

Dyck P 1987 Sciatic Pain Lumbar Discectomy and Laminectomy. Aspen, Rockville

Elvey R 1979 Brachial plexus tension tests and the pathoanatomical origin of arm pain. In: Idczak R (ed) Aspects of Manipulative Therapy. Lincoln Institute of Health Sciences, Melbourne, pp 105–110

Elvey RL 1985 Brachial plexus tension tests and the pathoanatomical origin of arm pain. In: Glasgow EF, Twomey LT, Scull ER, Kleynhans AM, Idczak RM (eds) Aspects of Manipulative Therapy, 2nd edn. Churchill Livingstone, Melbourne, pp 116–122

Elvey RL 1986 Treatment of arm pain associated with abnormal brachial plexus tension. Australian Journal of Physiotherapy 32: 225–230

Elvey RL 1998 Commentary: Treatment of arm pain associated with abnormal brachial plexus tension. In: Maher C (ed) Adverse Neural Tension Revisited. Australian Physiotherapy Association, Melbourne, pp 13–17

Elvey R, Hall T 1997 Neural tissue evaluation and treatment. In: Donatelli R (ed) Physical Therapy of the Shoulder, 3rd edn. Churchill Livingstone, New York, pp 131–152

Epstein JA, Epstein BS, Levine LS, Carras R, Rosenthall AD, Sumner P 1973 Lumbar nerve root compression at the intervertebral foramina caused by arthritis of the posterior facet. Journal of Neurosurgery 39: 362–369

Fahlgren Grampo J, Reynolds HM, Vorro J, Beal M 1991 3-D motion of the pelvis during passive leg lifting. In: Anderson PA, Hobart DJ, Danoff JV (eds) Electromyographical Kinesiology. Elsevier Science Publishers BV, pp 119–122

Fields HL 1987 Pain. McGraw Hill, New York

Goddard MD, Reid JD 1965 Movements induced by straight leg raising in the lumbo-sacral roots, nerves and plexus and in the intrapelvic section of the sciatic nerve. Journal of Neurology Neurosurgery Psychiatry 28: 12–18

Greening J, Lynn B 1998 Minor peripheral nerve injuries: an underestimated source of pain. Manual Therapy 3(4): 187–194

Hall T, Elvey RL, Davies N, Dutton L, Moog M 1997 Efficacy of manipulative physiotherapy for the treatment of cervicobrachial pain. In: Tenth Biennial conference of the MPAA, Manipulative Physiotherapists Association of Australia. Melbourne, pp 73–74

Hall T, Quintner J 1996 Responses to mechanical stimulation of the upper limb in painful cervical radiculopathy. Australian Journal of Physiotherapy 42(4): 277–285

Hall T, Zusman M, Elvey RL 1995 Manually detected impediments during the straight leg raise test. In: Jull G (ed) Clinical Solutions; Ninth Biennial Conference, Manipulative Physiotherapists Association of Australia. Gold Coast, Queensland, pp 48–53

Hall T, Zusman M, Elvey RL 1998 Adverse mechanical tension in the nervous system? Analysis of straight leg raise. Manual Therapy 3(3): 140–146

Henderson CM, Hennessy R, Shuey H 1983 Posterior lateral foraminotomy for an exclusive operative technique for cervical radiculopathy: a review of 846 consecutively operated cases. Journal of Neurosurgery 13: 504–512

Howe JF, Loeser JD, Calvin WH 1977 Mechanosensitivity of dorsal root ganglia and chronically injured axons: a physiological basis for the radicular pain of nerve root compression. Pain 3: 25–41

Hromada J 1963 On the nerve supply of the connective tissue of some peripheral nervous system components. Acta Anatomica 55: 343–351

Kleinrensink G, Stoeckart R, Vleeming A, Sjniders C, Mulder P 1995 Mechanical tension in the median nerve. The effects of joint positions. Clinical Biomechanics 10(5): 240–244

Kleynhans AM, Terrett AGJ 1986 The prevention of complications from spinal manipulative therapy. In: Glasgow EF Twomey LT (eds) Aspects of Manipulative Therapy. Churchill Livingstone, Melbourne, pp 171–174

Kuslich SD, Ulstrom CL, Cam JM 1991 The tissue origin of low back pain and sciatica: a report of pain responses to tissue stimulation during operations on the lumbar spine using local anaesthesia. Orthopaedic Clinics of North America 22(2): 181–187

Kwan MK, Wall EJ, Massie J, Garfin SR 1992 Strain, stress and stretch of peripheral nerve: rabbit experiments in vitro and in vivo. Acta Orthopaedica Scandinavica 63(3): 267–272

Laird JMA, Bennett GJ 1993 An electrophysiological study of dorsal horn neurons in the spinal cord of rats with an experimental peripheral neuropathy. Journal of Neurophysiology 69(6): 2072–2085

Lewis J, Ramot R, Green A 1998 Changes in mechanical tension in the median nerve: possible implications for the upper limb tension test. Physiotherapy 84(6): 254–261

Louis R 1981 Vertebroradicular and vertebromedullar dynamics. Anatomia Clinica 3: 1–11

Lundborg G, Rydevik B 1973 Effects of stretching the tibial nerve of the rabbit: a preliminary study of the intraneural

circulation and the barrier function of the perineurium. Journal of Bone and Joint Surgery 55B(2): 390–401

Madison Taylor J 1909 Treatment of occupation neuroses and neuritis in the arms. Journal of the American Medical Association 53(3): 198–200

Maitland GD 1991 Peripheral Manipulation, 3rd edn. Butterworth-Heinemann, London

Marshall J 1883 Nerve stretching for the relief or cure of pain. British Medical Journal 15: 1173–1179

McLellan DL, Swash M 1976 Longitudinal sliding of the median nerve during movements of the upper limb. Journal of Neurology, Neurosurgery, and Psychiatry 39: 566–570

O'Connell JEA 1951 Protrusions of the lumbar intervertebral disc. Journal of Bone and Joint Surgery 33B(1): 8–17

Ogato K, Naito M 1986 Blood flow of peripheral nerves: effects of dissection, stretching and compression. Journal of Hand Surgery 11: 10

Olmarker K, Rydevik B 1991 Pathophysiology of sciatica. Orthopaedic Clinics of North America 22(2): 223–234

Quintner J 1998 Peripheral neuropathic pain: a rediscovered clinical entity. In: Annual General Meeting of the Australian Pain Society. Australian Pain Society, Hobart

Rankine J, Fortune D, Hutchinson C, Hughes D, Main C 1998 Pain drawings in the assessment of nerve root compression: a comparative study with lumbar spine magnetic resonance imaging. Spine 23(15): 1668–1676

Reid S 1987 The Measurement of Tension Changes in the Brachial Plexus. In: Dalziel BA, Snowsill JC (Eds) Proceedings of the Fifth Biennial Conference of the Manipulative Therapists Association of Australia. Melbourne, pp 79–90

Sugimoto T, Bennett GJ, Kajanda KC 1989 Strychnine-induced transynaptic degeneration of dorsal horn neurons in rats with an experimental neuropathy. Neuroscience Letters 98: 139–143

Sugiura K, Yoshida T, Katoh S, Mimatsu M 1979 A study on tension signs in lumbar disc hernia. International Orthopaedics 3: 225–228

Sunderland S 1990 The anatomy and physiology of nerve injury. Muscle and Nerve 13: 771–784

Thomas PK, Berthold C-H, Ochoa J 1993 Microscopic anatomy of the peripheral nervous system. In: Dyck PJ, Thomas PK (eds) Peripheral Neuropathy, 3rd edn, Vol. 1. WB Saunders, Philadelphia, pp 28–91

Vicenzino B, Collins D, Wright A 1995 Cervical mobilisation: immediate effects on neural tissue mobility, mechanical hyperalgesia and pain free grip strength in lateral epicondylitis. In: Jull G (ed) Clinical Solutions. Manipulative Physiotherapists Association of Australia, Gold Coast, Queensland, pp 155–156

Wiesel SW, Tsourmas N, Feffer HL, Citrin CM, Patronas N 1984 A study of computer-assisted tomography: 1. The incidence of positive CAT scans in an asymptomatic group of patients. Spine 9: 549–551

Woolf CJ 1991 Generation of acute pain: central mechanisms. British Medical Bulletin 47: 523–533

Yuan Q, Dougherty L, Margulies S 1998 In vivo human cervical spinal cord deformation and displacement in flexion. Spine 23(15): 1677–1683

Zochodne D 1993 Epineural peptides: A role in neuropathic pain. Canadian Journal of Neurological Sciences 20: 69–72

Zusman M 1998 Irritability. Manual Therapy 3(4): 195–202

POSTSCRIPT

The evaluation and physical management of neural tissue pain disorders continues to be refined (Butler 2000; Gifford 2001; Hall & Elvey 2001) and there is evidence that this approach is increasingly being utilized by physiotherapists in their clinical practice (Milidonis et al 1997). Encouragingly, there has also been continued research into the scientific validation of neural examination techniques (Coppieters et al 2001a). However, outcome studies remain limited to small samples (Allison et al 2002; Cowell & Phillips 2002) and, unfortunately, there is still limited acceptance of this approach in the medical literature, wider medical community and even in some mainstream physiotherapy journals where the concept has been the subject of some justified criticism (Di Fabio 2001a, b). This may be because of a failure for the research to be presented in peer reviewed journals that are readily available to and read by, those who have criticized the concept (Coppieters 2001b). More needs to be done to bring this increasing body of research to the attention of a wider audience.

In the management of neuromusculoskeletal disorders, identification of specific diagnostic subgroups should be of particular importance. Patients classified into distinct subgroups, having common, readily identifiable disorders, can then be prescribed appropriate treatment strategies. It appears logical that specific treatment designed for a distinct category of pain will have a more favourable outcome when compared to a generic approach, and the literature appears to support this (O'Sullivan et al 1997; Jull & Moore 2000).

For most manual therapists a significant aspect of the examination procedure is to identify any possible physical cause, or the structural origin, of the patient's pain. It has been accepted that a primary lesion in the peripheral nervous system can cause persistent pain and other sensations (Quintner & Bove 2001) and that neural tissue syndromes are a significant subgroup of pain disorders (Spitzer 1987; Abenhaim et al 2000), but they can be difficult to define. As mentioned above, by far the most common clinical presentation, with regard to pain of nerve trunk origin, is that associated with increased neural tissue mechanosensitivity. Unfortunately this diagnosis can only be made on clinical grounds, and this may lead, in part, to difficulties with wider acceptance of the concept in the medical community. At present there is no gold standard laboratory test with which one can compare and corroborate the clinical evidence. There appears to have been some improvements in medical imaging to identify dysfunctional neural structures, particularly with the use of magnetic resonance neurography and diagnostic ultrasound, which shows further hope for the future (Maravilla & Bowen 1998; Dilley et al 2001; Greening et al 2001; Loewe 2001). With further developments in these imaging tools the sensitivity and specificity of clinical examination procedures can be identified. This will enable the true incidence of adverse neural tissue mechanosensitivity to be identified and hence appropriate management strategies provided.

REFERENCES

Abenhaim L, Rossignol M, Valat J, Nordin M, Avouac B, Blotman F, Charlot J, Dreiser RL, Legrand E, Rozenberg S, Vautravers P 2000 The role of activity in the therapeutic management of back pain: Report of the international Paris task force on back pain. Spine 25(4): 1S–33S

Allison GT, Nagy BM, Hall TM 2002 A randomised clinical trial of manual therapy for cervico-brachial pain syndrome — a pilot study. Manual Therapy. 7(2): 95–102

Butler D 2000 The sensitive nervous system. NoiGroup Publications, Adelaide

Coppieters MW, Stappaerts KH, Everaert DG, Staes FF 2001a Addition of test components during neurodynamic testing: Effect of range of motion and sensory responses. Journal of Orthopaedic and Sports Physical Therapy 31(5); 226–237

Coppieters MW, Butler DS 2001b In defence of neural mobilisation. Journal of Orthopaedic and Sports Physical Therapy. 31(9): 520–521

Cowell IM, Phillips DR 2002 Effectiveness of manipulative physiotherapy for the treatment of a neurogenic cervicobrachial pain syndrome: A single case study — experimental design. Manual Therapy 7(1): 31–38

Di Fabio RP 2001a Neural mobilisation: The impossible. Journal of Orthopaedic and Sports Physical Therapy 31(5): 224–225

Di Fabio RP 2001b Neural tension, neurodynamics, and neural mobilisation. Journal of Orthopaedic and Sports Physical Therapy 31(9): 522–522

Dilley A, Greening J, Lynn B, Leary R, Morris V 2001 The use of cross-correlation analysis between high-frequency ultrasound images to measure longitudinal median nerve movement. Ultrasound in Medicine and Biology. 27(9): 1211–1218

Gifford L 2001 Acute low cervical nerve root conditions: symptom presentations and pathobiological reasoning. Manual Therapy 6(2); 106–115

Greening J, Lynn B, Leary R, Warren L, O'Higgins P, Hall-Craggs M 2001 The use of ultrasound imaging to demonstrate reduced movement of the median nerve during wrist flexion in patients with non-specific arm pain. Journal of Hand Surgery 26(5): 401–406

Hall T, Elvey R 2001 Evaluation and treatment of neural tissue pain disorders. In: Donatelli RA, Wooden MJ (eds) Orthopaedic Physical Therapy, 3rd edn. Churchill Livingstone, Philadelphia

Jull G, Moore A 2000 Evidence based practices: The need for research directions. Manual Therapy 5(3): 131

Loewe J 2001 Ultrasonography and magnetic resonance imaging of abnormalities of the peripheral nerves. Canadian Association Radiology Journal 52(5): 292–301

Maravilla KR, Bowen BC 1998 Imaging of the peripheral nervous system: Evaluation of peripheral neuropathy and plexopathy. American Journal of Neuroradiology 19:1011–1023

Milidonis MK, Ritter RC, Sweeney MA, Godges JJ, Knapp J, Antonucci E 1997 Practical analysis survey: revalidation of advanced clinical practice in orthopaedic physical therapy. Journal of Orthopaedic and Sports Physical Therapy 25: 163–170

O'Sullivan P, Twomey, L, Allison G 1997 Evaluation of specific stabilising exercises in the treatment of chronic low back pain with radiologic diagnosis of spondylosis or spondylolisthesis. Spine 22: 2959–2967

Quintner JL, Bove G 2001 From neuralgia to peripheral neuropathic pain: Evolution of a concept. Regional Anaesthesia and Pain Medicine 26: 368–372

Spitzer W 1987 Scientific approach to the assessment and management of activity-related spinal disorders: a monograph for clinicians, report of the Quebec Task Force on spinal disorders. Spine 12: 9–54

7

Patient positioning and spinal locking for lumbar spine rotation manipulation

P. Gibbons   P. Tehan
School of Health Sciences, Faculty of Human
Development, Victoria University, Melbourne,
Australia

High-velocity low-amplitude (HVLA) thrust techniques are widely used by many manual therapists to treat low back pain. There is increasing evidence that spinal manipulation produces positive patient outcomes for acute low back pain. HVLA thrust techniques are associated with an audible release in the form of a pop or cracking sound that is widely accepted to represent cavitation of a spinal zygapophyseal joint. This audible release distinguishes these techniques from other manual therapy interventions. When using long lever HVLA thrust techniques spinal locking is necessary to localize forces and achieve cavitation at a specific vertebral segment. A critical factor in applying lumbar spine manipulation with minimal force is patient positioning and spinal locking. A knowledge of coupled movements of the lumbar spine aids an understanding of the patient positioning required to achieve spinal locking consistent with maximal patient comfort and cooperation. Excessive rotation can result in pain, patient resistance and failed technique. This article presents a model of patient positioning for the lumbar spine that minimizes excessive use of rotation to achieve spinal locking prior to the application of the thrust.
Manual Therapy (2001) **6(3)**, 130–138

INTRODUCTION

HVLA thrust techniques of the spine are widely used by many manual therapists. HVLA thrust techniques are also known by a number of names, e.g. manipulation, adjustment, high velocity thrust, manipulation with impulse, grade V mobilization. Despite the different nomenclature, the common feature in techniques of this type is that they achieve a pop or cracking sound within synovial joints. The cause of this audible release (pop or crack) is open to some speculation but is widely accepted to represent cavitation of a spinal zygapophyseal joint (Brodeur 1995). The audible release distinguishes HVLA thrust techniques from other manual therapy interventions.

Spinal locking is necessary for long lever HVLA thrust techniques to localize forces and achieve cavitation at a specific vertebral segment (Stoddard 1972; Downing 1985; Beal 1989; Kappler 1989; Nyberg 1993; Greenman 1996; Hartman 1997). Short lever HVLA thrust techniques do not require locking of adjacent spinal segments. Locking can be achieved by either facet apposition or the utilization of ligamentous myofascial tension or a combination of both (Stoddard 1972; Downing 1985; Beal 1989; Nyberg 1993; Greenman 1996; Hartman 1997). The principle used in these approaches is to position the spine in such a way that leverage is localized to one joint without undue strain being placed upon adjacent spinal segments. The principle of facet apposition locking is to apply leverages to the spine that cause the facet joints of uninvolved segments to be apposed and consequently locked. To achieve locking by facet apposition the spine is placed in a position opposite to that of normal coupling behaviour. The vertebral segment at which the therapist wishes to produce cavitation should never be locked.

Lumbar spine rotation manipulation is commonly used in the treatment of low back pain with increasing evidence of efficacy for acute low back pain (Waddell 1998). To maximize positive outcomes from HVLA thrust techniques it is essential that their use be preceded by a thorough patient history and physical assessment and that due attention has been given to clinical indications and contraindications. The use of HVLA thrust techniques must be considered within the context of a comprehensive patient management plan, which may include the application of other manual therapy and adjunctive techniques.

Patient comfort is a prerequisite for successful HVLA thrust technique. Excessive lumbar spine rotation may exacerbate back pain. This results in loss of patient cooperation, patient resistance and failed technique. Procedures to minimize lumbar spine rotation leverage can reduce patient discomfort and enhance technique delivery. This article will review the 'pop' or 'crack' phenomena, clinical indications and contraindications associated with manipulation and focus upon a model of patient positioning and spinal locking that can assist in achieving the safe and effective application of HVLA thrust techniques in the lumbar spine. This model minimizes the amount of the rotation used in the build-up of leverages and spinal locking and enhances patient comfort and cooperation.

CAVITATION ASSOCIATED WITH HIGH-VELOCITY LOW-AMPLITUDE THRUST TECHNIQUES

Research involving the metacarpophalangeal joint indicates that the audible release is generated by a cavitation mechanism resulting from a drop in the internal joint pressure (Roston & Haines 1947; Unsworth et al 1972; Meal & Scott 1986; Watson & Mollan 1990). Following cavitation, there is an increase in the size of the joint space and gas is found within that space (Roston & Haines 1947; Unsworth et al 1972; Meal & Scott 1986; Mierau et al 1988; Watson & Mollan 1990). The gas bubble has been described as 80% carbon dioxide (Unsworth et al 1972), or having the density of nitrogen (Greenman 1996). The gas bubble remains within the joint for between 15 and 30 min (Roston & Haines 1947; Unsworth et al 1972; Meal & Scott 1986; Mierau et al 1988; Greenman 1996), which is consistent with the time taken for the gas to be re-absorbed into the synovial fluid (Unsworth et al 1972).

An increased range of joint motion immediately following cavitation has been demonstrated (Mierau et al 1988; Surkitt et al 2000) with a number of studies reporting that thrust techniques are associated with a temporary increase in the range of spinal motion (Howe et al 1983; Nansel et al 1989; Nansel et al 1990; Cassidy et al 1992; Nansel et al 1992; Nilsson et al 1996; Surkitt et al 2000). Longer-term effects of HVLA thrust techniques have also been reported (Nordemar & Thorner 1981; Stodolny & Chmielewski 1989) and it is postulated these may be due to reflex mechanisms that either directly cause muscle relaxation or inhibit pain (Brodeur 1995).

Repeated 'cracking' or 'popping' associated with cavitation of the joints of the hand has not been shown to be linked with an increased incidence of degenerative change (Swezey & Swezey 1975; Castellanos & Axelrod 1990).

CLINICAL INDICATIONS FOR THE USE OF HIGH-VELOCITY LOW-AMPLITUDE THRUST TECHNIQUES

Within manual therapy there is an on-going debate about the specific effects of HVLA thrust techniques compared with other manual therapy interventions. If one accepts that cavitation is usually only associated with HVLA thrust techniques, an argument might be made that there are specific effects relating to thrust techniques that may not be evoked by other manual interventions. Various authors have described specific indications for the use of HVLA thrust techniques (Table 7.1).

It is recognized that the use of HVLA thrust techniques must be considered within the context of a comprehensive patient management plan, which includes the application of other manual techniques and adjunctive therapies. After considering safety issues and excluding contraindications, a number of treatment models use the diagnosis of somatic dysfunction as the basis for the selection of HVLA thrust techniques (DiGiovanna 1991; Bourdillon et al 1992; Kuchera & Kuchera 1994; Mitchell 1995; Greenman 1996; Kappler 1997).

DIAGNOSIS OF SOMATIC DYSFUNCTION

The accepted definition for Somatic Dysfunction is as follows.

Somatic dysfunction is an impaired or altered function of related components of the somatic (body framework) system: skeletal, arthrodial and myofascial structures, and related vascular, lymphatic, and neural elements (Glossary Review Committee of the Educational Council on Osteopathic Principles 1993).

Specific criteria in identifying areas of dysfunction have been developed. The diagnosis of somatic dysfunction is made on the basis of several positive findings and is identified by the A-R-T-T of diagnosis (Table 7.2).

Table 7.1. Specific indications for HVLA thrust techniques as listed by various authors.

Indication	Author(s)
Hypomobility	Kenna & Murtagh 1989 Bruckner & Khan 1994
Motion restriction	Lewit 1991 Maigne 1996 Brodeur 1995
Joint fixation	Eder & Tilscher 1990 Sammut & Searle-Barnes 1998
Acute joint locking	Gainsbury 1985 Bruckner & Khan 1994 Zusman 1994
Motion loss with somatic dysfunction	Kuchera & Kuchera 1992 Kappler 1997
Somatic dysfunction	Bourdillon et al 1992 Kimberly 1992 Greenman 1996
Restore bony alignment	Nyberg & Basmajian 1993 Maigne 1996
Meniscoid entrapment	Kenna & Murtagh 1989 Lewit 1991 Bogduk & Twomey 1991 Maigne 1996 Sammut & Searle-Barnes 1998
Adhesions	Stoddard 1969
Displaced disc fragment	Cyriax 1975
Pain modulation	Hoehler et al 1981 Terrett & Vernon 1984 Kenna & Murtagh 1989 Zusman 1994 Brodeur 1995
Reflex relaxation of muscles	Fisk 1979 Neumann 1989 Kenna & Murtagh 1989 Kuchera & Kuchera 1994 Brodeur 1995
Reprogramming of the central nervous system	Bourdillon et al 1992
Release of endorphins	Vernon et al 1986

- A relates to asymmetry
DiGiovanna (1991) links the criteria of asymmetry to a positional focus stating that the 'position of the vertebra or other bone is asymmetrical'. Greenman (1996) broadens the concept of asymmetry by including functional in addition to structural asymmetry.
- R relates to range of motion
Alteration in range of motion can apply to a single joint, several joints or a region of the musculoskeletal system. The abnormality may be either restricted or increased mobility and includes assessment of quality of movement and 'end feel'.
- T relates to tissue texture changes
The identification of tissue texture change is important in the diagnosis of somatic dysfunction. Palpable changes may be noted in superficial, intermediate and deep tissues. It is important for clinicians to recognize normal from abnormal.
- T relates to tissue tenderness
Undue tissue tenderness may be evident. Pain provocation and reproduction of familiar symptoms are often used to localize somatic dysfunction.

Somatic dysfunction is further classified as acute (Table 7.3) or chronic (Table 7.4).

It could be postulated that reflex changes resulting from the use of HVLA thrust techniques can produce more immediate benefits in cases with acute somatic dysfunction while spinal dysfunction of a more chronic nature would require an approach where the use of HVLA thrust techniques is accompanied by other manual therapy and rehabilitative approaches.

CONTRAINDICATIONS FOR THE USE OF LUMBAR SPINE HIGH-VELOCITY LOW-AMPLITUDE THRUST TECHNIQUES

There are risks and benefits associated with any therapeutic intervention. HVLA techniques are distinguished from other manual therapy techniques because the practitioner applies a rapid thrust or impulse. Thrust or impulse techniques

Table 7.2 Diagnosis of somatic dysfunction.

- A relates to asymmetry
- R relates to range of motion
- T relates to tissue texture changes
- T relates to tissue tenderness

Table 7.3 Acute somatic dysfunction of zygapophyseal joints. Key positive findings for the use of HVLA thrust techniques.

A. Asymmetry of adjacent vertebra at involved level	May or may not be present
R. Segmental restricted mobility	Present
End feel consistent with segmental hypertonia	Present
T. Palpable changes from normal texture in deep segmental soft tissues	Present
Palpable changes in intermediate and superficial segmental soft tissues	May or may not be present
T. Undue tenderness at involved segment	Present
Pain provocation	May or may not be present

Table 7.4 Chronic somatic dysfunction of zygapophyseal joints. Key positive findings for the use of HVLA thrust techniques.

A. Asymmetry of adjacent vertebra at involved level	May or may not be present
R. Segmental restricted mobility	Present
End feel consistent with soft tissue contracture	Present
T. Palpable changes from normal texture in deep segmental soft tissues	Present
Palpable changes in intermediate soft tissues	Present
Palpable changes in superficial soft tissues	May or may not be present
T. Undue tenderness at involved segment	May or may not be present
Pain provocation	May or may not be present

are considered to be potentially more dangerous than non-impulse mobilization. Most published literature relating to the incidence of injury resulting from manipulative techniques focuses upon serious sequelae resulting from cervical spine manipulation. Adverse reactions have been reported by patients receiving lumbar spine manipulation but this needs to be contrasted with the national clinical guidelines on acute and recurrent low back pain which indicate that the risks of manipulation for low back pain are very low provided patients are assessed and selected for treatment by trained practitioners (RCGP 1996; Waddell 1998). Transient side-effects resulting from manipulative treatment may be more common than one might expect and may remain unreported by patients unless information is explicitly requested. A study of common side-effects resulting from chiropractic treatment indicated that 55% of patients reported at least one unpleasant reaction during a course of treatment (Senstad et al 1997). These side-effects generally disappear within 24 hours.

Whenever a practitioner applies a therapeutic intervention due consideration must be given to the risk–benefit ratio. The benefit to the patient must outweigh any potential risk associated with the intervention. Traditionally contraindications have been classified as absolute and relative (Gibbons & Tehan 2000). Absolute contraindications preclude the use of HVLA thrust techniques. Some of the circumstances listed under relative contraindications may become absolute contraindications dependent upon factors such as the skill, experience and training of the practitioner, the type of technique selected, the amount of leverage and force used and the age, general health and physique of the patient. Safety and patient comfort are critically linked to the appropriate use of spinal positioning and locking prior to the application of the thrust.

ABSOLUTE CONTRAINDICATIONS

Bone

Any pathology that has led to significant bone weakening:

- Tumour, e.g. metastatic deposits

- Infection, e.g. tuberculosis
- Metabolic, e.g. osteomalacia
- Congenital, e.g. dysplasias
- Iatrogenic, e.g. long-term corticosteroid medication
- Inflammatory, e.g. severe rheumatoid arthritis
- Traumatic, e.g. fracture.

Neurological

- Cord compression
- Cauda equina compression
- Nerve root compression with increasing neurological deficit.

Vascular

- Aortic aneurysm
- Bleeding into joints, e.g. severe haemophilia.

Lack of a diagnosis

Lack of patient consent

Patient positioning cannot be achieved because of pain or resistance.

RELATIVE CONTRAINDICATIONS

Certain categories of patients have an increased potential for adverse reactions following the application of an HVLA thrust technique. Special consideration should be given prior to the use of HVLA thrust techniques in the following circumstances:

- Adverse reactions to previous manual therapy
- Disc herniation or prolapse
- Inflammatory arthritides
- Pregnancy
- Spondylolysis
- Spondylolisthesis
- Osteoporosis
- Anticoagulant or long-term corticosteroid use
- Advanced degenerative joint disease and spondylosis

- Psychological dependence upon HVLA thrust technique
- Ligamentous laxity
- Arterial calcification.

The above list is not intended to cover all possible clinical situations. Patients who have pathology may also have coincidental spinal pain and discomfort arising from mechanical dysfunction that may benefit from manipulative treatment.

The use of manipulation techniques under general anaesthesia for low back pain is associated with an increased risk of serious neurological damage (Haldeman & Rubinstein 1992). There is no evidence that this approach for the treatment of low back pain is effective (CSAG 1994).

PATIENT POSITIONING AND SPINAL LOCKING

A critical factor in achieving lumbar spine cavitation with minimal force is patient positioning and spinal locking. The principle of facet apposition locking is to apply leverages to the spine that cause the facet joints of uninvolved segments to be apposed and consequently locked. To achieve locking by facet apposition the spine is placed in a position opposite to that of normal coupling behaviour. The vertebral segment at which you wish to produce cavitation should never be locked.

The osteopathic profession developed a nomenclature to classify spinal motion based upon the coupling of sidebending and rotation movements. This coupling behaviour will vary dependent upon spinal positioning.

- Type 1 Movement — Sidebending and rotation occur in opposite directions. (Fig. 7.1)
- Type 2 Movement — Sidebending and rotation occur in the same direction. (Fig. 7.2)

LUMBAR SPINE

In broad terms, facet apposition locking uses combinations of sidebending and rotation. An under-

standing of the biomechanics associated with coupled movements of the lumbar spine in different postures allows the practitioner to decide on optimal pre-thrust positioning. Primary and secondary joint leverages are required to facilitate effective localization of forces to a specific segment of the spine prior to application of the thrust (Gibbons & Tehan 2000).

Evidence supports the view that spinal posture and positioning alters coupling behaviour (Fryette 1954; Panjabi et al 1989; Vicenzino & Twomey 1993). Coupling behaviour is different in the flexed position when compared to the neutral/extended position. This has implications for joint locking in the lumbar spine.

There is evidence to support the view that, in

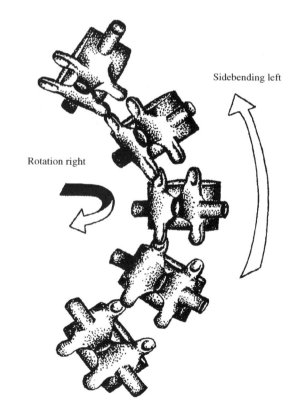

Sidebending left

Rotation right

Figure 7.1 Type 1 movement — sidebending and rotation occur to opposite sides. (Reproduced with permission from Gibbons and Tehan 1998, Muscle energy concepts and coupled motion of the spine. Manual Therapy 3(2): 95–101.

the flexed position, the coupling of sidebending and rotation is to the same side (Fryette 1954; Stoddard 1969; Panjabi et al 1989; Vicenzino & Twomey 1993) whereas, in the neutral/extended position, the coupling of sidebending and rotation occurs to opposite sides (Fryette 1954; Stoddard 1969; Vicenzino & Twomey 1993).

The following model for patient positioning and spinal locking is a safe and effective starting point upon which practitioners can build basic and then more refined technical skills in the use of lumbar spine HVLA thrust techniques (Table 7.5). Practitioners using this model can minimize the degree of rotation required to achieve spinal locking in both the neutral/extension and flexed positions.

NEUTRAL/EXTENSION POSITIONING

The patient's lumbar and thoracic spine is positioned in a neutral/extended posture (Fig 7.3). Using the model outlined, the normal coupling behaviour of sidebending and rotation in the neutral/extension position is Type 1 motion. Facet apposition locking will be achieved by introducing a Type 2 movement, i.e. sidebending and rotation to the same side.

Trunk rotation to the right is introduced by gently pushing the patient's upper shoulder away from the operator. Rotation and sidebending to the same side achieves facet apposition locking in the neutral or extended position, in this instance with sidebending and rotation to the right (Fig. 7.4).

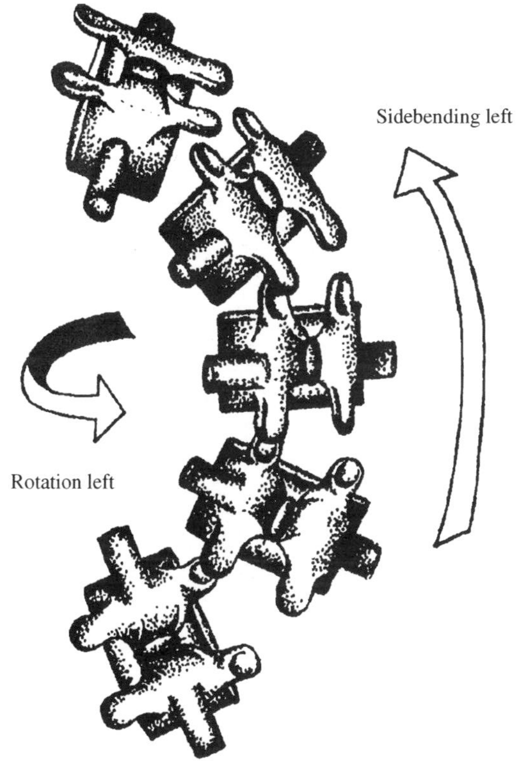

Sidebending left

Rotation left

Figure 7.2 Type 2 movement — sidebending and rotation occur to the same side. (Reproduced with permission from Gibbons and Tehan 1998, Muscle energy concepts and coupled motion of the spine. Manual Therapy 3(2): 95–101.

Table 7.5 Patient positioning and spinal locking.

Position of spine L1–L5	Coupled motion	Facet apposition locking
Neutral/extension	Type 1 motion	Type 2 locking with sidebending and rotation to the same side
NeuFlexion	Type 2 motion	Type 1 locking with sidebending and rotation to the opposite side

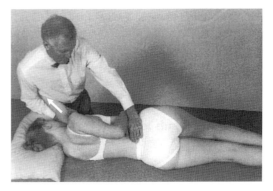

Figure 7.3 Neutral/extension positioning. (Reproduced with permission from Gibbons and Tehan 2000, Manipulation of the Spine, Thorax and Pelvis: An Osteopathic Perspective. Churchill Livingstone, Edinburgh (Fig. B3.3.3, p214.))

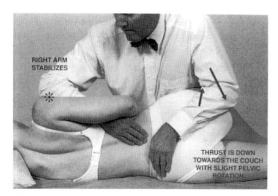

Figure 7.4 Neutral/extension positioning. Type 2 locking — rotation and sidebending to the same side, i.e. sidebending right and rotation right. (Reproduced with permission from Gibbons and Tehan 2000, Manipulation of the Spine, Thorax and Pelvis: An Osteopathic Perspective. Churchill Livingstone, Edinburgh (Fig. B3.3.5, p216.))

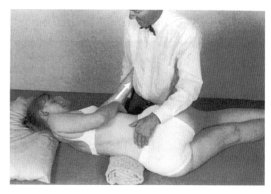

Figure 7.5 Flexion positioning. (Reproduced with permission from Gibbons and Tehan 2000, Manipulation of the Spine, Thorax and Pelvis: An Osteopathic Perspective. Churchill Livingstone, Edinburgh (Fig. B3.4.1, p220.))

FLEXION POSITIONING

The patient's lumbar and thoracic spinal regions are positioned in a flexed posture (Fig. 7.5). The normal coupling behaviour of sidebending and rotation in the flexed position is Type 2 motion. Facet apposition locking will be achieved by introducing a Type 1 movement, i.e. sidebending and rotation to opposite sides.

To achieve facet apposition locking of the spine, in the flexed posture, the trunk must be rotated and sidebent to opposite sides. The operator introduces trunk sidebending to the left by placing a rolled towel or pillow under the patient's thoracolumbar spine.

Trunk rotation to the right is introduced by gently pushing the patient's upper shoulder away from the operator (Fig. 7.6).

The principles of patient positioning and spinal locking are also valid with HVLA thrust techniques applied in the sitting position, e.g. neutral/extension positioning (Figs 7.7 & 7.8).

While rotation and sidebending are the principal leverages used, the more experienced manipulator may include elements of flexion, extension, translation, compression or traction to enhance localization of forces and patient comfort.

The model described identifies two distinct components for safe and effective HVLA thrust techniques in the lumbar spine.

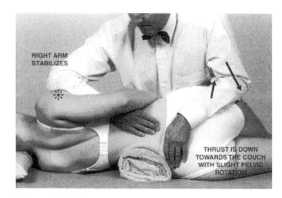

Figure 7.6 Flexion positioning. Type 1 locking — rotation and sidebending to opposite sides, i.e. sidebending left and rotation right. (Reproduced with permission from Gibbons and Tehan 2000, Manipulation of the Spine, Thorax and Pelvis: An Osteopathic Perspective. Churchill Livingstone, Edinburgh (Fig. B3.4.3, p222.))

1. Patient position and spinal locking
2. Direction of manipulation.

Once facet apposition locking has been achieved in either the flexed or neutral extended position the practitioner can, if appropriate, thrust in directions other than that for rotation.

Many factors such as facet tropism, vertebral level, intervertebral disc height, back pain and spinal position can affect coupling behaviour and there will be occasions when the model outlined needs to be modified to suit an individual

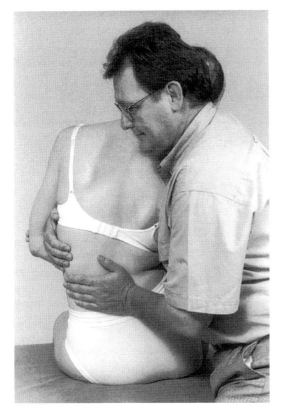

Figure 7.7 Neutral/extension positioning. Trunk sidebending to the right. (Reproduced with permission from Gibbons and Tehan 2000, Manipulation of the Spine, Thorax and Pelvis: An Osteopathic Perspective. Churchill Livingstone, Edinburgh (Fig. B3.5.2, p227.))

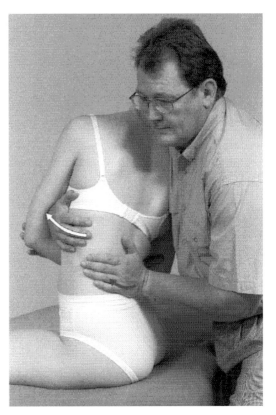

Figure 7.8 Neutral/extension positioning. Type 2 locking — rotation and sidebending to the same side, i.e. sidebending right and rotation right. (Reproduced with permission from Gibbons and Tehan 2000, Manipulation of the Spine, Thorax and Pelvis: An Osteopathic Perspective. Churchill Livingstone, Edinburgh (Fig. B3.5.3, p228.))

patient. In such circumstances the operator will need to adjust patient positioning to facilitate effective localization of forces. To achieve this, the operator must develop the palpatory skills necessary to sense appropriate pre-thrust tension and leverage prior to delivering the HVLA thrust.

TECHNIQUE FAILURE AND ANALYSIS

Many clinicians achieve high levels of expertise and competence in the use of HVLA thrust techniques. The nature of manipulative practice is such that there are many different ways to achieve joint cavitation at any given spinal segment.

Inability to achieve cavitation with minimal force may arise for a number of different reasons and can be evaluated under three broad headings (Gibbons & Tehan 2000):

1. General technique analysis
2. Practitioner and patient variables
3. Physical and biomechanical modifying factors.

GENERAL TECHNIQUE ANALYSIS

Incorrect selection of technique

- Practitioner too small and patient too large
- Practitioner has physical limitations that limit effective delivery of technique

- Practitioner inexperience with selected technique
- Inability to position patient due to pain, discomfort or physical limitations
- Patient apprehension.

Inadequate localization of forces

- Incorrect application of primary leverage
- Incorrect application of secondary leverages
- Inability to recognize appropriate pre-thrust tension.

Ineffective thrust

- Loss of contact point pressure
- Poor bimanual coordination
- Incorrect direction of thrust
- Inadequate velocity of thrust
- Incorrect amplitude of thrust
- Incorrect force of thrust
- Loss of leverage at time of thrust
- Poor practitioner posture
- Practitioner not relaxed
- Failure to arrest thrust and leverage adequately
- Lack of practitioner confidence.

PRACTITIONER AND PATIENT VARIABLES

Common faults

- Patient not comfortably positioned
- Patient not relaxed
- Rough patient handling
- Rushing technique
- Poor practitioner posture
- Lack of practitioner confidence.

PHYSICAL AND BIOMECHANICAL MODIFYING FACTORS

Common faults

- Insufficient primary leverage

- Too much secondary leverage — locking often results from the over-application of secondary leverages; this can occur during the build up of leverages or at the point of thrust
- Loss of contact point pressure immediately pre-thrust
- Not identifying appropriate pre-thrust tension and leverage prior to thrust — if in doubt about optimum pre-thrust tension attempt multiple light thrusts
- Incorrect direction of thrust — the thrust should be in a direction that is appropriate and comfortable for the patient; multiple light thrusts can assist in the identification of the appropriate direction of thrust
- Insufficient velocity of thrust
- Too much amplitude — this is often a consequence of too much force and/or poor control
- Too much force
- Insufficient arrest of technique — this is often a consequence of poor practitioner coordination and control.

CONCLUSION

Safe and effective HVLA thrust techniques require that the patient has been thoroughly assessed, contraindications have been excluded and informed consent has been obtained. The patient should be in a comfortable position and spinal locking should be pain free before the thrust is applied. Successful manipulation of the lumbar spine using HVLA thrust techniques demands precision in the application of the biomechanical forces involved. Excessive lumbar spine rotation can result in pain, patient resistance and failed technique. This article has focused on a model of patient positioning that minimizes excessive use of lumbar spine rotation and maximizes patient comfort to achieve spinal locking prior to the application of the thrust.

REFERENCES

Beal MC 1989 Teaching of basic principles of osteopathic manipulative techniques. In: Beal MC (ed) The principles of Palpatory Diagnosis and Manipulative Technique. American Academy of Osteopathy, Newark

Bogduk N, Twomey L 1991 Clinical Anatomy of the Lumbar Spine, 2nd edn. Churchill Livingstone, Melbourne

Bourdillon J, Day E, Bookhout M 1992 Spinal Manipulation, 5th edn. Butterworth–Heinemann, Oxford

Brodeur R 1995 The audible release associated with joint manipulation. Journal of Manipulative and Physiological Therapeutics 18(3): 155–164

Bruckner P, Khan K 1994 Clinical Sports Medicine. McGraw-Hill, Sydney

Cassidy JD, Quon J A, Lafrance L J, Yong-Ying K 1992 The effect of manipulation on pain and range of motion in the cervical spine: A pilot study. Journal of Manipulative and Physiological Therapeutics 15(8): 495–500

Castellanos J, Axelrod D 1990 Effect of habitual knuckle cracking on hand function. Annals of Rheumatic Disease 49: 308–309

CSAG 1994 Back pain. Clinical Standards Advisory Group Report. HMSO, London

Cyriax J 1975 Textbook of Orthopaedic Medicine, Vol 1, 6th edn. Balliere Tindall, London

DiGiovanna E 1991 Somatic dysfunction. In: DiGiovanna E, Schiowitz S (eds) An Osteopathic Approach to Diagnosis and Treatment. Lippincott, Philadelphia

Downing CH 1985 Principles and Practice of Osteopathy. Tamor Pierston Publishers, London

Eder M, Tilscher H 1990 Chiropractic Therapy. Diagnosis and Treatment. Aspen Publications, Maryland

Fisk J 1979 A contolled trial of manipulation in a selected group of patients with low back pain favouring one side. New Zealand Medical Journal 90(645): 288–291

Fryette H 1954 (Re-print 1990) Principles of Osteopathic Technic. American Academy of Osteopathy, Newark

Gainsbury J 1985 High-velocity thrust and pathophysiology of segmental dysfunction. In: Glasgow E, Twomey L, Sculle E, Kleynhans A, Idczak R (eds) Aspects of Manipulative Therapy, 2nd edn. Churchill Livingstone, Melbourne

Gibbons P, Tehan P 2000 Manipulation of the Spine, Thorax and Pelvis: An Osteopathic Perspective. Churchill Livingstone, Edinburgh

Glossary Review Committee of the Educational Council on Osteopathic Principles 1993 Glossary of osteopathic terminology. In: Allen TW (ed). AOA Yearbook and Directory of Osteopathic Physicians. American Osteopathic Association, Chicago

Greenman PE 1996 Principles of Manual Medicine, 2nd edn. Williams and Wilkins, Baltimore

Haldeman S, Rubinstein S 1992 Cauda equina syndrome in patients undergoing manipulation of the lumbar spine. Spine 17: 1469–1473

Hartman L 1997 Handbook of Osteopathic Technique, 3rd edn. Chapman & Hall, London

Hoehler F, Tobis J, Buerger A 1981 Spinal manipulation for low back pain. Journal of the American Medical Association 245: 1835–1838

Howe DH, Newcombe RG, Wade MT 1983 Manipulation of the cervical spine: A pilot study. Journal of the Royal College of General Practitioners 33(254): 574–579

Kappler RE 1989 Direct action techniques. In: Beal MC (ed) The Principles of Palpatory Diagnosis and Manipulative Technique. American Academy of Osteopathy, Newark

Kappler R 1997 Thrust techniques. In: Ward R (ed) Foundations for Osteopathic Medicine. Williams and Wilkins, Baltimore

Kenna C, Murtagh J 1989 Back Pain and Spinal Manipulation, 2nd edn. Butterworth Heinemann, Oxford

Kimberly P 1992 Formulating a prescription for osteopathic manipulative treatment. In: Beal M (ed) The Principles of Palpatory Diagnosis and Manipulative Technique. American Academy of Osteopathy, Ohio

Kuchera W, Kuchera M 1992 Osteopathic Principles in Practice. KCOM press, Kirksville, Missouri

Kuchera W, Kuchera M 1994 Osteopathic Principles in Practice. Greyden Press, Ohio

Lewit K 1991 Manipulative Therapy in Rehabilitation of the Locomotor System, 2nd edn. Butterworth Heinemann, Oxford

Maigne R 1996 Diagnosis and Treatment of Pain of Vertebral Origin. Williams and Wilkins, Baltimore

Meal G, Scott R 1986 Analysis of the joint crack by simultaneous recording of sound and tension. Journal of Manipulative and Physiological Therapeutics 9: 189–195

Mierau D, Cassidy J, Bowen V, Dupuis P, Noftall F 1988 Manipulation and mobilization of the third metacarpophalangeal joint: a quantitative radiographic and range of motion study. Manual Medicine 3: 135–140

Mitchell F 1995 The Muscle Energy Manual. MET Press, Michigan

Nansel D, Cremata E, Carlson J, Szlazak M 1989 Effect of unilateral spinal adjustments on goniometrically assessed cervical lateral-flexion end-range asymmetries in otherwise asymptomatic subjects. Journal of Manipulative and Physiological Therapeutics 12(6): 419–427

Nansel D, Peneff A, Carlson J, Szlazak M 1990 Time course considerations for the effects of unilateral lower cervical adjustments with respect to the amelioration of cervical lateral-flexion passive end-range asymmetry. Journal of Manipulative and Physiological Therapeutics 13(6): 297–304

Nansel D, Peneff A, Quitoriano D 1992 Effectiveness of upper verses lower cervical adjustments with respect to the amelioration of passive rotational verses lateral-flexion end-range asymmetries in otherwise asymptomatic subjects. Journal of Manipulative and Physiological Therapeutics 15(2): 99–105

Neumann H 1989 Introduction to Manual Medicine. Springer-Verlag, Berlin

Nilsson N, Christenson HW, Hartrigson J 1996 Lasting changes in passive range of motion after spinal manipulation: A randomised, blind, controlled trial. Journal of Manipulative and Physiological Therapeutics 19(3): 165–168

Nordemar R, Thorner C 1981 Treatment of acute cervical pain: a comparative group study. Pain 10: 93–101

Nyberg R 1993 Manipulation: Definition, types, application In: Basmajian J, Nyberg R (eds) Rational Manual Therapies. Williams and Wilkins, Baltimore

Nyberg R, Basmajian J 1993 Rationale for the use of spinal manipulation. In: Basmajian J, Nyberg R (eds) Rational Manual Therapies. Williams and Wilkins, Baltimore

Panjabi M, Yamamoto I, Oxland T, Crisco J 1989 How does posture affect coupling in the lumbar spine? Spine 14(9): 1002–1011

Roston J, Haines R 1947 Cracking in the metacarpophalangeal joint. Journal of Anatomy 81: 165–173

Royal College of General Practitioners 1996 Clinical guidelines on acute and recurrent low back pain. RCGP, London

Sammut E, Searle-Barnes P 1998 Osteopathic Diagnosis. Stanley Thornes, Cheltenham

Senstad O, Leboeuf-Yde C, Borchgrevink C 1997 Frequency and characteristics of side effects of spinal manipulative therapy. Spine 22(4): 435–440

Stoddard A 1969 Manual of Osteopathic Practice. Hutchinson Medical Publications, London

Stoddard A 1972 Manual of Osteopathic Technique, 2nd edn. Hutchinson Medical Publications, London

Stodolny J, Chmielewski H 1989 Manual therapy in the treatment of patients with cervical migraine. Manual Medicine 4: 49–51

Surkitt D, Gibbons P, McLaughlin P 2000 High velocity low amplitude manipulation of the atlanto-axial joint: effect on atlanto-axial and cervical spine rotation asymmetry in asymptomatic subjects. Journal of Osteopathic Medicine 3(1): 13–19

Swezey R, Swezey S 1975 The consequences of habitual knuckle cracking. Western Journal of Medicine 122: 377–379

Terrett A, Vernon H 1984 Manipulation and pain tolerance. A controlled study on the effect of spinal manipulation on paraspinal cutaneous pain tolerance levels. American Journal of Physical Medicine 63: 217–225

Unsworth A, Dowson D, Wright V 1972 Cracking joints: a bioengineering study of cavitation in the metacarpophalangeal joint. Annals of Rheumatic Disease 30: 348–358

Vernon H, Dharmi I, Howley T, Annett R 1986 Spinal manipulation and beta-endorphin: a controlled study of the effect of a spinal manipulation on plasma beta-endorphin levels in normal males. Journal of Manipulative and Physiological Therapeutics 9: 115–123

Vicenzino G, Twomey L 1993 Side flexion induced lumbar spine conjunct rotation and its influencing factors. Australian Journal of Physiotherapy 39(4): 299–306

Waddell G 1998 The Back Pain Revolution. Churchill Livingstone, Edinburgh

Watson P, Mollan R 1990 Cineradiography of a cracking joint. British Journal of Radiology 63: 145–147

Zusman M 1994 What does manipulation do? The need for basic research. In: Boyling J, Palastanga M (eds) Grieve's Modern Manual Therapy, 2nd edn. Churchill Livingstone, New York

8

The management of low back pain in pregnancy

S. E. Sandler

The Expectant Mothers Clinic, London; The British
School of Osteopathy, London, UK

Low back pain is a common condition seen in pregnancy. The treatment of low back pain in pregnant patients is essentially different from the treatment of the non-pregnant patient. These differences arise when it comes to understanding the reasons why pregnant patients get back pain and the differential diagnostics relating to obstetrics. The techniques are different as the patient cannot be treated prone, and manual techniques are better than mechanical ones because the palpatory response to the changing tissues is very important in this group of patients. *Manual Therapy* (1996) **1(4)**, 178–185

INTRODUCTION

Low back pain during pregnancy is now recognized as a universal phenomenon, so much so that it is often quoted as a common minor disorder during pregnancy in standard obstetric textbooks such as *Fundamentals of Obstetrics and Gynaecology* (1986).

The size of the problem varies according to different authorities. It can be as high as 82%, as found in one study by Bullock et al (1987) and as low as 50%, as found in other studies by Mantle et al (1977) and Moore et al (1990).

However, most authorities agree that nearly all pregnant women can expect to suffer from a degree of back pain. In the majority of cases the problem is benign and temporary and with good care should disappear after the pregnancy. This article is focused on the work carried out at The British School of Osteopathy Expectant Mothers Clinic.

DIAGNOSIS

The diagnostic rationale is based on case history analysis, postural analysis and specific segmental analysis of the joints throughout the spine and pelvis, as well as the supporting muscles and ligaments, so as to devise a treatment programme based on the individual and her specific needs.

CASE HISTORY ANALYSIS

Patients coming into the Expectant Mothers Clinic are referred by their GP, consultant or midwife, or

Table 8.1 Differential diagnosis of lumbar spine pain and sacroiliac joint (SIJ) pain.

Disc disease has the following characteristics in relation to pain:

Morning pain and stiffness
Weight-bearing component
Age of the patient
Increased abdominal pressure provokes pain
Sleep not usually disturbed
Eases as day progresses and then gets worse again
History of repeated micro-trauma
Movement eases pain but not for long, i.e. fidgets
Going up hill provokes pain
Sitting too long provokes pain, especially in low chairs
Getting out of a chair provokes pain
Dawdling-type walking provokes pain, again because of the prolonged weight-bearing and overuse of fatigued postural muscles
Cocktail party back syndrome

Facet joint involvement has the following characteristics in relation to pain:

Not weight-bearing
Related to movement, specifically rotation
Does not like lateral compression
History of minor injury in relation to major symptoms
Pain is not usually referred to an extremity
Eased by rest
Not affected by coughing or sneezing

SIJ involvement has the following characteristics in relation to pain:

There is a definite laterality to pain
Pain does not cross midline
Can refer pain to the leg
Turning in bed provokes pain
Getting into the bath lifting leg over the sill is very painful
Getting out of the car provokes pain
Going upstairs, i.e. taking the whole of the body weight and then lifting it against gravity will provoke pain
Pain is referred to the groin or genitals
Pain goes over the hip not to the hip
Pain is related to menstruation prior to pregnancy because of the effects of cyclic hormones on pre-pregnant SIJ ligaments

are self-referred. A differential diagnosis is essential as not all back pain in pregnancy is of mechanical origin. A full and comprehensive medical history, as well as an obstetric case history, is taken at the first visit to exclude any cases that might be unsuitable for treatment. At the clinic there have been patients with pre-eclampsia complaining of headaches, patients with back pain that were false labours or urinary tract infections, and even one case of a primiparous woman at 30 weeks, who had not seen her midwife for a fortnight, who had oedema presenting as pain in the hand and finger, which were so swollen the patient was unable to open the door without assistance.

Otherwise, the case history analysis at this stage is very similar to the standard case history that one might expect in any practice that specializes in manual therapy. Table 8.1 illustrates some common differential diagnostic questions. Practitioners should remember, however, that patients may suffer from more than one complaint at a time, often giving rise to mixed symptom pictures.

Once the musculoskeletal questions have been asked, specific obstetric questions relating to the current pregnancy and previous pregnancies are asked to ascertain the likelihood of the pain being non-musculoskeletal in nature; if it is, it lies outwith the scope of this article.

POSTURAL ANALYSIS

The patient is assessed in both standing and sitting positions, and her posture in the anteroposterior (A/P) and lateral planes is assessed and compared with the expected findings of a patient of this weight, age, height, and build at this stage of her pregnancy. Her postures are drawn on the chart and this information is then checked and compared at second and subsequent visits to anticipate the change in posture and the problems she might develop (Fig. 8.1). From a postural point of view there are a number of factors that lead directly into treatment which have to be taken into account.

At the end of a pregnancy, 75% of patients will have a posterior posture with a posterior carriage where weight falls behind the normal A/P centre of gravity line, and 25% will have an anterior

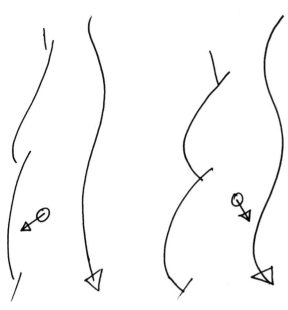

The anterior posture
The weight of the gravid
uterus is carried anterior
to the normal centre of
gravity

The posterior posture
The weight of the gravid
uterus is carried posterior
to the normal centre of
gravity

Figure 8.1 The postures of late pregnancy.

posture with an anterior carriage where the weight falls on the vertebral bodies or the discs. Sometimes with an anterior carriage the weight falls on the pubic symphysis causing pubalgia and, in really severe cases, a diastasis of the pubis.

The spine is in a dynamic state during pregnancy because of the hormonal changes, and the hyperlaxity of the ligaments is not restricted to the lumbar spine and pelvis alone. With the increase in size and weight of the breast tissues there is an increase in the expected thoracic kyphosis, with a corresponding increase in cervical lordosis to compensate. The arms and shoulders are medially rotated and protracted, giving a greater potential for thoracic outlet syndromes, which should not be confused with carpal tunnel syndromes caused by oedema.

The factors that control which sort of posture the subject will develop include the following.

The patient's morphology. Taller, thinner women are more prone to develop an anterior posture and shorter, fatter women a lordosis.

The pre-pregnancy state and fitness. The presence or absence of factors such as osteochondrosis or spondylosis can prevent the change in posture from taking place by causing a hypomobility of the areas of the spine where the change is expected.

The relative weight and size of the developing foetus compared to the available abdominal space. Diabetic mothers usually give birth to larger babies (Dunnihoo 1992). If there is a smaller pelvis than normal the baby will not only have problems passing through the birth canal, but during the pregnancy the foetus will be carried anteriorly, thus causing a lordotic posture as the body attempts to compensate.

The integrity of the abdominal muscles. If the patient has had previous abdominal operations the scar tissue will be resistant to stretch and this could prevent the lordosis from developing. Also, if the patient has had several children in a short space of time her abdominal muscles are more likely to have lost tone and thus not support the weight of the growing foetus. This could lead to the establishment of the lordosis too early with all of the attendant problems.

Previous traumas and low back pain. If the patient had a history of low back pain before her pregnancy, the resultant state of the musculoskeletal system, plus the presence or absence of scar tissue, will again compromise the ability of her posture to change during the pregnancy. The facet joints in the lumbar spine are usually orientated in a sagittal direction and not designed to carry body weight. However, sometimes they lie coronally and are thus weight-bearing and predisposed to degenerative changes. If the subject had weight-bearing facets in her lower lumbar spine before she became pregnant, the posterior centre of gravity and lordosis will provoke symptoms fairly early on. Likewise, if she has a grade 1 spondylolisthesis and is carrying anteriorly, this might well provoke the situation and produce a slippage with all of the attendant clinical signs and symptoms.

All of these factors are variable and the extent of any or all of them in any individual patient will determine her ability to adapt during her pregnancy. It naturally follows that they will also determine the ability of the patient to form a lordosis or an anterior posture.

Investigations by Moore, Dumas and Reid (1990) suggest that the accepted view of lordosis formation is wrong. Bullock et al (1987) does not support the theory that the lordosis has any part to play in the evolution of back pain at all. Ostgaard et al (1993) suggest that the lordosis is one part of the problem involving the production of back pain in pregnancy, but biomechanical factors alone cannot explain the problem in full.

It is this author's opinion, having seen over 1000 cases since the Expectant Mothers Clinic was established, that the development of this lordosis depends on the many and various factors within the individual previously mentioned. Some are predictable and some are not. It may be how the body compensates for change which will determine whether the pregnant woman develops symptoms.

OTHER DIAGNOSTIC TESTS

Standard orthopaedic and neurological tests, including reflexes, power and sensory testing, are all employed as part of the diagnostic routine in the clinic. Dipsticks are also used if the patient has a suspected urinary tract infection or possible proteinuria, etc.

PALPATION TESTING

The palpatory examination is performed sidelying and sitting for lumbar and thoracic spines, and supported at 45 degrees for cervical and sacroiliac joint (SIJ) assessment. Skin tone and superficial and deep muscle tone, together with deeper palpatory responses, all give clues as to the nature of the pain and the location of the tissue in question. Specific segmental analysis looking at different qualities of 'end feel' might indicate facet locking (abrupt end feel), ligamentous and muscular hypertonia (normal end feel but earlier than expected) and muscle spasms. Spasm is rare and often protective and, if encountered, is usually a contraindication without further investigation.

COMMON PROBLEMS

The common problems that are encountered include:

- Postural back pain of muscular and ligamentous origin
- SIJ strain with or without referred pain to the leg
- Pubalgia
- Cervicothoracic pain
- Outlet syndromes both thoracic and lumbar.

A survey of the first 400 patients seen at the Expectant Mothers Clinic (Sandler 1996) showed that most patients have pain for 4–6 weeks before they seek help and the commonest time to present with back pain is at the start of the third trimester. The pain is usually chronic and dull in nature, but can be very acute confining the patient to bed. The usual advice offered by the GP is rest, heat and paracetamol, but most mothers are reluctant to take drugs during their pregnancy and prefer to seek other ways of dealing with the pain.

TREATMENT OF PAIN OF LUMBAR ORIGIN

The treatment stems from the diagnosis. This statement, whilst apparently obvious, is worthy of examination itself. When treating pregnant patients the clinician should be aware that the changes in the tissues produced by changes in cyclical hormones can be very profound. Levels of oestrogens, progesterone and relaxin all rise dramatically during pregnancy. Much has been written about the effects of oestrogen withdrawal after the menopause and its effects on collagen. The huge rise in oestrogens during pregnancy contributes much to the growing elasticity of ligamentous tissues. The hormone relaxin is probably the most important hormone of all from a musculoskeletal point of view (Maclennan 1991; Bryant-Greenwood 1991; Dunnihoo 1992).

The purpose of the softening is to allow for separation of the bones of the pelvis and passage of the presenting part. However, clinical experience shows that the joints can start to become mobile very early on in the pregnancy, long before this physiological need arises. Just why this occurs is one of the many questions that needs to be solved before we fully understand why women suffer low back pain in pregnancy.

The aim of treatment therefore should be to relieve symptoms in the short term and to prevent long-term dysfunction.

It is best to treat the patient in sidelying or sitting positions during pregnancy to avoid too much pressure by the gravid uterus on the vena cava. In the short term, treatment is aimed at relieving the acute painful situation. This usually involves facet or joint locking with accompanying muscular hypertonia, and ligamentous overstrain.

HIGH-VELOCITY THRUST TECHNIQUES FOR THE LUMBAR SPINE

The treatment of choice for a locked facet is a manipulation or high-velocity thrust (HVT). An HVT is a short-amplitude, high-velocity manoeuvre aimed at breaking facet restriction and relaxing intrinsic muscle tone. The technique works via a neuromuscular reflex arc locally. If the joint concerned is palpated before and after the manoeuvre, the change in range of motion should determine if the manoeuvre has achieved its objective.

It is important to comment on the safety of the HVT during pregnancy. Before the Expectant

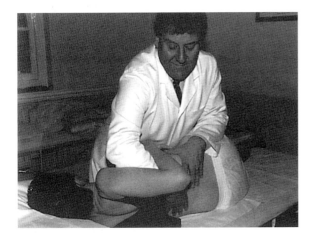

Figure 8.2 Modified lumbar roll.

Mothers Clinic was opened, this author spent many hours researching the effects of the HVT particularly during pregnancy. Unfortunately, there is very little written in the literature. There has not been one reported case, in the literature, of miscarriage caused by the use of a manipulation during pregnancy. However, there are times when spontaneous abortion is more common. According to standard obstetric tables, weeks 12 and 16 are the times of highest risk for spontaneous abortion; therefore, it is probably best to withhold any manual treatment at this time in order to minimize any possible risk that might occur. In addition, the trauma of a miscarriage is one that affects the therapist as well as the patient and there is no evidence to warrant self-blame for a condition that would have occurred naturally.

Some patients present with a history of threatened miscarriage or repeated spontaneous abortions. These patients are best treated after the start of week 20 when the potential risk is very small indeed.

From a practical point of view, the standard lumbar roll techniques are made very difficult because of the size of the gravid foetus, especially in the last trimester when this sort of mechanical back pain is so common (Fig. 8.2).

The problem with the standard technique is that it uses rotation to impart a force to move the inferior facet in question away from the superior facet. Take for example a manoeuvre designed to reduce facet fixation at L4/5 on the right. The patient lies on her left side with the painful facet joint uppermost. The mobility of pregnancy plus the bulk of the gravid uterus dictates that the minimum of leverage should be used, and the thrust should be in the midrange of the joint's possible motion. The direction of the thrust is all-important. One of the initial parameters used is flexion and extension, which is designed to focus the force at the joint in question. The legs are set with the bottom leg straight and the top leg crossed at the ankle. Care is taken to palpate the joint with the left hand whilst the right imparts a small amount of flexion to the trunk via the lower arm just sufficient to reach the point of tension at the palpating hand. The minimum of force must be used here because with too much flexion, the localization of forces becomes unachievable. Rotation of the bottom lever is impossible because of the bulk of the abdomen, and so the rotation and sidebending to focus the forces must come from above. The upper lever is fixed by the right forearm of the therapist against the right anterior axillary fold of the patient. A small downward force with the right arm towards the patient's chest reduces the risk of upper lever torsion. Gentle shifting of the therapist's body weight, arms, especially the right arm, and the position of the patient's head and trunk are used to bring the point of tension under the palpating hand. When the tissue tension is felt, a sharp, low-amplitude, high-velocity thrust with the back of the right forearm against the axilla of the patient in a direction away from the baby, i.e. backwards, will affect the manoeuvre at the point of tissue tension.

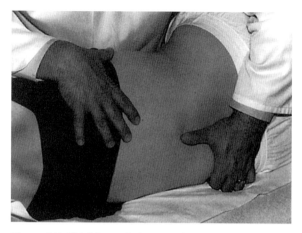

Figure 8.3 Sidelying soft tissue technique using the thenar eminence.

Many years of teaching in the clinical situation have shown this author that the common errors that arise will be:

1. Not focusing the point of tissue tension with the left hand.
2. Not using the mid-range of ligamentous tension, but instead overlocking the facet joints, which pushes them towards each other and not away from each other.
3. Not having sufficient speed in the thrust to carry out the joint separation.

SOFT TISSUE MASSAGE TECHNIQUES FOR THE LUMBAR SPINE

Other procedures used in the clinic include soft tissue massage techniques to relax tight and strained spinal musculature. These techniques are performed with the patient lying on her side.
There are many different ways of performing these manoeuvres. To relax the tissues nearest the table, the operator uses the thenar eminence (Fig. 8.3).

To relax the tissues on the opposite side, an eight-fingered soft tissue stretch technique is employed (Fig. 8.4).

These techniques are used right up into the thoracic spine, moving across the fibres of the erector spinae muscles to stretch them. The inferior attachment of these powerful muscles derives

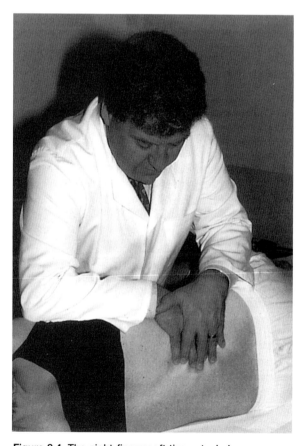

Figure 8.4 The eight-finger soft tissue technique.

from the sacrum and iliac crests, and good inhibitory preparatory work at the muscle attachments will enhance the success of the technique.

LIGAMENTOUS STRETCH TECHNIQUES FOR THE LUMBAR SPINE

The patient lies on her side, usually with the most painful side uppermost. The therapist flexes the top leg and holds it against the front of their thighs. The technique is performed with a slow rocking movement of the top hip into flexion, the right hand palpating between the spinous processes of the lumbar spine, and the left forearm pulling along the length of the spine via a hold on the sacrum so as to reinforce the technique from below (Fig. 8.5).

This technique is particularly helpful in cases of tight ligaments caused by shortening of the posterior structures or weight-bearing facets brought about by a lordotic posture.

SACROILIAC JOINT STRAINS

Sacroiliac joint (SIJ) strains are common in pregnancy as the ligaments of the pelvis soften under the action of the hormones mentioned previously.

It should be remembered that the joint is described classically as a deeply corrugated joint with irregular surfaces and very strong interosseous ligaments. Berg et al (1988) have found a correlation between low back pain in a previous pregnancy and subsequent SIJ pain. SIJ pain must be differentially diagnosed from the pain of lumbar and hip joints (see Table 8.1).

The location of SIJ pain is usually specific and lateral to the spine. It can radiate down a leg to the thigh, or over the iliac crest and into the groin where it may be mistaken for pubalgia.

Specific tests have been described in the texts and the author will not elaborate on them here except to say that palpation of bony points in the standing position is a very inaccurate way of judging the position of the posterior superior iliac spines and as a test it should not be employed without the back-up of at least three

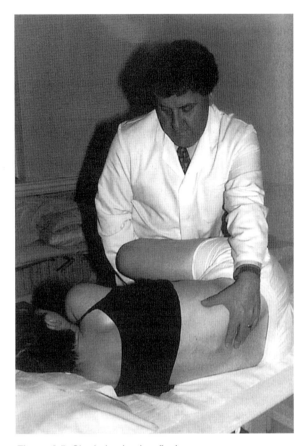

Figure 8.5 Single leg lumbar flexion.

other tests. These might include any of the following:

1. Standing shearing test between the sacrum and innominate
2. Supine shearing test for the interosseous ligaments
3. Supine shearing test for the anterior and posterior ligaments
4. Supine gapping test with the foot on the table so as to differentially diagnose pain arising from the lumbar spine
5. Supine leg length test
6. Supine abduction test.

All of these tests can be found in any standard osteopathic text, for example *An Osteopathic Approach to Diagnosis and Treatment* (1991).

TREATMENT OF SACROILIAC JOINT PAIN SYNDROMES

If the SIJ is locked and painful the treatment of choice is an HVT. The contraindications mentioned before apply here too.

The problems relating to positioning the patient, again mean that when treating the pregnant patient the operator has to find ways of imparting the thrust through the joint without using a force that might put excess pressure on the patient's abdomen. The three techniques of choice are sidelying from behind, sitting and supine, the so-called Chicago technique.

THE SIDELYING TECHNIQUE

The purpose of the technique is to impart a thrust against the innominate to relieve the fixation at the SIJ between the innominate and the sacrum. It is not possible for the innominate to move and get stuck anteriorly or posteriorly, as is described in classic osteopathic literature. This sort of dislocation is prevented by the very strong posterior and interosseous ligaments, as well as by the keystone shape of the sacrum itself. However, with a slight slackening of the ligaments there is an increase in play in the joints and thus locking can occur causing pain.

The patient lies on her side with the painful side up as before. The upper leg is crossed at the ankle. In this technique the therapist palpates at the L5/S1 segment until the tension is felt as flexion from above is introduced (Fig. 8.6).

Making sure that the patient is stable and comfortable, the therapist moves to the other side of the table and stands facing the feet of the patient. Reaching over the patient the therapist pulls the lower arm forwards and round the chest to impart rotation down to the level of L5/S1, fixing that joint but being careful not to overlock it. Using the left arm in contact with the axilla of the patient the therapist rotates her trunk backwards, thus taking pressure away from the abdomen. The thrust is given with the right palm against the posterior superior iliac spine in a direction towards the table so as to break adhesion. This might be accompanied by a pop or crack noise.

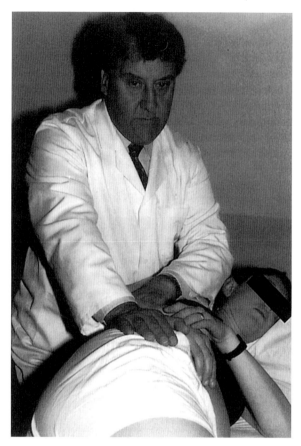

Figure 8.6 The SIJ HVT sidelying from behind.

Two other techniques found to be very useful here are the sitting and Chicago techniques for the SIJs (Figs 8.7 & 8.8). For a full description of these techniques the reader is referred to *A Handbook of Osteopathic Technique* (1985).

SOFT TISSUE TECHNIQUES SPECIFIC FOR THE SACROILIAC JOINT

There are no muscles that act directly over the SIJ. However, the muscles of the buttock that pass over the joint, including the gluteal muscles, can become very painful and will respond well to cross-fibre massage techniques.

The piriformis muscle originates from the capsule of the inferior pole of the SIJ and is often

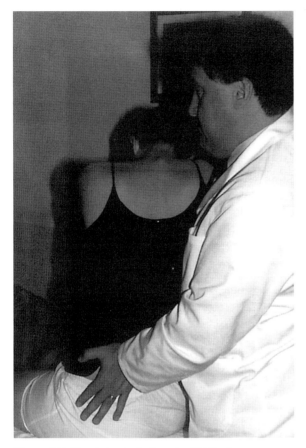

Figure 8.7 The sitting technique for SIJ fixation.

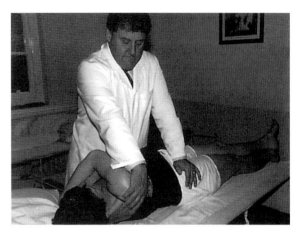

Figure 8.8 The Chicago technique for SIJ fixation.

found to be hypertonic in cases of SIJ pain. The best technique for relaxing this muscle is a combination of muscle energy or isometric contraction together with direct cross-fibre stretch (Fig. 8.9).

ARTICULATION TECHNIQUES FOR THE SIJ

These are best done supine with the patient supported on pillows. The point of the technique is to stretch the posterior SI ligaments using a flexed thigh. The therapist specifically palpates the joint with their left hand whilst employing the right to perform the technique. The force is transmitted down the flexed thigh via the hip joint to the SIJ and it is a very powerful technique (Fig. 8.10).

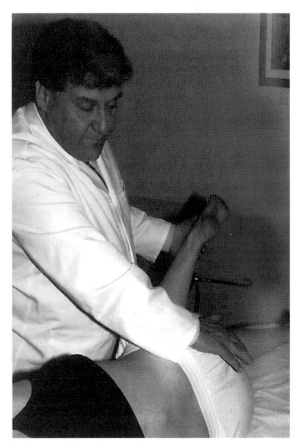

Figure 8.9 Soft tissue technique for the buttock muscles.

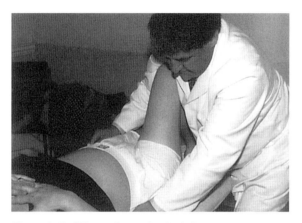

Figure 8.10 SIJ gapping and articulation.

CONCLUSION

This article has attempted to discuss some of the more common problems that can occur during pregnancy, together with the diagnostic regimes and treatment techniques used. Manual treatment during pregnancy is safe and effective and should be available to the vast numbers of our patients who demand a way of coping with their problems that does not include drug therapy.

REFERENCES

Berg G, Hammer M, Moller-Neilson J, Linden U, Thornblad J 1988 Low back pain during pregnancy. Acta Obstetrica Gynaecologica 71: 71–75

Bullock JE, Jull G, Bullock MI 1987 The relationship of low back pain to the postural changes of pregnancy. Australian Journal of Physiotherapy 33: 11–17

Bryant-Greenwood GD 1991 Human decidual and placental relaxins. Reproduction Fertility and Development 3(4): 385–389

DiGiovanna E L, Schiowitz S 1991 An Osteopathic Approach to Diagnosis and Treatment. Lippincott, Philadelphia

Dunnihoo D 1992 Fundamentals of Obstetrics and Gynaecology. 3rd edn, Lippincott Philadelphia, p. 503(a), p. 348(b)

Hartman L S 1985 A Handbook of Osteopathic Technique. 2nd edn. Hutchinson, London

Llewelyn Jones D 1986 In: Fundamentals of Obstetrics and Gynaecology, 4th edn, Faber and Faber, London. p. 182

Maclennan A H 1991 The role of the hormone Relaxin in human reproduction and pelvic girdle relaxation. Scandinavian Journal of Rheumatology Supplement 88: 7–15

Mantle MJ, Greenwood RM, Currey HCF 1977 Backache in pregnancy. Rheumatology and Rehabilitation 16: 95–101

Mantle MJ, Holmes J, Currey HCF 1981 Backache in pregnancy II: Prophylactic influence of back care classes. Rheumatology and Rehabilitation 20: 227–232

Moore K, Dumas GA, Reid JG 1990 Postural changes associated with pregnancy and their relationship to low back pain. Journal of Clinical Biomechanics. 5: 169–174

Ostgaard HC, Anderson GB, Schultz AB, Miller JA 1993 Influence of some biomechanical factors in low back pain in pregnancy. Spine 18(1): 61–65

Sandler SE 1996 A survey of the first 400 cases seen in The Expectant Mothers Clinic at The British School of Osteopathy. Unpublished data

9

Recalcitrant chronic low back and leg pain — a new theory and different approach to management

J. McConnell

McConnell & Clements Physiotherapy, Mosman, Sydney, New South Wales, Australia

The management of chronic low back and leg pain has always provided a challenge for therapists. This paper examines the influence of a repetitive movement such as walking as a possible causative factor of chronic low back pain (LBP). Diminished shock absorption and limited hip extension and external rotation are hypothesized to affect the mobility of the lumbar spine. These compensatory changes can result in lumbar spine dysfunction. Treatment must, therefore, be directed not only at increasing the mobility of the hips and thoracic spine, but at the stability of the lumbar spine. Sometimes, however, the symptoms can be exacerbated by treatment, so the neural tissue needs to be unloaded to optimize the treatment outcome. This can be achieved by taping the buttock and down the leg, following the dermatome to shorten the inflamed tissue. *Manual Therapy* (2002) **7(4):** 183–192

INTRODUCTION

LBP is a major problem in our society, costing millions of dollars per year. Eighty per cent of the population will suffer a disabling episode of LBP at least once during their lives and at any one time 35% will be suffering from LBP (Waddell 1987; Frymoyer & Cats-Baril 1991). Risk factors for first time LBP sufferers have recently been investigated in a prospective study of 403 health-care workers over a 3-year period (Adams et al 1999). Over 85% had reported having some back pain with 22% experiencing serious back pain. The most consistent predictors were decreased lateral flexion range, a long back, reduced lumbar lordosis, increased psychological distress and previous nonserious LBP (Adams et al 1999). Despite extensive research in the area of prevention and management of LBP, the effectiveness of the treatment has, on the whole, been quite poor. Treatment success is more common with acute LBP, but as highlighted in the literature, the majority of LBP sufferers will spontaneously recover within a month of the episode, regardless of the type of treatment. However, it has been found on MRI that multifidus muscle atrophy is present in 80% of patients with LBP (Kader et al 2000) and the multifidus seems to remain atrophied even though spontaneous recovery from LBP has occurred (Hides et al 1996).

Chronic LBP seems to be a quite different scenario. It has been described as a 'complex disorder that must be managed aggressively with a multidisciplinary approach that addresses physical, pyschological and socioeconomic aspects of the illness' (Wheeler 1995). In fact, all the recent literature examining chronic LBP has attributed this condition to primarily psychosocial factors (Cats-Baril & Frymoyer 1991; Feuerstein & Beattie 1995; Zusman 1998; Andersson 1999; Kendall 1999; Lundberg 1999; Hadjistavropoulos & LaChapelle 2000; Maras et al 2000). This is probably because chronic LBP usually does not respond to treatment directed locally at the site of symptoms, so the patient is often blamed for treatment failure. Physiotherapists examine spinal movements in detail, but often fail to examine other dynamic activities, such as walking, getting out of a chair and lifting the arms. Patients with chronic back and leg pain frequently complain of increasing pain not only with prolonged sitting, but with walking and standing. In many situations, patients are reluctant to seek further treatment as they are concerned that their symptoms will be exacerbated. The practitioner therefore, needs to employ strategies that will minimize the aggravation of the symptoms and facilitate the rehabilitation of the patient. It may be difficult for the clinician to determine the cause and origin of the back pain as there may be confounding hyper/hypomobility problems of the surrounding soft tissues. Chronic low back and leg pain could therefore be seen as the result of habit-ual imbalances in the movement system where spinal level/s develop increasing mobility as compensation for restrictions in adjacent areas. (Comerford & Mottram 2001b; Sahrmann 2002). This article will examine the effects of hip stiffness, lower limb loading and thoracic spine restriction as a precursor to lumbar spine dysfunction (instability) and pain. Some new directions in treatment will also be offered.

NEUTRAL ZONE, INSTABILITY AND SYMPTOM PRODUCTION

Spinal stability requires the interaction of three systems — passive (the vertebrae, ligaments, fascia and discs), active (the muscles acting on the spine) and neural (central nervous system and nerves controlling the muscles) (Panjabi 1992a). Theoretically, the most vulnerable area of the spine (the neutral zone) occurs around the neutral position of a spinal segment, where little resistance is offered by the passive structures (Panjabi 1992b). If decreased passive stability occurs, the active and neural systems can compensate by providing the spine with dynamic stability. Stability around the neutral zone can be increased by muscle activity of as little as 1–3% (Cholewicki et al 1997). Uncompensated dysfunction, however, will ultimately cause pathology (Panjabi 1992a).

How long will it take before uncompensated movement causes symptoms? The answer to this question is probably best determined by Dye's model of tissue homeostasis of a joint (1996). Dye contends that symptoms will only occur when an individual is no longer operating inside his/her envelope of function (see Fig. 9.1), reaching a particular threshold thereby causing a complex biological cascade of trauma and repair which is manifested clinically as pain and swelling. The threshold, which varies from individual to individual, depends on the amount and the frequency of the loading (Dye 1996; Novacheck 1997; Schache et al 1999). Breaching the threshold will diminish the patient's envelope of function, causing activities that initially were not painful for a patient to become painful. Four factors (anatomic,

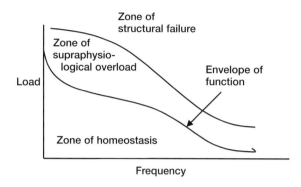

Figure 9.1 Homeostasis of a joint (adapted from Dye's Homeostasis of the Knee, 1996).

kinematic, physiological and treatment) are pertinent in determining the size of the envelope of function (Dye 1996, 1999). The anatomical factors involve the morphology, structural integrity and biomechanical characteristics of tissue (Panjabi's passive subsystem). The kinematic factors include the dynamic control of the joint involving proprioceptive sensory output, cerebral and cerebellar sequencing of motor units, spinal reflex mechanisms, muscle strength and motor control (the active and neural subsystems described by Panjabi). The physiological factors involve the genetically determined mechanisms of molecular and cellular homeostasis that determine the quality and rate of repair of damaged tissues. Treatment factors include the type of rehabilitation or surgery received.

The therapist can have a positive influence on the patient's envelope of function by minimizing the aggravation of the inflamed tissue and can even increase the patient's threshold of function by improving the control over the mobile segments (O'Sullivan 2000), and the movement of the stiff segments.

JOINT STIFFNESS AND STARTING POSITION

Therapists often consider joint stiffness and soft tissue tightness, be it muscle, fascial or neural, as restricting range of motion, but the amount of joint mobility in any one direction needs to be carefully interpreted as often the joint is not in its neutral position when the assessment is made. A conclusion is therefore made about the overall range of movement (either hyper- or hypomobility) regardless of where the movement started. An obvious example would be the patient with a ruptured posterior cruciate ligament: when an anterior draw test is performed, an increased draw movement would be demonstrated. In this situation would demonstrate, the therapist would not conclude that the anterior cruciate ligament is ruptured, but would examine the resting position of the tibia before deciding that the increased anterior movement was a consequence of the starting position rather than a pathological increase in movement.

HIP INVOLVEMENT IN SPINE MOVEMENTS

During forward bending of the trunk not only does the spine flex, but the hips must flex and internally rotate (see Fig. 9.2). A patient who has internally rotated femurs often demonstrates a decrease in forward bending because the femurs are at the end of range of rotation at the beginning of movement and cannot rotate further during the forward bending. Movement will have to increase elsewhere (usually in the lumbar spine), if the forward bending range is going to be maintained. This contention has been supported in part by the work of Hamilton and Richardson (1998), who found that individuals with LBP used more lumbar spine movement than individuals with no LBP during forward leaning in sitting, indicating an increase in relative spinal flexibility in these individuals.

It has been observed clinically that a large number of LBP sufferers have internally rotated femurs. Internal rotation of the femurs not only affects forward bending of the spine but reduces the range of hip movement into extension and external rotation. This causes an increase in the rotary movement required in the lumbar spine when the patient walks. The internal rotation in the hip also causes tightness in the iliotibial band and diminished activity in the gluteus medius

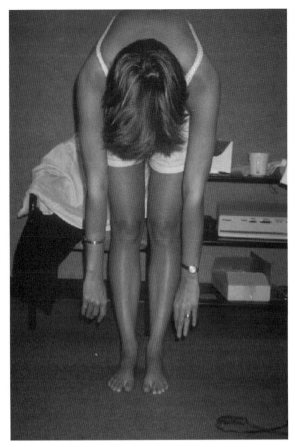

Figure 9.2 Forward bending: notice the internal rotation of the femurs.

posterior fibres (Sahrmann 2002). The patient will, therefore, demonstrate diminished pelvic muscular control. This lack of control around the pelvis may further increase the movement of an already mobile lumbar spine segment. It has been established that excessive movement, particularly in rotation, is a contributory factor to disc injury and the torsional forces may irrevocably damage fibres of the annulus fibrosus (Farfan et al 1970; Kelsey et al 1984). Therefore, an excessive amount of movement about a lumbar spine segment because of limited hip movement and control, in combination with poor abdominal support and diminished load dissipation in the lower extremity, may possibly be a significant factor in the development of LBP, particularly if the repetitive nature of the loading is considered. It has been estimated that if an individual walks for about 80 min in a day,

then each limb will go through 2500 stance and swing cycles per day, which equates to one million cycles per year (Dananberg 1997). By age 30, each limb has performed almost 30 million cycles so if there is any asymmetry in the system there will be a greater propensity for tissue overload and hence pain.

SHOCK ABSORPTION DURING GAIT

Lumbopelvic movement is further increased during gait if adequate shock absorption has not occurred at the knee or the foot, or if dorsiflexion of the great toe is inadequate at push off, reducing the available ankle range of plantar flexion and hip extension (Dananberg 1997).

Initial shock absorption occurs with knee flexion of 10–151, because the foot is supinated when the heel first strikes the ground (Perry 1992). As soon as the heel hits the ground, the foot rapidly pronates and the lower leg internally rotates. If the knee is hyperextended or the subtalar joint is stiff, there will be increased rotation and/or lateral tilting of the pelvis which will manifest as excessive motion in the spine. If the patient has an anteriorly tilted pelvis, then an increase in pelvic rotation occurs during walking, because that individual lacks hip extension and external rotation. If the patient has a posteriorly tilted pelvis, he/she presents with a 'Trendelenberglike' gait, indicating weak gluteal musculature. The individual with a sway back posture walks with a combination of increased tilt and rotation. The optimal amount of pelvic movement is reported to be 101 for rotation, 41 for lateral tilt and 71 for anteroposterior tilt (Perry 1992).

Saunders and colleagues (1953) described six components essential to normal gait. These were pelvic rotation, pelvic tilt, lateral pelvic displacement, hip flexion, knee flexion and knee and ankle interaction. They felt that when an individual lost one of these essential gait components, compensation was reasonably effective, with exaggerated motions occurring at the unaffected levels to preserve as low a level of energy consumption as possible. This contention has been supported in a recent study examining the long-term effect of hip arthrodesis on gait in adolescents. All subjects showed excessive motion in the joint above and below the arthrodesis, that is the ipsilateral knee and the lumbar spine, which the authors hypothesized led to the high incidence of LBP in these individuals (Karol et al 2000). Further evidence of the interrelationship of hip muscle control and lumbar spine function surfaced recently when it was found that hip muscle imbalance was predictive of the development of LBP in female athletes (Nadler et al 2001).

It has been postulated that the sacroiliac joint (SI) also has a role in the control of locomotion and body posture (Indahl et al 1999). Indahl and colleagues (1999) found that stimulation of the porcine SI joint capsule elicited activity in the multifidus muscle, whereas stimulation of the anterior aspect of the joint elicited responses in quadratus lumborum and gluteus maximus. Interestingly, it has been found that the activity of the gluteus maximus is shorter in duration in back pain patients during trunk flexion and extension than in controls. However, activation patterns in the lumbar paraspinals and biceps femoris muscles were similar in both order and duration in back pain patients and controls (Leinonen et al 2000).

To further understand the effect over time of repetitive torsional forces at one or two lumbar segments, some relevant anatomy and biomechanics must be explored.

ANNULAR MECHANICS

During twisting movements all points on the lower surface of one vertebra will move circumferentially in the direction of the twist; this has a unique effect on the annulus fibrosus. Because of the alternating direction of orientation of the collagen fibres in the annulus, only those fibres inclined in the direction of the movement will have their points of attachment separated. Those inclined in the opposite direction will have their points of attachment approximated. Thus, at any one time the annulus resists twisting motion with half of its complement of collagen fibres. This is one of the major reasons why twisting movements are the most likely to injure the annulus. The max-

imum range of rotation of an intervertebral disc without injury is about 31(Bogduk & Twomey 1991). Beyond this the fibre will undergo micro injury. After 121 of rotation overt failure occurs. The disc contributes 35% resistance to torsion; the remainder (65%) comes from the posterior elements (Bogduk & Twomey 1991). As the distance between the zygapophyseal joint (ZAJ) and the axis of rotation is about 30 mm, for every 11 of rotation 0.5 mm of compression must occur. The articular cartilages of the ZAJ are about 2 mm thick and articular cartilage is about 75% water, so to accommodate 31 of rotation the cartilages must be compressed to about 62% of their resting thickness and must lose over half of their water (Bogduk & Twomey 1991).

Therefore, the annulus is protected from injury by the ZAJ. Impaction of the ZAJ occurs before the fibres of the annulus undergo more than 4% strain (Bogduk & Twomey 1991). However, it is possible that the excessive movement at one lumbar segment occurring with every step an individual takes may cause a permanent elongation of the annular fibres so these fibres are unable to provide adequate restraint when a sudden twisting motion occurs. Alternatively, the excess mobility of a particular lumbar segment may affect the recovery from compression of the ZAJ and hence hysteresis. Passive structural changes will affect the neutral zone and hence the stability of the lumbar segments.

Hysteresis is a phenomenon in which there is a loss of energy when a structure is subjected to repetitive load and unload cycles (White & Panjabi 1978). Restoration of a collagenous structure to its initial length occurs at a lesser rate and to a lesser extent than would otherwise be the case because of the original deformation. When a structure is deformed the energy applied to it goes into deforming the structure and straining the bonds within it. For collagenous tissues, some of the energy goes into displacing proteoglycans and water, and rearranging some of the bonds between collagen fibres. Once used in this way, the energy is not immediately available to restore the structure to its original shape. Displaced water, for example, does not remain in the structure and exerts a form of back pressure in an attempt to regain its original format. It is squeezed out of the structure and the energy used is no longer available to the system. If chemical bonds are broken, they cannot act to restore the form of the structure. The tissue is, therefore, vulnerable to injury during this restoration period (White & Panjabi 1978).

MECHANICAL FINDINGS IN CHRONIC LOW BACK PAIN

Patients with chronic low back and leg pain who lack hip extension and external rotation in gait, will present with tight anterior hip structures, particularly the adductor muscles. Adductor longus and brevis activity will increase flexion and internal rotation of the hip whereas the posterior fibres of adductor magnus will encourage extension and external rotation (Basmajian & De Luca 1985). Although the adductors forcibly adduct the thigh, this is not a common activity, so they are essentially synergists supporting the pelvis during gait (Williams & Warwick 1980; Basmajian & De Luca 1985). When the adductor longus is tight, there seems to be an associated painful trigger point, which, if palpated, often reproduces posterior buttock pain.

Anterior hip tightness is tested in prone with the patient in a figure of four position (see Fig. 9.3). Ideally, the pelvis should be flat on the table. Usually, the hip on the painful side is higher off the plinth than the non-painful side. As the patient's condition improves this hip lies closer to the plinth. If the adductors are tight and painful, the patient cannot get into this position until the trigger point in the adductor is released (see Fig. 9.4).

Additionally, many patients with chronic LBP have associated stiffness in the thoracic spine. The thoracic spine is inherently stiff as it is constrained by the ribs and possesses long spinous processes. Increased stiffness in the thoracic region may result in compensatory changes in the passive and active structures in the regions above and below, in this case the lumbar spine, which may, in turn, cause an increased stiffness in the thoracic region, thereby increasing the segmental mobility in the lumbar spine and so forth. Increased mobility (instability) in the lumbar segment, which can be

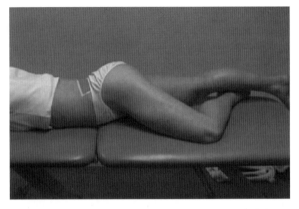

Figure 9.3 Testing the flexibility of the anterior hip joint structures.

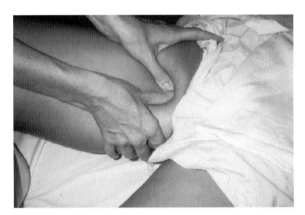

Figure 9.4 Releasing the adductor trigger point. Leg is supported in external rotation.

examined using accessory or physiological movements, is often in nonphysiological direction/s.

If the palpation is being performed in prone and the patient has an increased lumbar lordosis, the segment may actually feel stiff, unless the spine has been placed in a neutral position prior to the commencement of palpation. Thus, the starting position of the joint is critical in the decision-making process.

Increased lumbar spine mobility is often accompanied by poor segmental muscle recruitment/control (Hodges & Richardson 1996; Richardson et al 1999). A variety of strategies are used to control spinal stability at different levels. The deep intrinsic muscles of the spine are recruited to control translation and rotation at the intervertebral level, enabling spine stiffening, while the long multisegmental muscles prevent buckling of the spine (Bergmark 1989). However, in LBP sufferers, changes in the recruitment pattern of the local muscles of the trunk have been found, compromising intervertebral stability (King et al 1988; Hodges & Richardson 1996; Wilder et al 1996). In contrast, a delayed offset of activity when a load is released from the trunk has been found in the global muscles such as the oblique abdominals and erector spinae, possibly indicating an attempt by these superficial muscles to compensate for poor deep muscle function (Radebold et al 2000). It has not yet been established whether the muscle control problem causes the back pain or whether the back pain triggers the muscle control problem (Hodges 2000).

The situation may be quite different with chronic pain as some of the alteration in motor control may be due to the neuroplastic changes that have occurred in the nervous system (Coderre et al 1993). Changes may occur because of altered proprioceptive input, either locally, by damage to receptors and surrounding structures, or centrally, by changes in the interpretation of proprioceptive input, where non-noxious stimuli are perceived as pain (Flor et al 1997). In this situation, the normal proprioceptive input is either misinterpreted, the appropriate motor response therefore not being elicited or the internal motor planning model is faulty (Hodges 2000). Motor performance may also be affected by changes in attentional demands, whereby people with chronic pain perform poorly in tasks demanding attention (Kewman et al 1991; Eccleston 1994) and are less able to be focus away from pain (Dufton 1989). Therefore, there is a need to decrease the pain input from the periphery so that treatment does not aggravate the condition.

UNLOADING PAINFUL STRUCTURES

The concept of minimizing the aggravation of inflamed tissue is certainly central to all interventions in manual therapy. Therapists have a number of weapons in their armoury to manage pain and reduce inflammation. It is in the chronic state that pain is more diffcult to settle and sometimes symptoms seem to be increased by the very treatment that is designed to diminish them. The patient with chronic back and leg pain who can only flex to his knees is often given a slump stretch as part of his treatment, but increased pain indicates an adverse reaction to treatment. This patient is then reluctant to have further treatment, limits his movement even more, becomes stiffer and experiences increases in pain. Key to the success of management of this patient is to unload the inflamed soft tissues so that the clinician can address the issues of lack of flexibility and poor dynamic control (McConnell 2000). Unloading the soft tissue structures, particularly the neural tissues, will allow the physiotherapist to mobilize the appropriate stiff segments without inadvertently stretching mobile tissues.

The principle of unloading is based on the premise that inflamed soft tissue does not respond well to stretch (Gresalmer & McConnell 1998; McConnell 2000). For example, clinical experience has demonstrated that if a patient presents with a sprained medial collateral ligament, applying a valgus stress to the knee will aggravate the condition, whereas a varus stress will decrease the symptoms. The same principle applies for patients with an inflamed nerve root, producing leg pain. The inflamed tissue needs to be shortened or unloaded. Tape can be used to unload (shorten) the inflamed neural tissue, which will, in turn, decrease the pain. Initially the buttock is unloaded, which should decrease the proximal symptoms but may increase the distal symptoms (see Fig. 9.5A). Next a diagonal strip of tape is placed mid-thigh over the appropriate dermatome (posterior thigh for S1; lateral aspect of the thigh for L5 and so forth; see Fig. 9.5B). The soft tissues are lifted up towards the buttock. The direction of the tape is dependent on symptom response. If there is a local increase in symptoms then the direction of the diagonal should be reversed. Another diagonal piece of tape is commenced mid calf/shin (following the dermatome), again lifting the skin towards the buttock (see Fig. 9.5C). The patient should experience an immediate 50% decrease in symptoms. The tape is kept on for a week before it is renewed and usually only needs two or three applications before the symptoms have settled sufficiently.

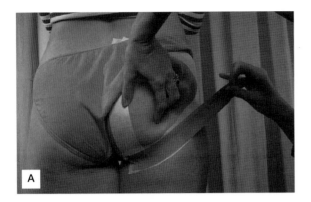

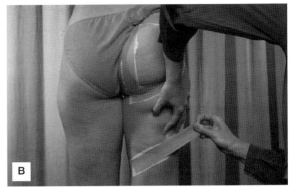

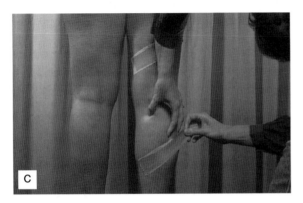

Figure 9.5 (A) Unloading the buttock to decrease leg symptoms. The tape must be sculptured into the gluteal fold. (B) For S1 distribution of pain, the posterior thigh is taped, with the skin being lifted to the buttock. If the proximal symptoms worsen, the tape diagonal should be reversed. (C) Unloading the calf to further decrease S1 symptoms.

EFFECT OF TAPE

The effect of tape on pain, particularly patellofemoral pain, has been fairly well established in the literature (Conway et al 1992; Bockrath et al 1993; Cushnagan et al 1994; Cerny 1995; Powers et al 1997; Gilleard et al 1998; Cowan et al 2001). Although there have been no studies investigating the effect of tape on LBP, it can be surmised that there would be a similar measurable pain reduction effect. The mechanism causing pain reduction for patellofemoral patients is still debated in the literature. It has been found that taping the patella of symptomatic individuals such that the pain is decreased by 50% results in an earlier activation of the vastus medialis oblique (VMO) relative to the vastus lateralis (VL) on ascending and descending stairs (Gilleard et al 1998; Cowan et al 2001). Patellar taping has also been associated with increases in loading response knee flexion, as well as increases in quadriceps

muscle torque (Conway et al 1992; Powers et al 1997; Handfield & Kramer 2000). Whether taping the back causes a change in the timing in the spinal musculature, enhancing segmental stability, is still speculative.

So far as the effect of the unloading tape is concerned, the mechanism is yet to be investigated. Clinically it works. The tape on the posterior thigh could be inhibiting an overactive hamstring muscle, which is a protective response to mechanical provocation of neural tissue (Hall et al 1995). It has been found that firm taping across the muscle belly of VL of asymptomatic individuals significantly decreases the VL activity during stair descent (Tobin & Robinson 2000). The tape could have some effect on changing the orientation of the fascia or could just have a proprioceptive effect, affecting the gating mechanism of pain (Garnett & Stephens 1981; Jenner & Stephens 1982). The unloading tape does, however, enable the patient to be treated without an increase in symptoms, so in the long term, treatment is more efficacious.

TREATMENT

Once the soft tissues have been unloaded, treatment should be directed at increasing hip and thoracic spine mobility (Fig. 9.6) as well as improving the stability of the relevant lumbar segments. The patient may need to practise walking with the knees slightly bent to improve the shock absorption through the lower leg — small range eccentric quadriceps control is needed for stability around the knee. Shock absorption can also be improved by mobilizing a stiff subtalar joint. If there is a problem with push-off the first metatarsophalangeal joint may need to be mobilized to minimize the possibility of compensatory lumbar spine movement.

At the same time as increasing the mobility of adjacent areas, the therapist needs to commence stability work on the unstable areas. Segmental stability training involves muscle control of the multifidus and transversus abdominis and the posterior fibres of the gluteus medius. Specific exercises for these muscles must be carefully supervised by the therapist, so the appropriate muscles are recruited during the exercise. If there has been habitual disuse of the muscles, activation will be difficult. Feedback to the patient must be precise to achieve the desired outcome (Sale 1987). Precise training of the transversus abdominis and multifidus has been quite adequately described by Richardson et al (1999), O'Sullivan (2000), Comerford and Mottram (2001a) and others. As the multifidus, transversus abdominis and gluteus medius muscles all have a stabilizing function, endurance training should be emphasized in treatment. Decreased activity of the obliques and transversus abdominis has been reported when subjects perform rapid ballistic sit up exercises (Richardson et al 1991). Thus, exercises should be performed in a slow, controlled fashion. The number of repetitions performed by the patient at a training session will depend upon the onset of muscle fatigue. The long-term aim is to increase the number of repetitions before the onset of fatigue. Patients should be taught to recognize fatigue so that they do not train through fatigue and risk, exacerbating their symptoms.

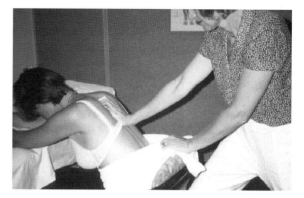

Figure 9.6 Mobilizing a stiff thoracic spine in sitting. The lumbar spine is stabilized with the towel.

Muscle training to control mobile segments dynamically may take many months to achieve. O'Sullivan (2000) has described a three-stage model for training local trunk muscles. The training process may be accelerated by the addition of firm tape across the lumbar mobile segment, minimizing the amount of movement and enhancing the proprioceptive input to the stabilizing muscles (Fig. 9.7). It has been found that taping is effective in preventing ankle sprains and improving proprioception in the ankle (Robbins et al 1995; Verhagen et al 2000), as well as preventing the lateral shift of the patella that occurs with exercise (Larsen et al 1995), so there could be a similar proprioceptive effect on an unstable segment in the spine.

Pelvic stability training should not be overlooked, as poor pelvic control can undermine the progress of the muscle training of the spine. If possible, gluteus medius training should be performed in weight bearing, simulating the stance phase of gait (Fig. 9.8). This can be done with the patient standing with the foot and hip of the exercising leg parallel to the wall and the knee slightly flexed. The other knee is flexed to 60° and is resting on the wall for balance. The patient externally rotates the standing knee without moving the hips or the feet. This contraction is held for 15 seconds and should be repeated often to effect an automatic change in the motor programme. If the patient experiences pain or has poor 'core' stability then a more stable position such as sidelying or prone should be chosen initially. However, muscle

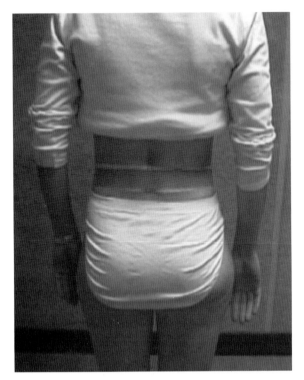

Figure 9.7 Stabilizing an unstable lumbar segment.

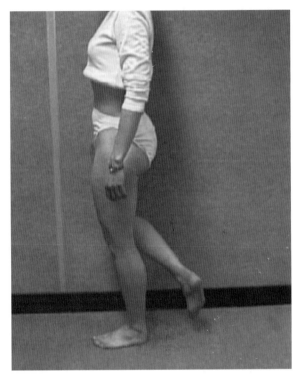

Figure 9.8 Training posterior gluteus medius. Knee slightly flexed, weight back through the heel, hips and foot facing the front, external rotation of the standing leg thigh.

training is very specific to limb position, joint angle and velocity, type and force of contraction [see Herbert (1993) and Sale & MacDougall (1981) for excellent reviews on specificity of training], so for training to be effective, a return to functional positions should occur as soon as possible.

CONCLUSION

Management of chronic low back and leg pain requires a multifactorial approach. The therapist needs to examine the way the patient walks so the effect of any uneven loading through the lower extremity on the lumbar spine can be observed.

The inflamed soft tissue should be unloaded so the symptoms are not increased when there is an attempt, in treatment, to gain range. Flexibility needs to be gained in the anterior hip structures and thoracic spine, while stability is required at the mobile lumbar segment/s and pelvis. There is also a need, in the management of chronic pain problems in general, for therapists to review patients every 6 or 12 months to ensure patients still know how to manage their symptoms, as chronic problems are never cured, only managed. If patients are empowered to manage their own symptoms, the burden of chronic musculoskeletal problems on the health-care system could possibly be reduced.

REFERENCES

Adams MA, Mannion AF, Dolan P 1999 Personal risk factors for first time LBP. Spine 24(23): 2497–2505

Andersson GB 1999 Epidemiological features of chronic low back pain. Lancet 14, 354(9178): 581–585

Basmajian J, De Luca C 1985 Muscles Alive. 5th edn. Williams & Wilkins, Baltimore

Bergmark A 1989 Stability of the lumbar spine. A study in mechanical engineering. Acta Orthopedica Scandinavica 60(Suppl 230): 1–54

Bockrath K, Wooden C, Worrell T, Ingersoll C, Farr J 1993 Effects of patella taping on patella position and perceived pain. Medicine and Science in Sports and Exercise 25(9): 989–992

Bogduk N, Twomey L 1991 Clinical Anatomy of the Lumbar Spine. Churchill Livingstone, Edinburgh

Cats-Baril WL, Frymoyer JW 1991 Identifying patients at risk of becoming disabled because of low-back pain. The Vermont Rehabilitation Engineering Center predictive model. Spine 16(6): 605–607

Cerny K 1995 Vastus medialis oblique/vastus lateralis muscle activity ratios for selected exercises in persons with and without patellofemoral pain syndrome. Physical Therapy 75(8): 672–683

Cholewicki J, Panjabi MM, Khachatryan A 1997 Stabilizing function of trunk flexor–extensor muscles around a neutral spine posture. Spine 22(19): 2207–2212

Coderre TJ, Katz J, Vaccarino AL, Melzack R 1993 Contribution of central neuroplasticity to pathological pain: Review of clinical and experimental evidence. Pain 52(3): 259–285

Comerford MJ, Mottram SL 2001a Functional stability retraining: Principles and strategies for managing mechanical dysfunction. Manual Therapy 6(1): 3–14

Comerford MJ and Mottram SL 2001b Movement and stability dysfunction — contemporary developments. Manual Therapy 6(1): 15–26

Conway A, Malone T, Conway P 1992 Patellar alignment/tracking alteration: Effect on force output and perceived pain. Isokinetics and Exercise Science 2(1): 9–17.

Cowan SM, Bennell KL, Crossley KM, Hodges PW, McConnell J 2001 Physiotherapy treatment changes motor control of the vastii in patellofemoral pain syndrome (PFPS): A randomised, double-blind, placebo controlled trial. Medicine and Science in Sports and Exercise 33(5): S89

Cushnaghan J, McCarthy R, Dieppe P 1994 The effect of taping the patella on pain in the osteoarthritic patient. British Medical Journal 308(6931): 753–755

Dananberg H 1997 Lower back pain as a gait related repetitive motion injury. In: Vleeming A, Mooney V, Dorman T, Snijders C, Stoeckart R (eds) Movement and Stability & Low Back Pain — The Essential Role of the Pelvis. Churchill Livingstone, Edinburgh

Dufton BD 1989 Cognitive failure and chronic pain. International Journal of Psychiatry in Medicine 19(3): 291–297

Dye S 1996 The knee as a biologic transmission with an envelope of function: A theory. Clinical Orthopaedics (325):10–18

Dye S 1999 Invited commentary. Journal Orthopaedic Sports Physical Therapy 29(7): 386–387

Eccleston C 1994 Chronic pain and attention: A cognitive approach. British Journal of Clinical Psychology 33(Part 4): 535–547

Farfan HF, Cossette JW, Robertson GH, Wells RV, Kraus H 1970 The effects of torsion on lumbar intervertebral joints: The role of torsion in the production of disc degeneration. Journal of Bone and Joint Surgery 52A: 468–497

Feuerstein M, Beattie P, 1995 Biobehavioral factors affecting pain and disability in LBP: Mechanisms and assessment. Physical Therapy 75(4): 267–280

Flor H, Braun, C, Elbert T, Birbaumer N 1997 Extensive reorganization of primary somatosensory cortex in chronic back pain patients. Neuroscience Letters 224(1): 5–8

Frymoyer JW, Cats-Baril WL 1991 An overview of the incidences and costs of LBP. Orthopaedic Clinics of North America 22(2): 263–271

Garnett R, Stephens JA 1981 Changes in recruitment threshold of motor units produced by cutaneous stimulation in man. Journal of Physiology 311: 463–473

Gilleard W, McConnell J, Parsons D 1998 The effect of patellar taping on the onset of vastus medialis obliquus and vastus lateralis muscle activity in persons with patellofemoral pain. Physical Therapy 78(1): 25–32

Gresalmer R, McConnell J 1998 The Patella: A Team Approach. Aspen Publishers, Gaithersburg, MD

Hadjistavropoulos HD, LaChapelle DL 2000 Extent and nature of anxiety experienced during physical examination of chronic LBP. Behavioural Research Therapy 38(1): 13–29

Hadjipavlou AG, Simmons JW, Yang JP, Bi LX, Ansari GA, Kaphalia BS, Simmons DJ, Nicodemus CL, Necessary JT, Lane R, Esch O 1998 Torsional injury resulting in disc degeneration: I. An in vivo rabbit model. Journal of Spinal Disorders 11(4): 312–317

Hall T, Zusman M, Elvey R 1995 Manually Detected Impediments During the Straight Leg Raise Test. Proceedings 9th Biennial Conference of the Manipulative Physiotherapists Association of Australia, Gold Coast, pp 48–53

Hamilton C, Richardson C (1998) Active control of the neutral lumbopelvic posture: A comparison of LBP and non LBP subjects. In: Vleeming A, Mooney V, Tilsher H, Dorman T, Snijders C (eds) Proceedings of the 3rd Interdisciplinary World Congress on Low Back and Pelvic Pain, Vienna, Austria

Handfield T, Kramer J 2000 Effect of McConnell taping on perceived pain and knee extensor torques during isokinetic exercise performed by patients with patellofemoral pain syndrome. Physiotherapy Canada, Winter: 39–44

Herbert R 1993 Human strength adaptations — implications for therapy. In: Crosbie J, McConnell J (eds) Key Issues in Musculoskeletal Physiotherapy. Butterworth-Heinemann, Oxford

Hides JA, Jull GA, Richardson CA 1996 Multifidus muscle recovery is not spontaneous after resolution of acute first episode low back pain. Spine 21(23) 2763–2769

Hodges PW 2000 The role of the motor system in spinal pain: Implications for rehabilitation of the athlete following lower back pain. Journal of Science and Medicine in Sport; 3(3): 243–253

Hodges PW Richardson CA 1996 Inefficient muscular stabilization of the lumbar spine associated with LBP. A motor control evaluation of transversus abdominis. Spine 15; 21(22): 2640–2650

Hutten MM, Hermens HJ, Ijzerman MJ, Lousberg R, Zilvold G 1999 Distribution of psychological aspects in subgroups of chronic LBP patients divided on the score of physical performance. International Journal of Rehabilitation Research 22(4): 261–268

Indahl A, Kaigle AM, Reikeras O, Holm SH 1999 Sacroiliac joint involvement in activation of the porcine spinal and gluteal musculature. Journal of Spinal Disorders 12(4): 325–330

Jenner JR, Stephens JA 1982 Cutaneous reflex responses and their central nervous system pathways studied in man. Journal of Physiology 333: 405–419

Kader D, Wardlaw D, Smith F 2000 Correlation between MRI changes in the lumbar multifidus muscle and leg pain. Clinical Radiology 55(2): 145–149

Karol LA, Halliday SE, Gourineni P 2000 Gait and function after intra-articular arthrodesis of the hip in adolescents. Journal of Bone and Joint Surgery 82(4): 561–569

Kelsey JL, Githens PB, White AA 1984 An epidemiological study of lifting and twisting on the job and the risk for acute prolapsed lumbar intevertebral disc. Journal of Orthopaedic Research 2: 61–66

Kendall NA 1999 Psychosocial approaches to the prevention of chronic pain: The low back paradigm. Baillieres Best Practice Research Clinical Rheumatology 13(3): 545–554

Kewman DG, Vaishampayan N, Zald D, Han B 1991 Cognitive impairment in musculoskeletal pain patients. International Journal of Psychiatry in Medicine 21(3): 253–262

King JC, Lehmkuhl DL, French J, Dimitrijevic M 1988 Dynamic postural reflexes: Comparison in normal subjects and patients with chronic LBP. Current Concepts in Rehabilitation Medicine 4: 7–11

Larsen B, Andreasen E, Urfer A, Mickleson MR, Newhouse KE 1995 Patellar taping: A radiographic examination of the medial glide technique. American Journal of Sports Medicine 23: 465–471

Leinonen V, Kankaanpaa M, Airaksinen O, Hanninen O 2000 Back and hip extensor activities during trunk flexion/extension: Effects of low back pain and rehabilitation. Archives of Physical Medicine and Rehabilitation 81(1): 32–37

Lundberg U 1999 Stress responses in low-status jobs and their relationship to health risks: Musculoskeletal disorders. Annals of the New York Academy of Science 896: 162–172

McConnell J 2000 A novel approach to pain relief pre-therapeutic exercise. Journal of Science and Medicine in Sport 3(3): 325–334

Nadler SF, Malanga GA, Feinberg JH, Prybicien M, Stitik TP, DePrince M 2001 Relationship between hip muscle imbalance and occurrence of LBP in collegiate athletes: A prospective study. American Journal of Physical Medicine and Rehabilitation; 80(8): 572–577

Novacheck TF 1997 The biomechanics of running and sprinting. In: Guten GN (ed) Running Injuries. WB Saunders, Philadelphia, PA, pp 4–19

O'Sullivan PB 2000 Lumbar segmental 'instability': Clinical presentation and specific stabilizing exercise management. Manual Therapy 5(1): 2–12

Panjabi M 1992a The stabilising system of the spine. Part I. Journal of Spinal Disorders 5(4): 383–389

Panjabi M 1992b The stabilising system of the spine. Part I. Journal of Spinal Disorders 5(4): 390–397

Perry J 1992 Gait Analysis. McGraw-Hill, New York

Powers C, Landel R, Sosnick T, Kirby J, Mengel K, Cheney A, Perry J 1997 The effects of patellar taping on stride characteristics and joint motion in subjects with patellofemoral pain. Journal of Orthopaedic and Sports Physical Therapy 26(6): 286–291

Radebold A, Cholewicki J, Panjabi MM, Patel TC 2000. Muscle response pattern to sudden trunk loading in healthy individuals and in patients with chronic low back pain. Spine 25(8): 947–954

Richardson CA, Jull GA, Hodges PW, Hides JA 1999 Therapeutic Exercise for Spinal Segmental Stabilisation in LBP: Scientific Basis and Clinical Approach. Churchill Livingstone, Edinburgh

Richardson C, Jull G, Wohlfahrt D 1991 Ballistic Exercise: Can it Undermine the Protective Stability Role of the Lumbar Musculature. Proceedings MPAA 7th Biennial Conference, NSW, Australia

Robbins S, Waked E, Rappel R 1995 Ankle taping improves proprioception before and after exercise in young men. British Journal of Sports Medicine 29(4): 242–247

Sahrmann S 2002 Diagnosis and Treatment of Movement Impairment Syndromes. Mosby, St Louis

Sale D 1987 Influence of exercise and training on motor unit activation. Exercise & Sports Science Review 5: 95–151

Sale D, MacDougall D 1981 Specificity of strength training: A review for coach & athlete. Canadian Journal of Applied Sports Sciences 6(2): 87–92

Saunders J, Inman V, Eberhart H 1953 The major determinants in normal and pathological gait. Journal of Bone and Joint Surgery 35A: 543–558

Schache AG, Bennell KL, Blanch PD, Wrigley TV 1999 The coordinated movement of the lumbo-pelvic hip complex during running: A literature review Gait Posture 10(1): 30–47

Tobin S, Robinson G 2000 The effect of McConnell's vastus lateralis inhibition taping technique on vastus lateralis and vastus medialis activity. Physiotherapy 86(1): 174–183

Verhagen EA, van Mechelen W, de Vente W 2000 The effect of preventive measures on the incidence of ankle sprains. Clinical Journal of Sport Medicine 10(4): 291–296

Waddell G 1987 Volvo award in clinical sciences. A new clinical model for the treatment of low-back pain. Spine 12(7): 632–644

White A, Panjabi M 1978 Clinical Biomechanics of the Spine. Lippincott, Philadelphia, PA

Wheeler A 1995 Diagnosis and management of LBP and sciatica. American Family Physician 52(5): 133–141

Wilder DG, Aleksiev AR, Magnusson ML, Pope MH, Spratt KF, Goel VK 1996 Muscular response to sudden load. A tool to evaluate fatigue and rehabilitation. Spine 21(22): 2628–2639

Williams P, Warwick R 1980. Gray's Anatomy, 36th edn. Churchill Livingstone, London

Zusman M 1998 Structure-oriented beliefs and disability due to back pain. Australian Journal of Physiotherapy 44: 13–20

10

Use of real-time ultrasound imaging for feedback in rehabilitation

*J. A. Hides   C. A. Richardson
G. A. Jull*
Department of Physiotherapy, The University of
Queensland, Brisbane, Australia

Real-time ultrasound imaging is currently used extensively in medicine. It provides a safe, cost-effective and readily accessible method of examination of various organs and tissues. One area where ultrasonography has proved to be useful is investigation of musculoskeletal pathology. Tissues that can be imaged include muscles, tendons, joints, ligaments and bursae. One of the most useful features of real-time ultrasound imaging is that movement of anatomical structures can be observed as it actually occurs. This has allowed development of a new application of real-time ultrasound imaging for rehabilitation that involves observation of muscle contraction to provide feedback. An ability to image deep muscles is an advantage of the technique, and use of ultrasound imaging has been successfully incorporated in assessment and facilitation strategies for the transversus abdominis and multifidus muscles in low back pain (LBP) patients. The objective of this article is to provide a brief review of the principles, advantages and disadvantages of ultrasound imaging and to discuss this new application of real-time ultrasound to rehabilitation. The current use of real-time ultrasound imaging in LBP patients will be described, and future uses in rehabilitation and limitations discussed. *Manual Therapy* (1998) **3(3)**, 125–131

INTRODUCTION

Over the past 40–50 years, ultrasound technology has developed to a stage where it has found widespread application. In medicine, real-time ultrasound imaging allows rapid evaluation of morphology and pathomorphological changes in a number of organs and tissues. It is used extensively in gynaecology and obstetrics (where it has been of special value due to the fact that it does not involve exposure to ionizing radiation), internal medicine, surgery, orthopaedics, sports medicine, neurology and paediatrics.

A review of the applications of ultrasonography in medicine is beyond the scope of this article. The usefulness of ultrasonography for evaluation of the musculoskeletal system has been shown (Fornage & Rifkin 1988; Harcke et al 1988; Kaplan et al 1990; Laine & Peltokallio 1991; van Holsbeeck & Introcaso 1992; Chhem et al 1994). One example of the use of ultrasound imaging in this field is diagnosis of muscle lesions commonly seen in sports medicine (partial and complete muscle tears and haematomas). Ultrasound imaging has been used to determine the presence, location and severity of anatomic damage in these lesions (Laine & Peltokallio 1991; Chhem et al 1994). Similarly, joints, ligaments and bursaes at the knee, shoulder and ankle joints have been examined for diagnostic purposes (Laine & Peltokallio 1991; van Holsbeeck & Strouse 1993). However, tendons are the most frequently studied structures in musculoskeletal ultrasound to identify partial or complete tears or post-traumatic tenosynovitis (Fornage & Rifkin 1988). The most commonly evaluated tendons are the rotator cuff, achilles tendon and patellar tendon (Chhem et al 1994). The reason that these techniques are so useful is because dynamic studies (observing movement of tendons) can be performed. It is in fact this ability to image moving structures that is attractive to physiotherapists because real-time ultrasound can also be used as a feedback tool during muscle contraction.

Ultrasound imaging has previously had two main applications in rehabilitation: measurement of muscle size and more recently, imaging of muscle movement. Measurement of muscle size is possible as ultrasound imaging allows generation of measurements in cross-section, thus providing a method of direct assessment of muscle atrophy and hypertrophy. Various muscles have been measured including quadriceps, anterior tibial muscles and the lumbar multifidus (Stokes & Young 1986; Loo & Stokes 1990; Martinson & Stokes 1991; Hides et al 1992, 1994, 1995a, 1996; Sipila & Suominen 1993). Real-time ultrasound imaging has been used for observation of muscle contraction in research on the pelvic floor (Berstein et al 1991; Wijma et al 1991) and abdominal muscle contraction both under functional load (Kogut et al 1990) and during a submaximal Valsalva manoeuvre (Cresswell et al 1992). It has been described for feedback in rehabilitation of the lumbar multifidus (Hides et al 1995b, 1996; Stokes et al 1997) and our current work also involves assessment and rehabilitation of the transversus abdominis. The latter highlights a potentially important application for physiotherapy research and practice, i.e. imaging the action of deep muscles.

BASIC PRINCIPLES AND INSTRUMENTATION

Ultrasound imaging involves sending short pulses of ultrasound into the body and using reflections received from tissue interfaces to produce images of internal structures. Pulsed ultrasound is described by frequency, propagation speed, intensity, attenuation and pulse length (Kremkau 1983). Frequencies from 1 to 10 MHz are used. The lower frequencies are used when greater depths of imaging are required and the higher frequencies for visualizing more superficial structures.

As sound encounters boundaries between different tissues, it can be reflected and scattered. The distance from the transducer to the tissues causing scattering and reflection is determined by travel time (Kremkau 1983). Similar to therapeutic ultrasound, transducers used in ultrasound imaging convert electrical voltages into ultrasound (and vice versa) by piezo-electricity. For ultrasound imaging, the same transducer is used to both send pulses and receive echoes reflected back to it. To receive echoes, the transducer must be positioned so that the sound beam is perpendicular to the tissue interface being imaged (Saunders & James 1985).

Imaging systems consist of a pulser, transducer, receiver, memory and display (Kremkau 1983).

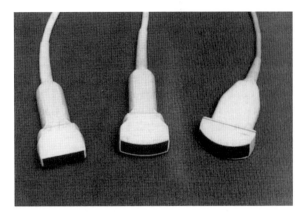

Figure 10.2 Examples of different ultrasound transducers used in musculoskeletal imaging. From left to right are a 10 MHz linear transducer, and 5 MHz and 3.5 MHz curvilinear transducers.

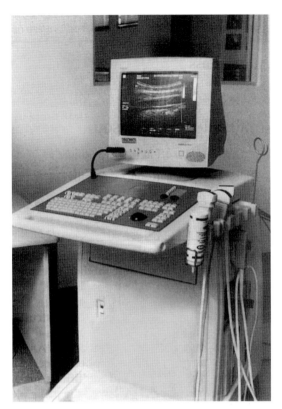

Figure 10.1 An example of real-time ultrasound imaging apparatus.

An example of real-time ultrasound apparatus and its components is shown in Figure 10.1. The process of how pulse echo imaging systems use intensity, direction and arrival time of echoes to produce cross-sectional B-mode images has been described by Kremkau (1983). The pulser applies voltages to the transducer, resulting in the production of ultrasound pulses. Echoes received from the tissues are converted into voltages that are amplified in the receiver. Numbers corresponding to echo strengths are stored in the digital memory at locations corresponding to the positions of tissues causing reflection and scattering of pulses. After a cross-sectional number representation is built up in the memory, the stored numbers are converted to brightness dots on the display, resulting in a cross-sectional anatomic image.

Various types of transducers are available for real-time ultrasound imaging. Multi-element transducers are usually used and transducer selection for musculoskeletal imaging is determined by the part of the body and the type of tissue being imaged. Straight linear and curvilinear array transducers are most commonly used (Fig. 10.2). For imaging the multifidus muscle, a 5 MHz convex array transducer was found to be appropriate (Hides et al 1995b). It produces a well-defined image of the complex fascial planes of this muscle. This transducer is also suitable for imaging the muscles of the abdominal wall. A linear array transducer is also suitable, and for larger patients a 3.5 MHz transducer can be used.

For a more detailed review of principles of ultrasound imaging, see Fish (1990) and Rumack et al (1991).

USE OF REAL-TIME ULTRASOUND IMAGING FOR BIOFEEDBACK IN REHABILITATION

NEED FOR VISUALIZATION OF DEEP MUSCLE ACTION

Research into muscle impairment in LBP has found that there is a specific impairment in the deep muscles of the trunk, notably the transversus abdominis and the segmental multifidus (Hides et al 1994, 1996; Hodges et al 1996; Hodges & Richardson 1996, 1997, 1998). Furthermore, randomized clinical trials have evaluated the efficacy of specific rehabilitation that focuses on co-activation of these deep muscles (Hides et al 1996; O'Sullivan et al 1997). Evidence suggests that it is very important that these deep muscles are targeted specifically in rehabilitation, i.e. that their action is ensured separately from other trunk muscles (Hodges & Richardson 1997). In the case of the multifidus, research has shown that the effect on the muscle following injury is rapid and very specific to the injured vertebral segment (Hides et al 1994). The approach to exercise therapy needs to be very precise because the unaffected parts of the multifidus and other muscles, such as the thoracic components of the erector spinae, will be more easily activated when rehabilitation is attempted. In the case of the transversus abdominis, it is apparent that if separate control of the muscle is lost, a generalized activation of more superficial abdominal muscles will ensue. Care and precision with facilitation is needed.

Currently, transversus abdominis is tested in the clinical situation through assessment of its action of drawing in the abdominal wall (Richardson & Jull 1995; Richardson et al 1998). This action is performed principally by the transversus abdominis (Lacote et al 1987) and can be described as a corset-like action. An indirect method of quantification of the action presently used is with use of the pressure biofeedback unit and testing in the prone position. If the patient is unable to do the action, the attempt is analysed by the physiotherapist through observation of the abdominal wall, palpation of the lower abdominal quadrant for a deep tensioning of muscle fibres and, if the muscles such as obliquus abdominis externus are overactive, this is monitored by surface electromyograph (EMG). The clinical assessment of multifidus is palpation of muscle size and consistency of activation. Comparisons can be made between sides and between vertebral levels. To assess multifidus activation in line with its stability role, the segmental multifidus is palpated as the patient attempts a slow, gentle and subtle isometric contraction. Considerable clinical skill is required to interpret the different strategies adopted by LBP patients who have difficulty activating the multifidus in this way. Surface EMG is

not very useful for providing feedback from the multifidus due to its depth and the cross-talk from the adjacent muscles. It can be used to provide feedback and to teach relaxation of the thoracic components of the erector spinae muscles if they are overactive.

While these methods are used clinically with much success, there is the drawback that the muscles are deep and, therefore, assessment strategies are to some extent indirect. Real-time ultrasound imaging is potentially an advantageous modality because it allows immediate visualization of contraction of the deep muscles such as the transversus abdominis and the multifidus. Furthermore it is non-invasive and could be useful for both assessment and facilitation of these muscles.

For the transversus abdominis muscle, real-time ultrasound imaging allows observation of the pattern of activation of the abdominal muscles during performance of the abdominal drawing-in action. The corset-like action can be observed as can unwanted contraction of the more superficial muscles. Each side can be examined separately for symmetry of contraction. For facilitation of the subtle corset-like action of transversus abdominis in relative isolation, visual verification that the correct facilitation strategy has been used by the physiotherapist and the correct activation has been achieved by the patient is of benefit to patient and

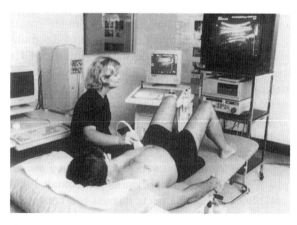

Figure 10.3 Patient positioned in supine lying observing the pattern of activation of the muscles of the anterolateral abdominal wall in transverse section as they attempt to isolate the subtle drawing in action of the transversus abdominis muscle.

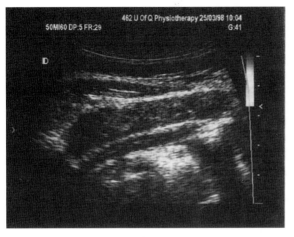

Figure 10.4A Sonographic appearance of the muscles of the anterolateral abdominal wall in transverse section.

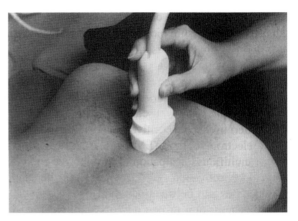

Figure 10.5 Position of 5 MHz curvilinear transducer to image the lumbar multifidus muscle in parasagittal section. The transducer is placed lateral to the spinous processes, in the plane of the zygapophyseal joints.

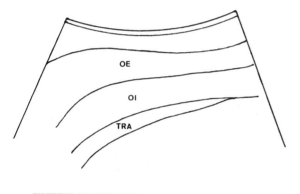

Figure 10.4B The skin layer is most superficial and the dark area superior to OE is subcutaneous tissue. Note the well defined fascia separating the muscles (white on the actual image). OE = obliquus externus abdominis muscle; OI = obliquus intermus abdominis muscle: TrA = transversus abdominis muscle.

physiotherapist alike. Figure 10.3 illustrates the use of ultrasound imaging with the patient in the supine position and an image of the muscles of the anterolateral abdominal wall is shown in Figures 10.4A and B.

For imaging of the multifidus the transducer is placed in a parasagittal orientation (Fig. 10.5). The patient is instructed in the subtle isometric contraction of the multifidus and the result is observed on the monitor. The pattern of activation can be observed at different vertebral levels on one side at a time and, importantly successful, contraction of the deep part of the muscle can be observed. The sonographic appearance of the multifidus in parasagittal section is shown in Figure 10.6. Real-time ultrasound imaging can also be used for feedback of multifidus activation. This may initially be performed in sidelying and later progressed to weight-bearing positions. Again, a parasagittal image is used for facilitation. Co-activation with the transversus abdominis can be palpated for, or alternatively contraction of the multifidus can be facilitated while the abdominal wall is imaged to observe for co-activation with the transversus abdominis (Fig. 10.7).

It is advocated that the use of real-time ultrasound imaging as feedback may enhance motor relearning of specific muscles by providing knowledge of performance. Feedback or information about performance is known to be critical for learning (Newell 1976) and how feedback is provided influences motor learning (Schmidt 1988). Knowledge of performance consists of information concerning the movement itself (such as demonstrated by real-time ultrasound imaging) and this form of feedback methodology has been advocated as most effective (Gentile 1972). Another form of feedback consist of knowledge of results. Knowledge of results equates to information supplied to the subject following task performance (Salmoni et al 1984). An example, in the

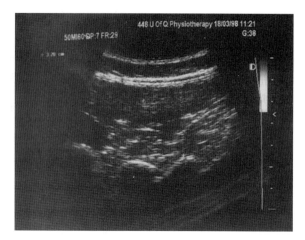

Figure 10.6A Sonographic appearance of the multifidus muscle in parasagittal section.

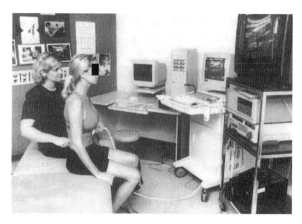

Figure 10.7 In sitting, a multifidus contraction is facilitated while the co-activation of the transversus abdominis muscle is observed for on the monitor while imaging the muscles of the anterolateral abdominal wall.

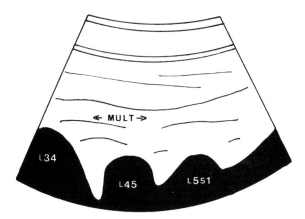

Figure 10.6B Superiorly are the skin and subcutaneous tissue. The multifidus fibres are seen running in a longitudinal direction (←MULT→). Inferiorly are the zygapophyseal joint and sacrum, from L3–4 (on the left side) to L5–S1 and the sacrum on the right. The depth of the muscle from its superior border to the dorsal surface of the L5–S1 zygapophyseal joint is 3.28 cm in this example.

context of real-time imaging of the multifidus, would be provision of the actual increase in depth in millimetres of the multifidus on isometric contraction or the length of time in seconds that the contraction was adequately held. This provides opportunities for further research into the effectiveness of different motor learning strategies on performance.

FUTURE USES OF ULTRASOUND IMAGING IN PHYSIOTHERAPY PRACTICE

ASSESSMENT AND BIOFEEDBACK TOOL FOR REHABILITATION

The use of ultrasound imaging as a biofeedback tool is an attractive application of real-time ultrasound imaging in rehabilitation. An ability to visualize the contraction of deep muscles in conjunction with the more superficial overlying muscles allows the physiotherapist to assess and problem-solve the patient's impairment. It can also assist to facilitate, or can provide evidence of, the effectiveness of a therapist's strategies in rehabilitation. The noninvasiveness of the technique, user friendliness and speed and ease of application are all appealing features.

There is now a focus in rehabilitation on the deep muscles that protect and support joints. Real-time ultrasound imaging could potentially be used to assist assessment and facilitation of various deep muscles of the body, including those of peripheral joints. To implement this technique, the first step is to identify the normal cross-sectional anatomy. As there are several artefacts that can occur while imaging, collaborative work between ultrasonographers and physiotherapists when exploring new areas is ideal. Also, due to the varying mechanics and orientation of muscle fascicles in different muscles, individual muscles will appear differently on imaging when they contract. Some deep muscles will be inaccessible, and for others acoustic windows may be found. For example, the obturator internus muscle can be observed by imaging diagonally from the anterior aspect through the bladder. In rehabilitation, for optimal benefit to be gained from imaging in the observation of deep muscles, research into the best sites and techniques is first required.

PREPARING A RESEARCH QUESTION

Research ideas and hypotheses usually originate in the clinic, from observations and interpretations made by the clinician. Often these ideas and hypotheses are difficult to test, especially in the case of rehabilitation of the deep muscles. Real-time ultrasound imaging is very useful in this situation to help prepare a research question. When a clinician has a theory on a particular dysfunction or a technique that possibly targets a particular muscle, ultrasound imaging gives the clinician an opportunity to test this quickly and noninvasively. Such pilot observations may speed up and refine a research question or send the researcher off to rethink the question.

LIMITATIONS OF THE USE OF REAL-TIME ULTRASOUND IMAGING

A MACHINE DOES NOT REPLACE CLINICAL SKILLS

While ultrasound imaging is an attractive modality for physiotherapists, simply visualizing muscles contracting will not by itself improve the patient's condition. For benefit to be obtained, real-time ultrasound imaging must be used in conjunction with good clinical skills, both in assessment and facilitation. It should be considered as an adjunct to physiotherapy assessment and treatment, not as a treatment method.

LIMITED FIELD OF VIEW

Ultrasound imaging is limited in its field of view to the area directly beneath the ultrasound transducer. This means that the field of view is much more restricted than in imaging techniques, such as magnetic resonance imaging and computed tomography scanning. For large muscles, such as the transversus abdominis, only a small part of the muscle can be imaged at one time. Furthermore what is happening simultaneously in other regions of the body cannot be assessed.

OBSERVATION OF MOVEMENT IS NOT AN OBJECTIVE MEASURE

While observation of movement is useful in assessment and powerful in treatment, observation of the contraction itself is not an objective measure. To derive measures of contraction, parameters of, for example depth of a muscle, can be measured and compared in the relaxed and contracted state. To use measures such as this for muscles that have not previously been measured, repeatability, reliability and validity studies need to be performed for use in research.

DIFFERING PATIENT BODY TYPES

Very large patients are sometimes difficult to image due to the depth of the subcutaneous tissue. Transducer selection can help to some degree in this case, but sometimes adequate resolution of images will not be possible. Also, some patients are 'ultrasound unfriendly' and are more difficult to image due to different tissue types.

COST

Cost of ultrasound imaging apparatus may be prohibitive to some. Overall, as technology improves, the price of ultrasound equipment is decreasing. There are now a greater number of less expensive portable ultrasound units on the market, and also there is a second-hand market. Often these units are suitable for physiotherapists, as we do not require nearly as high resolution of images for our purposes of muscle imaging when compared with obstetricians who are performing invasive procedures, such as amniocentesis and chorionic villus sampling.

SAFETY ISSUES

Use of ultrasound for feedback may raise some issues relating to safety, as this application is slightly different from many other assessments used in medicine. For example, obstetric imaging would not commonly be performed once or possibly twice per week for consecutive weeks, which is how this application might be used in rehabilitation. Ultrasound imaging is thought to be a safe modality and there are no known adverse effects of ultrasound imaging. However, as ultrasound is a form of energy, there is a risk (however small) that a biological effect could be produced on tissue (Docker & Duck 1991; Kremkau 1991; Preston 1991). As physiotherapists, we are familiar with the potential of therapeutic ultrasound (at much higher intensities) to induce thermal effects and cavitation caused by high acoustic pressures (Preston 1991), but damage of tissues has not been documented with diagnostic imaging. The output (intensity or acoustic power) is usually preset on ultrasound imaging equipment and not adjustable. When output is adjustable, safety principles would suggest that the lowest available setting, which provides an adequate image, be selected. Guidelines for minimizing risk during clinical application of ultrasound imaging have been provided (Docker & Duck 1991), with one of the main points being that the operator should be aware of the output

levels of the equipment and use minimal exposure levels possible to provide adequate images (Preston 1991).

CONCLUSION

Real-time ultrasound imaging is a modality that has great potential to be very useful in rehabilitation. Its uses in deep muscle assessment and facilitation are yet to be fully explored and realized. These techniques have been successfully applied to the abdominal and multifidus muscles in LBP patients for assessment and feedback, and the results of integration of this modality with other assessment techniques and good clinical skills are very encouraging. For integration into mainstream physiotherapy practice, the main emphasis must be on ultrasound imaging being an adjunct to assessment and treatment, with good clinical skills remaining of paramount importance. Real-time ultrasound imaging has the potential to be of tremendous benefit to the physiotherapy profession. The challenge for our profession is to introduce and implement it in such a manner that it is used judiciously and appropriately, to gain the credibility and acceptance that it deserves.

Acknowledgements

We wish to thank Dr D.H. Cooper for his continued assistance and guidance with ultrasound imaging and for reading the manuscript and providing useful feedback, and Mr Quentin Scott for assistance with illustrations and feedback.

REFERENCES

Berstein I, Juul N, Gronvall S, Bonde B, Klarskov P 1991 Pelvic floor muscle thickness measured by perineal ultrasonography. Scandinavian Journal of Urology and Nephrology Supplementum 137: 131–133

Chhem RK, Kaplan PA, Dussault RG 1994 Ultrasonography of the musculoskeletal system. Radiologic Clinics of North America 32(2): 275–289

Cresswell AG, Grundstrom A, Thorstensson A 1992 Observations on intrabdominal pressure and patterns of abdominal intramuscular activity in man. Acta Physiologica Scandinavica 144: 409–418

Docker MF, Duck FA 1991 The Safe Use of Diagnostic Ultrasound. British Institute of Radiology, London

Fish P 1990 Physics and Instrumentation of Diagnostic Medical Ultrasound. Wiley and Sons, London

Fornage BD, Rifkin MD 1988 Ultrasound examination of tendons. Radiologic Clinics of North America 22: 87–107

Gentile AM 1972 A working model of skill acquisition with application to teaching. Quest 17: 3–23

Harcke HT, Grissom LE, Finkelstein MS 1988 Evaluation of the musculoskeletal system with sonography. American Journal of Roentgenology 150: 1253–1261

Hides JA, Cooper DH, Stokes MJ 1992 Diagnostic ultrasound imaging for measurement of the lumbar multifidus muscle in normal young adults. Physiotherapy Theory and Practice 8: 19–26

Hides JA, Richardson CA, Jull GA 1995a Magnetic resonance imaging and ultrasonography of the lumbar multifidus muscle: Comparison of two different modalities. Spine 20: 54–58

Hides JA, Richardson CA, Jull GA, Davies SE 1995b Ultrasound imaging in rehabilitation. Australian Journal of Physiotherapy 41: 187–193

Hides JA, Richardson CA, Jull GA 1996 Multifidus muscle recovery is not automatic following resolution of acute first episode low back pain. Spine 21: 2763–2769

Hides JA, Stokes MJ, Saide M, Jull GA, Cooper DH 1994 Evidence of lumbar multifidus muscle wasting ipsilateral to symptoms in patients with acute/subacute low back pain. Spine 19(2): 165–172

Hodges PW, Richardson CA 1996 Inefficient muscular stabilisation of the lumbar spine associated with low back pain: a motor control evaluation of transversus abdominis. Spine 21: 2640–2650

Hodges PW, Richardson CA 1997 Feedforward contraction of transversus abdominis is not influenced by the direction of arm movement. Experimental Brain Research, 114: 362–370.

Hodges PW, Richardson CA 1998 Delayed postural contraction of transversus abdominis in low back pain associated with movement of the lower limbs. Journal of Spinal Disorders 11(1): 46–56

Hodges PW, Richardson CA, Jull GA 1996 Evaluation of the relationship between the findings of a laboratory and clinical test of transversus abdominis function. Physiotherapy Research International 1: 30–40

Kaplan PA, Matamoros A, Anderson JC 1990 Sonography of the musculoskeletal system. American Journal of Roentgenology 155: 237–245

Kogut BM, Sanigurskii GI, Maneshin VN 1990 Possibilities of using ultrasonography for intravital study of topographic anatomy of the anterior abdominal wall in humans. Arkhiv Anatomii Gistologii Embriologii 99: 55–59

Kremkau FW 1983 Ultrasound instrumentation: physical principles. In: Callen PW (ed) Ultrasonography in Obstetrics and Gynaecology. WB Saunders, Philadelphia, pp 313–324

Kremkau FW 1991 Biological Effects and Safety. In: Rumack CM, Wilson SR, Charboneau JW (eds) Diagnostic Ultrasound. London, Mosby, pp 19–29

Lacote M, Clevalier AM, Miranda A, Bleton JP, Stevenin P 1987 Clinical Evaluation of Muscle Function. Churchill Livingstone, Edinburgh, pp 290–293

Laine HR, Peltokallio P 1991 Ultrasonographic possibilities and findings in most common sports injuries. Annales Chirurgiae et Gynaecologiae 80(2): 127–133

Loo A, Stokes MJ 1990 Diagnostic Ultrasound Scanning for Clinical Estimation of Quadriceps Size and Estimation of Strength. Proceedings of the Third International Physiotherapy Congress, Hong Kong, pp 655–660

Martinson H, Stokes MJ 1991 Measurement of anterior tibial muscle size using real-time ultrasound imaging. European Journal of Applied Physiology 63: 250–254

Newell KM 1976 Knowledge of results and motor learning. Exercises and Sports Sciences Reviews 4: 195–228

O'Sullivan PB, Twomey LT Allison GT 1997 Evaluation of specific stabilising exercises in the treatment of chronic low back pain with radiological diagnosis of spondylolysis or spondylolisthesis. Spine 22(24): 2959–2967

Preston RC 1991 Output Measurements for Diagnostic Ultrasound. Springer, London

Richardson CA, Jull GA 1995 Muscle control–pain control. What exercises would you prescribe? Manual Therapy 1: 2–10

Richardson CA, Jull GA, Hodges PW, Hides JA 1998 Therapeutic Exercise for Spinal Segmental Stabilisation in Low Back Pain, Churchill Livingstone, Edinburgh

Rumack CM, Wilson SR, Charboneau JW 1991 Diagnostic Ultrasound, Mosby, London

Salmoni AW, Schmidt RA, Walter CB 1984 Knowledge of results and motor learning: A review and critical appraisal. Psychological Bulletin 95(3): 355–386

Saunders RC, James AE 1985 The Principles and Practice of Ultrasonography in Obstetrics and Gynaecology, 3rd edn. Appleton-Century-Crofts, Norwalk pp 1–14

Schmidt RA 1988 Motor Control and Learning, 2nd edn. Human Kinetics, Illinois

Sipila S, Suominen H 1993 Muscle ultrasonography and computed tomography in elderly trained and untrained women. Muscle and Nerve 16: 294–300

Stokes MJ, Hides JA, Nassiri DK 1997 Musculoskeletal ultrasound imaging: Diagnostic and treatment aid in rehabilitation. Physical Therapy Reviews 2(2): 73–92

Stokes MJ, Young A 1986 Measurement of quadriceps cross-sectional area by ultrasonography: a description of the technique and its application in physiotherapy. Physiotherapy Theory and Practice 2: 31–36

van Holsbeeck M, Strouse PJ 1993 Sonography of the shoulder: Evaluation of the subacromial-subdeltoid bursa. American Journal of Roentgenology 160(3): 561–564

van Holsbeeck M, Introcaso JH 1992 Musculoskeletal ultrasonography. Radiology Clinics of North America 30(5): 907–925

Wijma J, Tinga DJ, Visser GH 1991 Perineal ultrasonography in women with stress incontinence and controls: The role of the pelvic floor muscles. Gynecologic and Obstetric Investigation 32: 176–179

POSTSCRIPT

The use of real-time ultrasound imaging in clinical physiotherapy practice and research has increased since the main article was first published in 1998.

In many physiotherapy practices and hospital departments in Australia, real-time ultrasound imaging is routinely used in the rehabilitation of low back pain (LBP) patients. It is used to provide biofeedback and visualization of muscle action for the local synergy muscles, including the lumbar multifidus, transversus abdominis and pelvic floor. The advantages of real-time ultrasound compared with other more expensive imaging modalities include user friendliness, availability, ease of application, lack of exposure to ionizing radiation and portability.

Research into the effectiveness of using real-time ultrasound imaging to provide visual feedback of muscle action in rehabilitation has been conducted. It would seem from clinical practice that the technique enhances learning. This has been examined in subjects without LBP for the multifidus muscle (Van et al 2002). Naïve subjects were taught how to isometrically contract the multifidus muscle. The intervention group received feedback of their muscle activation by watching the multifidus contraction on the ultrasound monitor as it occurred. The control group received only verbal feedback of their performance. The increase in depth of the muscle that occurs during isometric contraction was measured. Results showed that subjects who received visual feedback of the muscle contraction using real-time ultrasound performed better when retested that those who did not receive the feedback. While this is a promising and seemingly logical finding, the study should be repeated with LBP subjects. In addition, for best clinical practice, the use of real-time ultrasound as a feedback tool needs to be considered with reference to the stages of motor relearning. Ultrasound feedback is most appropriate in the cognitive phase of motor relearning. Ultimately, the subjects must be able to perform the contractions in the absence of visual feedback to progress to the automatic phases of motor relearning.

The relationship between levels of muscle activation and what is observed on the ultrasound monitor has been investigated by Hodges et al (2003). They studied isometric contractions of the abdominal muscles, using both fine wire EMG and measurements of muscle width changes that occur with isometric muscle contraction on ultrasound imaging. The muscles studied were the transversus abdominis, internal oblique and external oblique muscles. Comparison between EMG and ultrasound measurements revealed that the correlation was best for the deep transversus abdominis and least reliable for the superficial external oblique muscle. While this may well relate to orientation of the muscle fibres and architecture of the muscles, it is encouraging to know that linear measurements of increase in muscle thickness on ultrasound imaging (for the transversus abdominis and internal oblique) correlated well with EMG activity. This would suggest that a combination of ultrasound imaging for the deep abdominal muscles and surface EMG for the external oblique muscles would be optimal for research.purposes

This combination of real-time ultrasound imaging and EMG has been used in research to examine the mechanism of action of the local synergy muscles (transversus abdominis, multifidus and the pelvic floor) (Richardson et al 2001). Snijders et al (1998) proposed that these muscles stiffen the sacroiliac joint and, therefore, force closure. In Holland, the Snijders group used Doppler imaging of vibrations to measure the stiffness of the sacroiliac joint (Buyruk et al 1999). The effects of both a global activation pattern of the abdominal muscles and a gentle co-contraction of the local synergy muscles on the stiffness of the sacroiliac joints in asymptomatic subjects were compared. The activation of the local synergy muscles stiffened the sacroiliac joints more than the global pattern of activation. Here, ultrasound was used both to measure joint stiffness and verify patterns of abdominal activation (in conjunction with EMG).

Current research is being conducted at the University of Queensland in association with biomedical engineers to develop prototypic models of deep muscle function in asymptomatic and chronic low back pain patients. One of the limitations of real-time ultrasound imaging is the limited field of view. MRI is being used to observe the whole 'muscular corset', and the results are being compared with those from real-time ultrasound imaging. As in previous investigations (Hides et al 1995), MRI is still regarded as the gold standard for imaging muscles, with superior resolution and a wider field of view. In other projects, real-time ultrasound imaging is being used to look at patterns of multifidus atrophy and activation in chronic LBP patients and surgical patients.

Ultrasound imaging appears to be very useful in both research and clinical practice. It is currently taught at the University of Queensland at both undergraduate and postgraduate levels. My opinion is that its applications will be further developed and utilized elsewhere in the body. The ability to image moving structures is still one of the main advantages for our profession. More research is required in the future for its potential to be maximized.

REFERENCES

Buyruk HM, Stan HJ, Snijders CJ, Lamens JS, Holland WP, Stinen TH 1999 Measurement of sacroiliac joint stiffness in peripartum pelvic pain patients with Doppler imaging of vibrations (DIV). European Journal of Obstetrics, Gynecologym, and Reproductive Biology 83: 159–163

Hides JA, Richardson CA, Jull GA 1995 MRI and ultrasonography of the lumbar multifudus muscle. Spine 20: 54–58

Hodges PW, Pengel LHM, Herbert RD, Gandevia SC 2003 Measurement of muscle contraction with ultrasound imaging. Muscle and Nerve. (in press)

Richardson CA, Snijders CJ, Hides JA, Damen L, Pas MS, Storm J 2001 The relationship between the transversely oriented abdominal muscles, sacroiliac joint mechanics and low back pain. Spine 27(4): 399–405

Snijders CJ, Ribbers MTLM, Bakker JV de, Steockart R, Stam HJ 1998 EMG recordings of abdominal and back muscles in various standing postures: Validations of a biomechanical model on sacroiliac joint stability. Journal of Electromyography and Kinesiology 8: 205–214

Van K, Hides J, Richardson CA 2002 Real-time ultrasound imaging enhances learning of an isometric multifidus contraction (submitted for publication)

Sacroiliac Joint

SECTION CONTENTS

11

Sacroiliac dysfunction in dancers with low back pain

L. E. DeMann Jr
Manhattan Chiropractic Center, New York, USA

Low back pain is a common occurrence in dancers. Studies have shown its prevalence to be around 12% of all dance-type injuries. It is commonly thought by health professionals who specialize in dance medicine that sacroiliac (SI) dysfunction is one of the more common causes of low back pain in dancers. The aetiology of SI dysfunction in dancers is related to both the biomechanics of the SI joint and the physiological demands placed on the SI joint from the dynamics of dance. Injury to the SI joint can be due to a combination of a single traumatic incident from overuse factors involving repetitive microtrauma, or from emotional stress. Clinical manifestations could be pain in the back, buttock, hip and leg, and limitation of movement specific to dance. Diagnosis is based on the deviation from normal of both the static and kinetic functions of the lower back and pelvis in its relationship to the biomechanics of dance. Treatment is aimed at relieving pain, restoring the function of the SI joint and returning the dancer to full function. *Manual Therapy* (1997) **2(1)**, 2–10

INTRODUCTION

Low back pain is a common occurrence in dancers. Studies have shown the incidence of low back pain to be around 12% of all dance injuries, with one study reporting it to be as high as 23% (Table 11.1) (Quirk 1983; Stephens 1986; Reid 1987; Schafle et al 1990; Garrick & Requa 1993; Solomon et al 1995). The most common problems causing low back pain are listed in Table 11.2 while less common ones are listed in Table 11.3 (DeMann 1992). Although there is much latitude in the literature (Washington 1978), it is thought by many health professionals who specialize in dance medicine that SI dysfunction is the

Table 11.1 Percentage of low back injuries to total dance injuries in different studies.

Frequency of injury by site, a comparison of studies

Quirk	Stephens	Reid	Schafle et al	Garrick & Requa	Solomon et al	Average
(1983)	(1986)	(1987)	(1990)	(1993)	(1994)	
8.5%	9.4%	10.8%	12%	23%	8%	12%

Table 11.2 Common causes of low back pain in dancers.

- Sacroiliac dysfunction
- Lumbar derangements
- Disc syndromes
- Facet syndromes
- Stress fracture
- Spondylosis
- Muscular syndromes
  — Piriformis
  — Psoas
  — Gluteus maximus
  — Quadratus lumborum
  — Erector spinae
  — Hamstrings

Table 11.3 Less common causes of low back pain in dancers.

- Spondylolisthesis
- Scoliosis
- Osteoarthritis
- Periostitis (due to direct pressure over the dorsal aspect of the spinous process from working with the back against a hard floor surface)
- Compensatory responses to other injured areas (i.e. hip, knee, foot and ankle

most common cause of low back pain in dancers (Marshall 1995). To date there has been no study that has categorized the specific types of spinal problems nor any study quantifying these problems. A variation in the interpretation of the types of spinal problems may exist because of the wide variety and styles of dance and the different physiological influences that these varying styles of dance place on the body. The physiological demands of modern dance are different to those of classical ballet and those of Broadway dancing (musical theatre) are different to those of ballet and modern dance. Even within the context of ballet

there are many different styles of dance. Generally, it has not been shown that one particular type of dance is more likely to lead to injury than another. There are, however, differences in distribution of injuries to various regions of the body. Each system of dance, each technique, and each practice and performance schedule will have a different effect on the biomechanics of the body, translating into a slightly different usage factor, which, in turn, may lead to a slightly different injury profile. For the purposes of this article the focus will be specifically the SI joint and its relationship to classical dance — ballet.

Dysfunction of the SI joint has been extensively reported as a major cause of low back pain since the early part of this century (Brooke 1924; Cox 1927). It was not until the late 1930s that interest in the SI joint diminished, as focus shifted towards the lumbar disc and its role in back pain. Interest in the SI joint resurfaced again in the 1970s and continues today (Davis & Lentle 1978; Kirkaldy-Willis & Hill 1979).

The role that the SI joint plays in its relationship to dance is a vital one, as the dynamics of dance are intimately involved with the biomechanics of the spine and pelvis. A great many of the movements of dance, concerned with the lower extremity as well as the torso, are made possible by the muscles of the back and pelvis (Micheli 1983; Don Tigny 1985; Keller & West 1995; Laws 1995). Stabilization of almost any dance posture will involve the muscles and ligaments of the spine. Fundamental to dance is turnout, i.e. extreme external rotation of the hip, which is the foundation of ballet and from which all steps and all movements are performed (Warren 1989). Combined with the extreme range of hip extension (arabesque), the rapid movement of the leg in all directions, the jumps, leaps, twisting, turning and lifting and carrying of other dancers, it is easy to understand the tremendous forces involved in the workings of both the lower back and pelvis (see Figs 11.1, 11.2 & 11.3). During gait, the amount of accessory motion at the SI joint helps protect the lumbar intervertebral discs by decreasing torsional stresses associated with pelvic rotation. Movement at the SI joint also helps to decrease forward shearing at the L5/S1 junction during the hip extension phase of gait (Don Tigny 1990; Lindsay et al 1993). Dancers utilize this movement to its maximum and any restriction of the SI joint mobility will greatly enhance the possibility of disturbing the mechanics of the entire spine and pelvis. Given the tremendous forces involved in dance, this could put the dancer at risk of injury to the lower back.

ANATOMY/BIOMECHANICS OF THE SACROILIAC JOINT

Categorizing the SI joint as synovial or fibrous has always been a problem (Bowen & Cassidy 1981). However, the current accepted view is that of Williams (1995) who classifies it as synovial. The confusion is due to the nature of its cartilaginous surfaces. The SI surfaces are C shaped in appearance. They are irregular with marked depressions on the sacral side and elevations on the iliac side. These irregularities develop after puberty and vary in individuals. The sacral surface has a smooth, glistening appearance of hyaline cartilage, while the iliac surface is duller and darker, appearing more fibrous in nature. The fibrous cartilage on the iliac side of the joint has been shown to undergo degenerative changes at a young age (Mierau et al 1984), and these degenerative changes have been reported in dancers (Sammarco 1984). It is, however, not currently

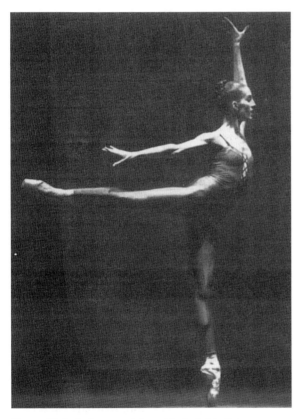

Figure 11.1 Arabesque. Integral to ballet is the arabesque where one leg is held in extension. Notice that both legs are in turnout position, the hip and leg being fully externally rotated. Turnout is fundamental to ballet and is a part of all ballet positions.

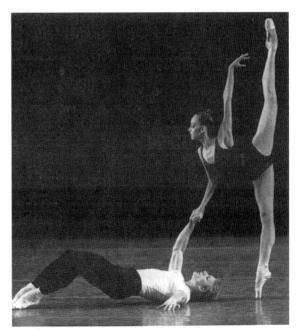

Figure 11.2 Arabesque penchee. This is similar to a straight arabesque except for being performed while bending forward. A great deal of strength is needed to sustain these balletic positions.

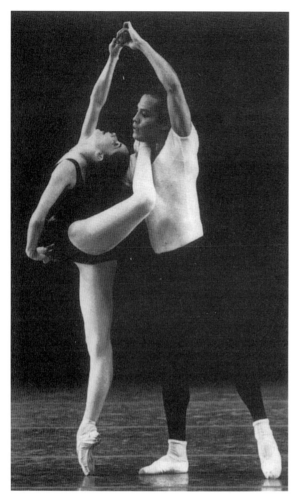

Figure 11.3 Extreme arabesque with attitude. It is easy to understand the tremendous amount of movement needed in the hips, back and pelvis and the forces used in maintaining these postures.

posterior superior spine to the lateral tubercles of the sacrum.

The function of the SI joint is partly that of a weight-bearing joint and also partly that of a joint with a role in energy absorption. Williams (1995) states that the function of the SI joint is to transmit the weight of the upper body to the lower limbs. A nutation movement occurs, which creates a small degree of sagittal rotation in the anterior–posterior direction (Lavignolle et al 1983). The centre of rotation is located posterior to the S2 tubercle.

The SI joint is innervated from the sacral plexus, the dorsal rami of S1 and S2, as well as from branches of the superior gluteal (L4, L5, S1) and obturator (L2, L3, L4) nerves. As with all synovial joints, nerve fibres are located in the periosteum of the bone, muscles, blood vessels, ligaments and joint capsule. These innervated structures comprise the pain-sensitive tissues that may give rise to joint pain. With such a wide overlap of innervation the SI joint is capable of referring pain into most parts of the back, groin, buttocks, thigh and leg (Norman & May 1956; McGregor & Cassidy 1983). Pain originating from the SI joint is capable of simulating a whole range of conditions.

DIAGNOSIS

Pain is accepted as a subjective complaint, and so the level and degree of pain each person feels will be different from one person to the next. Dancers generally have a very high tolerance of pain, as they are often accustomed to having some pain and discomfort in their body. There is a fine line separating pain from just overwork or fatigue and pain from overuse. Complicating matters somewhat is that dancers generally do not complain about pain unless it is interfering with their dancing (Krasnow et al 1994). They may be experiencing pain in their everyday life, such as in sitting or sleeping, but it is not until this pain and discomfort starts to interfere with their dancing that they will usually seek professional advice. It is likely that the pain threshold above which dancers seek professional advice is usually greater than that for non-dancers.

known whether these degenerative changes are of any clinical significance.

Based on anatomical knowledge, movement of the SI joint is restricted to a small range of motion, which decreases with increasing age (Don Tigny 1985). The joint is surrounded by large ligaments that bind the pelvic ring into a stable, weight-bearing structure. The three major ligaments are the anterior sacroiliac ligament, which is a short flat band; the interosseous ligament, which is a very strong band consisting of short stout fibres and thought to be the main stabilizing force; and the posterior sacroiliac ligament, extending from the

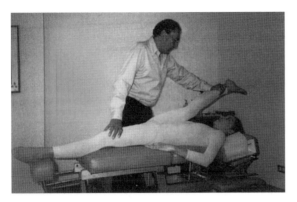

Figure 11.4 Straight leg raise. Assessment of the lower back via the SLR is often difficult and confusing because quite often the range of motion can approach and often exceed 180 degrees.)

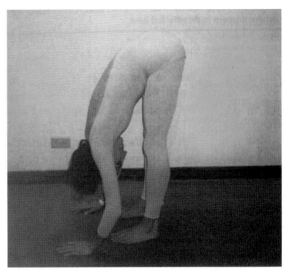

Figure 11.5 Forward flexion. Flexion of the lumbar spine and pelvis is effortless in dancers and its degree greatly exceeds that of non-dancers and other athletes.

As with any problem affecting the lower back, diagnosis is as much an art form as a science. The diagnosis of SI dysfunction is no exception. Given the complexities of the back, it is very difficult to accurately make a specific diagnosis (Porterfield & Derosa 1991). The difficulty exists because: (i) there is considerable overlapping of symptoms from one condition to another; (ii) rarely does one back problem exist in isolation, but rather as a complex, with one condition affecting another; and (iii) there is no one diagnostic test or group of tests that will conclusively differentiate one type of problem from another.

In evaluating the dancer with low back pain it is important to remember exactly the type of person being assessed. Many of the physical tests may be negative in the dancer, which otherwise may be positive in the non-dancer. A dancer's normal range of motion in the lumbar spine, hips and pelvis is often much greater than that of the non-dancer and for the most part other athletes as well (see Figs 11.4, 11.5 & 11.6). Their strength and their ability to hold posture throughout the entire range-of-motion arc is also much greater than in non-dancers and other athletes. Consequently many tests that have parameters in range of motion for producing pain or no pain have to be modified for the physiological joint ranges of the dancer (DeMann 1995). A test such as the straight leg raise, which is a standard test used in exami-

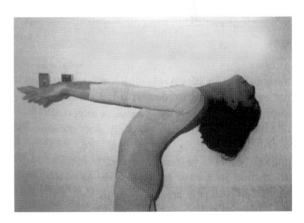

Figure 11.6 Backward extension. As with all movements of the spine and pelvis, movement again is effortless and its extent usually greater in the dancer.

nation of the lumbar spine, is virtually meaningless in the dancer as their passive range can often exceed 180 degrees.

The history and physical examination of the dancer complaining of low back pain will form the basic element for a working diagnosis. The diagnosis is based on evaluating the deviation from normal of both the static and kinetic functions of the low back and pelvis. It is also formed by an analysis of the mechanisms specific to dance and the involvement of the anatomy and its biomechanical applications (Sohl & Bowling 1990; Hald 1992).

Table 11.4 Diagnostic tests for sacroiliac dysfunction.

1. Static palpation of SI joint — posterior SI ligament
   The SI ligament is one of the main stabilizing components of the SI joint. If there is any dysfunction of this joint, this ligament will exhibit some degree of distress, usually pinpoint tenderness along the course of this ligament.

2. Kinetic palpation of SI joint with leg extension
   With the patient prone the palms of hands are gently placed over each SI joint. The patient is asked to extend each leg one at a time, while gentle pressure is applied downward with both hands. The patient with an SI joint dysfunction will either exhibit discomfort on extension of one leg or show compensatory signs by either trying to raise the pelvis off the table on the involved side, or increasing rotation/turnout of the extended leg.

3. Gillet standing flexion test
   With the patient standing, place the thumb of the right hand over the second sacral tubercle and the thumb of the left hand over the PSIS. Instruct the patient to flex the left hip and knee to 90°. In the normal joint the thumb of the left hand will move caudad. In the dysfunctional joint the thumb will move cephalad, thus evaluating the movement dynamics of the SI joint.

4. Supine distraction/iliac gapping test
   The patient lies supine, and the heels of the hands are placed on the ASIS of the ilium. Pressure is applied downward and laterally outward. The arms are crossed to increase the lateral component of force applied, creating strain on the SI ligaments. Discomfort is felt in the affected joint.

5. Supine single knee to chest torsion test (Gaenslen's Test)
   With the patient supine, the knee on the affected side is drawn up to the chest. The opposite hip and leg are kept fully extended. This manoeuvre produces rotatory stress and can increase pain in the presence of SI dysfunction.

6. SI compression test
   With the patient lying on their side, downward pressure applied on the lateral aspect of the pelvis can produce pain in the region of the affected SI joint.

7. Single leg stand
   Have the patient stand on the leg in the neutral position (not in turnout), with the opposite leg flexed 90° at the hip and knee. The patient may stabilize him/herself by lightly holding on to a stationary object. Have the patient remain in this position for 30–60 seconds. The standing leg will increase the weight-bearing properties of the affected SI joint, thereby producing pain in the affected joint.

SI joint dysfunction can exist by itself; however, it is more commonly seen in conjunction with some other structural or mechanical deficit, and/or with some type of soft tissue muscular involvement (Greenman 1989). SI joint dysfunction is usually unilateral, with no preference or dominance for either side (Alderink 1991; Fortin et al 1992). It can be acute or chronic.

X-ray analysis is usually negative, with no significant findings (Schuchman & Cannon 1986). Even if osteoarthritis is seen affecting the iliac portion of the SI joint, as stated earlier, it may be of no clinical significance.

In a pure SI dysfunction there are no neurological findings, no loss or diminution of reflexes, no muscle weakness, or any sensory loss (Le Blanc 1992). However, in combination with other back problems such as disc or piriformis involvement, neurological symptoms may exist.

Seven of the more common diagnostic tests used to isolate SI dysfunction are listed in Table 11.4. One or more of these tests may be positive while others may not be. There is also a great deal of tester subjectivity involved with these tests (Blower & Griffin 1984; Potter & Rothstein 1985; Cummings & Crowell 1988; Drefuss et al 1994; Laslett & Williams 1994).

Pain patterns run the spectrum of low back pain, ranging from localized pain over the SI joint, to pain across the low back, to pain radiating into the buttock and thigh (Beal 1989; Fortin et al 1992). The dancer might complain of pain or limitation of their arabesque (full leg extension), noticing that one side is higher than the other; to achieve the desired height they may have to compensate by rotating, turning out, or 'opening up' the pelvis more on the affected side. Since the SI joint absorbs concussion forces, jumping may become difficult, especially when a dancer lands on the leg of the affected side.

CLINICAL CONSIDERATIONS

Problems affecting the SI joint can be caused by a single traumatic incident, overuse factors arising from repetitive micro trauma, emotional stress and tension, or any combination of these.

Understanding the contributory factors involved in the dancer with low back pain will help greatly in the treatment of these dysfunctions.

CONTRIBUTORY FACTORS

There is often a synergistic relationship between SI dysfunction and other factors, most notably aberrant lumbar spine dynamics and lumbar pelvic muscular involvement (Bachrach 1988). The biomechanics of the lumbar spine are intimately involved with the lumbar pelvic region and alterations in this area can have an effect on the function of the SI joint. Problems involving the lumbar disc(s), facet syndromes and lumbar spine derangements (an alteration of the normal dynamics of a joint wherein there is an alteration to the structural and/or functional relationships) can all contribute to problems of the SI joint. Conversely, alterations in SI joint function can affect these and other areas. Muscle function, likewise, can not only be affected because of SI dysfunction or lumbar spine problems but it can cause problems in these areas. Strain on the muscles of the lower back from overuse (such as the erector spinae, quadratus lumborum and piriformis) can adversely alter SI function. Clinically, differential diagnosis of this 'chicken or egg' conundrum is a challenge.

Other contributory factors affecting the function of the SI joint in dancers are functional or structural abnormalities, such as leg length discrepancy, pelvic tilt and scoliosis. Scoliosis has been reported to be more prevalent in dancers than in non-dancers (Hamilton et al 1992), while leg length has been noted to be an important factor concerned with the dynamics of the spine and pelvis (Henry 1995).

Muscle imbalance is another important consideration with the dancer. Muscle balance in this instance refers to the strength and flexibility of opposing muscles relative to one another. A well-balanced ballet class will emphasize movement in all directions. As a result good training will develop muscles symmetrically and proportionally. However, in some instances excessive training and improper technique may cause imbalances in certain groups of muscles (Bachrach 1988). In ballet the

hip and pelvis are the most common sites for muscle imbalance, the most frequently affected being the piriformis, which is used in external rotation of the hip, the turnout position in dance. Overuse of this muscle, for example when the dancer tries to force their turnout, can directly contribute to problems with the SI joint (DeMann 1995).

PSYCHOLOGICAL AND EMOTIONAL FACTORS

It is commonly accepted today that emotional and psychological factors play a role in low back pain, yet to what extent and exactly how is still not known. Every dancer, no matter what their status or experience level, will suffer performance anxiety, peer pressure and self-criticism in their professional life. Anxiety is common before a performance and is heightened by participation in a new ballet or role. Even the most seasoned of veterans is not exempt from exhibiting some degree of anxiety before a performance. This 'self critique' evolves from the 'working in front of a mirror' attitude, whereby dancers are constantly striving to attain an ideal in both body image and movement that is, at best, elusive. Adding to this is the struggle of balancing their own artistic interpretations of dance with that of others. The late great choreographer George Balanchine often stated to his dancers 'don't think, just do!' (Martins, personal communication), implying that this expression is somehow to come from some intangible place mystically deep within themselves.

The role that emotional and psychological factors play in dancers is currently being explored (Hamilton et al 1989; Liederbach et al 1994). However, much is still not understood about the specific pathophysiology of low back pain and emotional stress, or indeed SI dysfunction and emotional stress. Hypothetically, emotional stress will cause tension within the body and body tissues, especially, but not limited to, the muscular system. Since the amount of movement in the SI joint is small, any further restriction of movement to this joint can adversely affect its function. The dancer, who needs maximum movement to perform, is thus susceptible to any restriction of SI movement. Not only can emotional stress and tension possibly act as a causative factor in SI joint dysfunction and low back pain, but it can act as a factor in the exacerbation of the dysfunction. There are times when a dancer with low back pain cannot dance due to the pain. They may feel that they are missing valuable (either financial or preparation) time if they are unable to rehearse or perform because of their injury. Not only does this add to their emotional stress and tension but it puts the dancer under pressure to return to work too soon.

WORK AND ENVIRONMENTAL FACTORS

It has been reported that the majority of ballet injuries are due to overuse factors (Ryan & Stephens 1987). The classic interpretation and application of overuse is such that the body or body part(s) used have their physiological capacity exceeded by the physical demands placed upon them. In dance this can happen in a number of ways: (i) the amount of time spent working and rehearsing; (ii) using the body in new and different ways from which it is accustomed; (iii) repetitive movements; (iv) working in different environments.

Practice and discipline, words often associated with a dancer, are essential because of the hard and lengthy work necessary not only to become a dancer but to maintain a dance career. The typical dancer begins their training at an early age, often at or before the age of 8 years, and will begin their professional career between the ages of 17 and 19 years. The professional dancer's schedule commonly starts in the morning with an hour and a half ballet class, followed by rehearsals lasting from 2 to 5 hours, and ending with a performance at night. During non-performance periods, rehearsal schedules may be longer. This rigid schedule is adhered to 6 days a week continuously for weeks or months depending on the company involved.

Repetition is a key factor in overuse injuries and the dancer is both vulnerable and susceptible to its effects and consequences. When rehearsing a ballet the dancer will repeat steps and movements in order to learn the ballet. When a new ballet is cho-

reographed, the choreographer will often ask the dancer to repeat steps many times, sometimes excessively, in order to see and evaluate the dance. Ballets, however, are often not new. More often they have been created earlier and usually for a specific dancer utilizing their specific and sometimes unique physical characteristics in order to create postures and movements for that dance. The dancer is expected to enter into a role in which their body dynamics may not be the same as the original dancer for which it was choreographed. This form of overuse is common in dance and is best expressed by Heather Watts, a former principal dancer with the New York City Ballet:

Every time I performed Violin Concerto, a very challenging ballet, I put my back out. This ballet was choreographed earlier on a different ballerina, whose body type was different than mine, and even though I had a great deal of artistic success with it, my back did not (Watts, personal communication).

Environmental factors will also play a large role in low back pain with the dancer. Different floor surfaces on which the dancer rehearses and performs can contribute to the concussive forces transmitted to the lower back. The ideal floor surface is a wood floor which is 'sprung', covered by a smooth synthetic rubberized surface. Often dancers do not have the opportunity of working on the ideal floor, but rather a much harder unforgiving surface. Climate control is another common contributor to dance-related lower back injuries. Dancers frequently complain of cold or draughty studios or theatres. In some cases classes or performances may be outdoors in pavilion tents or amphitheatres. Cool temperatures make it difficult to warmup properly or stay warmedup, creating a potentially harmful situation.

TREATMENT

The therapeutic goal of treatment of the SI joint in dancers is the relief of pain, restoring the biomechanics of the SI joint, normalizing any lumbar spine derangement as well as any muscular involvement in the back and pelvis, and having the dancer return to dance as soon as possible.

Treatment of the dancer with low back pain is a combination of both managing the patient and managing the functional or structural abnormality responsible for the condition.

In the treatment of SI dysfunction it is extremely helpful to evaluate the following.

1. Is it acute or chronic, or is it an acute exacerbation of a chronic condition?
2. Is the dysfunction either a primary or secondary involvement (either involving muscles or lumbar derangement)?
3. What are the functional or structural implications (e.g. leg length discrepancy, muscle imbalance, lumbar pelvic dysfunction)?
4. What are the social/psychological influences (the relationship of emotional stress and tension)?
5. What are the working conditions, technique and usage factors, e.g. type of floor surface, whether it is a hard surface or sprung floor, or a raked stage (a stage that has a slight incline from front to back) and the choreographic style?

The importance of movement in the dancer cannot be stressed enough. Dance is expression through movement. The role of the SI joint is vital not only in terms of the biomechanics of the spine and pelvis but in its relationship to the dynamics of dance. Dysfunction of the SI joint can have a disastrous effect in the dancer, as it can greatly impair their ability to move freely. SI joint trouble in dancers can quite simply be described as malfunction within the articular bed such that the joint is either hypomobile (fixated) or hypermobile. Both situations are problematic for the dancer, but because of (i) the architecture of the SI joint, (ii) the strength of the ligamentous support of the joint, and (iii) the dancer's need for full range of motion, the most common scenario is a fixated or hypomobile SI joint.

After the patient has been thoroughly evaluated, a comprehensive treatment programme can be set up. This author utilizes a combination of manipulation, exercise therapy and adjunctive therapy in the conservative management of this syndrome.

MANIPULATION

Manipulation has been reported to be very effective in patients with SI joint dysfunction (Bourdillon 1987). It is thought to work by stimulating the mechanoreceptors within the joint (Kirkaldy-Willis 1983). A manipulation is indicated when an SI joint is not properly functioning within its range of motion, most commonly seen as a fixated or hypomobile joint. There are numerous forms of manipulation that are effective with SI joint dysfunction. The goal for the use of any form of manipulation is to normalize the alignment and movement within the articular bed. This author prefers either a non-force technique, such as DeJarnette blocking (De Jarnette 1985) used when there is significant accompanying muscle spasms, or a more low force–high velocity sidelying technique, applied when there is little resistance with muscle tightness (see Figs 11.7 & 11.8).

EXERCISE THERAPY

There are many different types of exercises that can be effectively applied. It is, however, critical to identify the specific muscle imbalance and target the exercise to that imbalance. The most common muscles involved in SI dysfunction are:

- Piriformis
- Iliopsoas
- Hamstrings
- Quadratus lumborum
- Gluteus maximus.

Manual testing of muscles will give an indication of the muscles' strength. If weakness is demonstrated in a muscle tested then strengthening exercises are prescribed. If the muscles are short then lengthening exercises are prescribed.

The majority of muscle imbalance problems in dancers stem from improper training and work habits. In situations where this arises it is important to recognize the vital role that a dance teacher plays in the dancer's career. Most muscle imbalance problems can be corrected by the dancer taking proper classes under the guidance of a good teacher.

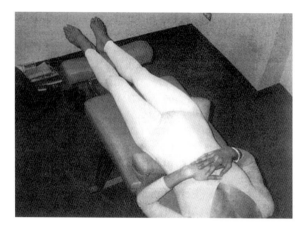

Figure 11.7 DeJarnette blocking procedure (category II). The patient is in the supine position. One wedge is placed under the iliac crest on the short leg side (posterior ilium) in the direction perpendicular to the body. The second wedge is placed under the gluteal fold in the direction facing the first wedge.

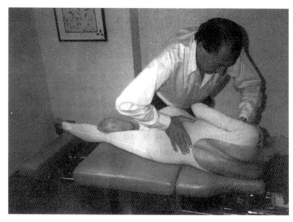

Figure 11.8 Sidelying SI joint reduction technique. The patient is in the sidelying position with the fixated SI joint lying up and their thigh flexed 90 degrees. The clinician applies downward pressure with their thigh on to the patient's flexed thigh. The contact hand is placed over and lateral to the SI joint. A quick short thrust is then delivered with the contact hand in the direction of posterior to anterior while applying greater downward pressure on the patient's thigh into adduction.

ADJUNCTIVE THERAPY

In the acute phase, ice is indicated to help control inflammation, while in the chronic phase heat may prove more beneficial in helping to promote an increase in circulation and relaxation. Basic modalities include electrical stimulation used in the acute phase to help relieve oedema and muscle spasm; ultrasound is used in the chronic phase to help relieve adhesions and promote healing. The use of bracing is ineffective with dancers, as it is virtually impossible to conceal it under leotards and tights and wearing it inhibits the dancer's movement. Nutritional support may also be considered. Oral administration of a protease mixture (proteolytic enzymes, which help reduce inflammation during the acute phase), a calcium/magnesium formula (needed for the repair of bone and connective tissue), an antioxidant mixture (destroys free radicals which are released during injury) and glucosamine sulphate (fundamental building blocks for the synthesis and repair of cartilage) can possibly be of help (Bucci 1994).

The general health and well being of a dancer is usually very good; they are generally in excellent physical condition and mostly are eager to resume work as quickly as possible. They have great discipline in their professional life, which helps greatly whenever they are rehabilitating an injury. The response to conservative treatment for SI dysfunction is usually excellent, especially when combined with successful patient management.

Acknowledgements

I would like to thank Diane Cordes for her support and help in preparing this manuscript, Lourdes Lopez and the New York City Ballet for use of photographs and Russell Iwami for his research help.

REFERENCES

Alderink GJ 1991 The sacroiliac joint: review of anatomy, mechanics and function. Journal of Orthopaedic and Sports Physical Therapy 13(2): 71–84

Bachrach RM 1988 Injuries to the low back/pelvic somatic dysfunction. Orthopaedic Review 17: 1037–1043

Beal MC 1989 The sacroiliac problem: review of anatomy, mechanics and diagnosis. Journal of the American Osteopathic Association 89(8): 1027–1035

Blower DW, Griffin AJ 1984 Clinical sacroiliac tests in ankylosing spondylitis and other causes of low back pain. Annals of the Rheumatic Diseases 43(2): 192–195

Bourdillon JF 1987 In: Spinal Manipulation, 4th edn. William Heinemann Medical Books Ltd, London, pp58–72

Bowen V, Cassidy JD 1981 Macroscopic and microscopic anatomy of the sacroiliac joint from embryonic life until the eighth decade. Spine 6: 620–628

Brooke R 1924 The sacroiliac joint. Journal of Anatomy 58: 298–305

Bucci LR 1994 Nutrition Applied to Injury Rehabilitation and Sports Medicine. CRC Press, Boca Raton, Florida

Cox HH 1927 Sacroiliac subluxation as a cause of backache. Surgery Gynaecology and Obstetrics 45: 637–649

Cummings GS, Crowell RD 1988 Source of error in clinical assessment of innominate rotation. Physical Therapy 68(1): 77–78

Davis P, Lentle B 1978 Evidence of sacroiliac disease as a common cause of low backache in women. Lancet 2: 496–497

De Jarnette MB 1985 In: Sacral-occipital technique, 2nd edn. Nebraska City NE

DeMann Jr LE 1992 Low back pain: a conservative approach to a common problem in dancers. Presented Medart World Congress on Arts Medicine, New York, March

DeMann Jr LE 1995 Piriformis involvement in dancers with low back pain — a conservation approach. Journal of Back and Musculoskeletal Rehabilitation 5: 247–257

Don Tigny RL 1990 Anterior dysfunction of the sacroiliac joint as a major factor in the aetiology of the idiopathic low back pain syndrome. Physical Therapy 70: 250–265

Don Tigny RL 1985 Function and pathomechanics of the sacroiliac joint. Physical Therapy 65(1): 35–44

Drefuss P, Dryer S, Griffin J, Hoffmann J, Walsh N 1994 Positive sacroiliac screening tests in asymptomatic adults. Spine 19(10): 1138–1143

Fortin JD, Dwyer AP, Aprill CN, West S, Pier J 1992 Sacroiliac joint: pain referral maps. Presented at the annual meeting of The North American Spine Society Boston, Massachusetts, July 9–11

Garrick JG, Requa RK 1993 Ballet injuries: an analysis of epidemiology and financial outcome. American Journal of Sports Medicine 21: 586–590

Greenman PE 1989 In: Principles of Diagnosis and Treatment of Pelvic Girdle Dysfunction. Principles of Manual Medicine. Williams and Wilkins, Baltimore, 220–270

Hald RD 1992 Dance injuries. Primary Care 19: 393–411

Hamilton LH, Hamilton WG, Meltzer JD, Marshall P, Molnar M 1989 Personality, stress, and injuries in professional ballet dancers. American Journal of Sports Medicine 17: 263–267

Hamilton WG, Hamilton LH, Marshall P, Molnar M 1992 A profile of the musculoskeletal characteristics of elite professional ballet dancers. American Journal of Sports Medicine 20(3): 267–273

Henry L 1995 Leg length discrepancy in the professional dancer. Journal of Back and Musculoskeletal Rehabilitation 5: 209–217

Keller K, West JC 1995 Functional movement impairment in dancers: an assessment and treatment approach utilising the biomechanical asymmetry corrector to restore normal mechanics of the spine and pelvis. Journal of Back and Musculoskeletal Rehabilitation 5: 219–233

Kirkaldy-Willis WH 1983 Manipulation. In: Kirkaldy-Willis WH. Managing Low Back Pain. Churchill Livingstone, New York, p. 177

Kirkaldy-Willis WH, Hill RJ 1979 A more precise diagnosis for low back pain. Spine 4: 102–109

Krasnow D, Kerr G, Mainwarms L 1994 Psychology of dealing with the injured dancer. Medical Problems of Performing Artists 9: 7–9

Laslett M, Williams M 1994 The reliability of selected pain provocation tests for sacroiliac joint pathology. Spine 19(11): 1243–1249

Lavignolle B, Vital JM, Senegas J 1983 An approach to the functional anatomy of the sacroiliac joints in vivo. Anatomia Clinica 5: 169–176

Laws K 1995 The physics and aesthetics of vertical movements in dance. Medical Problems of Performing Arts: 41–47

LeBlanc K 1992 Sacroiliac sprain: an overlooked cause of back pain. American Family Physician 46(5): 1459–1463

Liederbach M, Gleim GW, Nicholas JA 1994 Physiologic and psychological measurements of performance stress and onset of injuries in professional ballet dancers. Medical Problems of Performing Artists 9: 10–14

Lindsay DM, Meeuwisse WH, Vyse A, Mooney ME, Summersides J 1993 Lumbosacral dysfunctions in elite cross-country skiers. Journal of Orthopaedic and Sports Physical Therapy 18(5): 580–585

McGregor M, Cassidy D 1983 Post-surgical sacroiliac joint syndrome. Journal of Manipulative and Physiological Therapies March 6(1): 1–11

Marshall P 1995 Management adaptations for sacroiliac dysfunction in classical dancers. Journal of Back and Musculoskeletal Rehabilitation (5): 235–246

Micheli LJ 1983 Back injuries in dancers. Clinical Sports Medicine 2(3): 473–484

Mierau DR, Cassidy JD, Hamin T, Milne RA 1984 Sacroiliac joint dysfunction and low back pain in school aged children. Journal of Manipulative and Physiological Therapeutics 7(2): 81–84

Norman F, May A 1956 Sacroiliac conditions simulating intervertebral disc disease syndrome. Western Journal of Surgery 64: 461–462.

Porterfield A, Derosa C 1991 Functional assessment of the lumbopelvic region. In: Mechanical Low Back Pain —

Perspectives in Functional Anatomy. WB Saunders, Philadelphia, pp123–163

Potter NA, Rothstein JM 1985 Intertester reliability for selected clinical tests of the sacroiliac joint. Physical Therapy 65(11): 1671–1675

Quirk R 1983 Ballet injuries: the Australian experience. Clinical Sports Medicine 2: 507–514

Reid DC 1987 Preventing injuries to the young ballet dancer. Physiotherapy Canada 39: 231–236

Ryan A, Stephens RE 1987 The epidemiology of dance injuries. In: Ryan A, Stephens RE (eds) Dance Medicine: A Comprehensive Guide. Pluribus Press, Chicago, 3–15

Sammarco GJ 1984 Diagnosis and treatment in dancers. Clinical Orthopaedic Review 187: 176–187

Schafle M, Requa R, Garrick JG 1990 Comparison of patterns of injury in ballet, modern, and aerobic dance. In: Solomon R, Minton SC, Solomon J (eds) Preventing Dance Injuries: An Interdisciplinary Perspective. American Alliance for Health, Physical Education, Recreation and Dance, Reston, VA

Schuchman JA, Cannon C 1986 Sacroiliac strain syndrome: diagnosis and treatment. Texas Medicine 82(6): 33–36

Sohl P, Bowling A 1990 Injuries to dancers. Prevalence, treatment and prevention. Journal of Sports Medicine 9: 317–322

Solomon R, Micheli L, Solomon J, Kelley T 1995 The cost of injuries in a professional ballet company. Medical Problems of Performing Artists 3: 3–10

Stephens R 1986 The biomechanical aspects of injuries in elite dancers. In: Ryan AJ, Stephans RE (Eds.) Dance Medicine: A Comprehensive Guide, Pluribus Press, Chicago

Warren GN 1989 Classical Ballet Technique. The University of South Florida Press, Gainesville

Washington L 1978 Musculoskeletal injuries in theatrical dancers: site, frequency and severity. American Journal of Sports Medicine 6: 75–98

Williams PL (eds) 1995 Gray's Anatomy, 38th edn. Churchill Livingstone, New York, pp674–676

General

12

Functional stability re-training: principles and strategies for managing mechanical dysfunction

M. J. Comerford   S. L. Mottram
Kinetic Control, Southampton, UK

Functional stability is dependent on integrated local and global muscle function. Mechanical stability dysfunction presents as segmental (articular) and multisegmental (myofascial) dysfunction. These dysfunctions present as combinations of restriction of normal motion and associated compensations (give) to maintain function. Stability dysfunction is diagnosed by the site and direction of give or compensation that relates to symptomatic pathology. Strategies to manage mechanical stabililty dysfunction require specific mobilization of articular and connective tissue restrictions, regaining myofascial extensibility, retraining global stability muscle control of myofascial compensations and local stability muscle recruitment to control segmental motion. Stability retraining targets both the local and global stability systems. Activation of the local stability system to increase muscle stiffness along with functional low-load integration in the neutral joint position controls segmental or articular give. Global muscle retraining is required to correct multisegmental or myofascial dysfunction in terms of controlling the site and direction of load that relates to provocation. The strategy here is to train low-load recruitment to control and limit motion at the site of pathology and then actively move the adjacent restriction, regain through range control of motion with the global stability muscles and regain sufficient extensibility in the global mobility muscles to allow normal function. Individual strategies for integrating local and global recruitment retraining back into normal function are suggested. *Manual Therapy* (2001) **6(1)**, 3–14

INTRODUCTION

Over the past 20 years a greater understanding of movement and function has emerged. This has occurred from inter-linking anatomy, biomechanics, neurophysiology, motor control, pathology, pain mechanisms, and behavioural influences. The simplistic model of thinking that if something does not move well enough, it is tight and needs stretching or it is weak and needs strengthening no longer holds the answer to mechanical dysfunction.

Movement dysfunction can present as a local and/or global problem (Bergmark 1989), though both frequently occur concurrently. Poor movement habits, poor postural alignment (Janda 1978; Sahrmann 1992, 2000), and abnormal neurodynamic sensitization (Elvey 1995) can contribute to the development of imbalance between the global stability and mobility muscles. This imbalance presents in terms of alterations in the functional length and recruitment of these muscles and results in abnormal force contribution by the muscles around a motion segment. This places direction specific mechanical stress and strain on various structures which, if overloaded beyond tissue tolerance results in pain and related pathology. From the evidence to date, it appears the local stability system dysfunction only develops after the onset of pain and pathology (Richardson et al 1999; Comerford & Mottram 2001). This presents as dysfunction of the recruitment and motor control of the deep segmental stability system resulting in poor control of the neutral joint position. Although pain and dysfunction are related, the pain may resolve but the dysfunction may persist (Hides et al 1996; Hodges & Richardson 1996; Richardson et al 1999). This may cause an increased predisposition for recurrence, the early progression into degenerative change and maintenance of global imbalance (Comerford & Mottram 2001). Management strategies ideally should address rehabilitation of both the local and global systems concurrently.

Patients may present to the clinician complaining of symptoms in addition to dysfunction and disability (Fig. 12.1). The symptoms the patient describes relate to the pathology. Dysfunction can

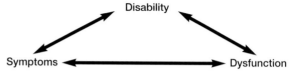

Figure 12.1 Management Goals. The priorities of management are different though they are inter-related.

be objectively measured, quantified and compared against a normal or ideal standard or some validated benchmark. Disability is the lack of ability to do what one wants or needs to do. Disability, therefore, is individual and one person's perceived disability may be exceptional function to another person. These three factors need to be assessed independently and their inter-relationships considered in the management of movement and stability dysfunction.

MUSCLE FUNCTION

All muscles have the ability to: (i) concentrically shorten and accelerate motion for mobility function; (ii) isometrically hold or eccentrically lengthen and decelerate motion for stability function; and (iii) provide afferent proprioceptive feedback to the central nervous system (CNS) for coordination and regulation of muscle function. Comerford and Mottram (2001) have proposed a classification system for muscle function. They have defined and characterized muscles as local stabilizers, global stabilizers and global mobilizers (Table 12.1).

STABILITY DYSFUNCTION

Movement dysfunction can present at a segmental level as abnormal articular translational movement at a single motion segment. Dysfunction can occur at a multi-segmental level in functional movements across several motion segments related to abnormal myofascial length and recruitment or abnormal patho-neurodynamic responses. These two components of the movement system are inter-related and consequently translational and myofascial dysfunctions often occur concurrently (Comerford & Mottram 2000).

Table 12.1 Muscle functional classification.

Local stabilizers	The functional stability role is to maintain low force continuous activity in all positions of joint range and in all directions of joint motion. This activity increases local muscle stiffness at a segmental level to control excessive physiological and translational motion, especially in the neutral joint position where passive support from the ligaments and capsule is minimal. Their activity often increases in an anticipatory action prior to load or movement, thus providing joint protection and support.
Global stabilizers	The functional stability role is to generate torque and provide eccentric control of inner and outer range of joint motion. They need to be able to (i) concentrically shorten into the full physiological inner range position; (ii) isometrically hold position and; (iii) eccentrically control or decelerate functional load against gravity. They should contribute significantly to rotation control in all functional movements.
Global mobilizers	Muscles that primarily have a mobilizing role are required to have adequate length to allow full physiological and accessory (translational) range of joint movement without causing compensatory overstrain elsewhere in the movement system. Their functional stability role is to augment stability under high load or strain, leverage disadvantage, lifting, pushing, pulling or ballistic shock absorption. These muscles are particularly efficient in the sagittal plane, but even though they can generate high forces they do not contribute significantly to rotation control and they cannot provide segmental control of physiological and translational motion.

Force couples act around all three axes of a joint. If the force vectors function ideally, there is a balance between the force vectors of synergistic and antagonistic muscles and there is equilibrium between the active and passive forces such that the axis of rotation or the path of the instantaneous centre of motion remains constant and stable. Imbalance of the force vectors acting around a joint may result in a displacement of the instantaneous axis of rotation (Fig. 12.2). There is 'give' or excessive uncontrolled joint motion in the direction of overactivity and restriction and a loss of joint motion in the direction of the underactivity. This characterizes an articular (segmental) give and restriction. The abnormal accessory glides that are the result of this faulty movement increase microtrauma in the tissues around the joint, which, if accumulative, leads to dysfunction and pain.

Multi-segmental dysfunction results in abnormal motion in functional movements between adjacent motion regions, which is largely due to changes in the myofascial system. When a lack of extensibility of myofascial tissue across one joint restricts normal motion at that joint, function can be maintained by increasing extensibility and decreasing activity in muscles across an adjacent joint. Sahrmann (2000) has referred to this as relative flexibility. Relative flexibility is a

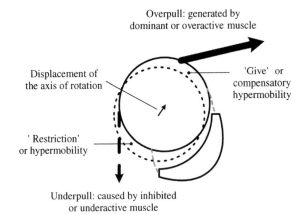

Figure 12.2 Imbalance of forces at a motion segment. Overactivity and underactivity in the muscles acting around a joint segment contribute to a net force that creates abnormal translation and displacement of the normal axis of rotation. Reproduced with kind permission of Kinetic Control.

concept that links movement dysfunction to pathology (Sahrmann 1992). The inability to dynamically control movement at a joint segment or region may present as a combination of uncontrolled movement or 'give', which is usually associated with a loss of motion or 'restriction'. This characterizes a myofascial (multi-segmental) give and restriction.

DIAGNOSIS OF STABILITY DYSFUNCTION

During functional movements, direction-specific hypermobility (give) is re-enforced and if repetitively loaded, tissue pathology results (Comerford & Mottram 2000) (Fig. 12.3). This may be the result of various contributing factors (Table 12.2). Give can be present without restriction (e.g. trauma) and restriction can be present without give or compensation (e.g. just losing function, though this is not common).

Mechanical stability dysfunction is identified by the site and direction of give or compensatory hypermobility. Two identifying features always qualify the diagnosis of stability dysfunction.

1. The site of dysfunction and pathology (site of symptoms)
2. The direction of give or compensation (direction or position of provocation).

The direction or plane of movement in which one joint is more flexible relative to its adjacent joint is diagnostic and is related to the direction of symptom-producing movement (Sahrmann 2000). For example, a segmental or multi-segmental give into excessive flexion under flexion load may place abnormal stress or strain on various tissues and result in flexion-related symptoms. Likewise,

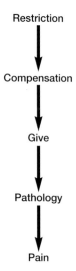

Figure 12.3 Sequelae of muscle imbalance.

Table 12.2 Contributing factors to dynamic stability dysfunction.

- Compensation for restriction to keep function (insidious)
- Over-facilitation: some muscle pulls too hard on a joint in a particular direction (insidious)
- Sustained passive postural positioning (lengthening strain or positional shortening)
- Trauma and damage to normal restraints of motion: traumatic laxity or restrictive scar tissue

Table 12.3 Primary elements of mechanical movement dysfunction

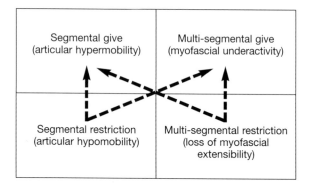

excessive give into extension under extension load produces extension-related symptoms, while excessive give into rotation or sidebend/sideshift under unilateral load produces unilateral symptoms.

A motion segment may have greater relative flexibility or give than its neighbour in one direction only or in multiple directions. One site can have stability dysfunction in more than one direction. Several different motion segments can have stability dysfunction at the same time, though usually in different directions. Adjacent sites can have stability dysfunction in different directions. Inappropriate motion may be shunted up or down the kinetic chain. The site of stability dysfunction is not always proximal — it may be distal to the site of the dysfunction (Comerford & Mottram 2000).

When a patient presents with chronic or recurrent pain several factors may contribute to the patient's symptoms. There may be articular (segmental) give and restriction and there may be myofascial (multi-segmental) give and restriction in any combination (Table 12.3), which constitute the mechanical component of movement dysfunction. There is an element of pathology that requires treatment and there may or may not be significant non-mechanical factors influencing the patient's symptoms and disability. All these elements present in varying proportions and as such need to be evaluated and managed accordingly (Fig. 12.4). It is important to relate the 'give' to symptoms and pathology and to the mechanism of provocation. This identifies the 'give' that is of clinical priority. 'Give' that may be evident, but does not relate to the mechanism of symptom provocation, is not a priority of management. However, it may indicate potential risk for the future.

When give and restriction are identified, four strategies must be developed to manage the relevant dysfunction.

1. When a segmental (articular) restriction identified with some form of manual palpation, then some specific joint mobilization techniques can be applied to mobilize the restriction.
2. When a multi-segmental (myofascial) restriction is identified by muscle

extensibility testing, some form of myofascial lengthening technique may be used to regain extensibility.
3. When movement analysis and specific muscle stability testing identifies a multisegmental give, the muscles that control range of motion (specifically the global stability muscles) can be retrained to control excessive range.
4. When a segmental give is identified by specific stability assessment, then the local stability muscles may be retrained to improve low threshold recruitment and increase segmental muscle stiffness to control excessive translation.

Regional pain or joint effusion has been shown to alter the normal recruitment processes of the local stability muscles around the joint (Stokes & Young 1984; Richardson & Bullock 1986; Hodges & Richardson 1996; Hides et al 1996; Richardson et al 1999; Jull et al 1999; Comerford & Mottram 2001). Because of this, the local stability muscles should be retrained if pain is a feature whether excessive segmental translation can be identified or not. Specific options familiar to most manual therapists are detailed in Table 12.4.

PRIORITIES AND PRINCIPLES OF STABILITY REHABILITATION

Several stages of rehabilitation in the management of movement dysfunction are proposed. Many patients will automatically integrate good stability retraining into higher-level activities if they have sufficient background stability.

LOCAL STABILITY SYSTEM: CONTROL OF NEUTRAL

I. CONTROL OF THE NEUTRAL JOINT POSITION

The aim is to retrain tonic, low-threshold activation of the local stability system to increase muscle stiffness and train the functional low-load

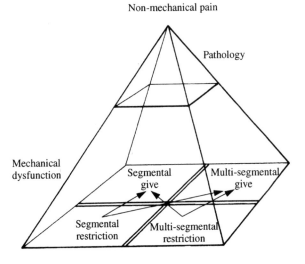

Figure 12.4 Model of mechanical movement dysfunction. Segmental and multi-segmental give and restriction make up the mechanical base of a pyramid of dysfunction. Pathology is always present on top of mechanical dysfunction and may provide a relatively smaller or larger contribution to the problem. There is often a significant, though variable, element of non-mechanical pain involved also. Reproduced with kind permission of Kinetic Control.

Table 12.4 Management strategies for mechanical dysfunction.

	Articular (segmental or translational)	Myofascicular (multi-segmental)
Give	• Facilitate tonic activation of the deep local stabilizers to increase muscle stiffness for control of the neutral joint position to provide dynamic stability when there is passive connective tissue laxity • Surgical reconstruction may attempt to augment stability but this is generally a salvage procedure • Immobilization may shorten lax connective structures but this has limited long-term effect	• Facilitate tonic activation of the monoarticular global stabilizers such that the muscle's active shortened position can control the joint's inner range motion (and hypermobile outer range motion) • Strengthening exercises can increase muscle stiffness and co-contraction rigidity to limit excessive motion — but it is difficult to maintain control during fast or large-range movements
Restriction	• Manual mobilization — end range accessory movements (oscillatory glides or thrust techniques) • Specific connective tissue mobilization or massage • Type II METs — muscle energy techniques or Facilitatory MAPs — myotatic activation procedures • SNAGs and localized mobilizations with movement	• Muscle lengthening techniques — sustained stretch, facilitatory stretches (contract–relax) and inhibitory stretches (active inhibitory restabilization and antagonist hold–relax) • Type I METs — muscle energy techniques or Inhibitory MAPs — myotactic activation procedures • Myofascial trigger point release or strain — counterstrain • Mobilizing exercises • Neurodynamic techniques

integration of the local and global stabilizer muscles to control the neutral joint position. Retraining should be facilitated in a pain-free posture or position. The neutral joint position is ideal because the local stability muscles primarily control this position. Retraining emphasizes the local stability muscles, though clinically it seems acceptable to allow some co-activation of the global stability muscles as they co-activate synergistically in normal function. However, it is important that the local stability muscles dominate the contraction and the global stability muscles only recruit with low-load, low-threshold coactivation. Also, there must be no significant increase in activation of the global mobility muscles.

The ability to sustain a consistent low force hold is paramount for rehabilitation of motor control deficits. High perceived effort is permissible initially, but as control and functional integration return low-effort activation should dominate. No fatigue or substitution should occur during the exercises. Motor control and recruitment are the priority (not strength and flexibility). The activation should be integrated through the entire range

Table 12.5 Clinical guidelines for local stabilizer retraining.

- Palpate for the correct activation
- Observe for:
  —Correct contraction pattern
  —Tonic (slow motor unit) recruitment (no fatigue under low load)
  —No substitution
- No Pain
- Breathe normally with a consistent, sustained contraction — no co-contraction rigidity
- Low–force sustained hold with normal breathing (10 seconds and repeat 10 times)
- Perform in a variety of different functional postures
  —Correct contraction pattern
  —Tonic (slow motor unit) recruitment (no fatigue under low load)

and into functional activities. Clinical guidelines for the assessment and retraining of local stabilizer recruitment are listed in Table 12.5.

Facilitation strategies for low-threshold slow motor unit training

Two categories of facilitation are suggested. The first category (the A list) uses very specific unloaded

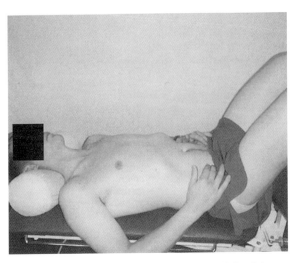

Figure 12.5 Specific unloaded transversus abdominis facilitation. Hollowing of the lower abdominal wall (especially the lateral aspect) without excessive overflow to the upper abdominal wall. This 'drawing in' action should be isolated to the lower muscular region and should attempt to minimize spinal or rib cage movement and should not cause lateral flaring of the waist. Palpate for transverses abdominis tensioning the low abdominal wall fascia without significant expansion of the internal obliques. (Richardson 1999) Reproduced with kind permission of Kinetic Control.

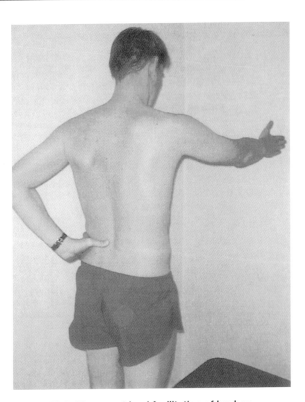

Figure 12.6 Movement load facilitation of lumbar multifidus. Palpate the dysfunctional multifidus with one hand and repetitively lift and lower the arm from neutral to 90° flexion and back to the side. The motor control challenge and therefore the retraining exercise is to try to sustain the contraction during the points when multifidus activity decreases. Maintain continual active muscle tension during slow, repetitive arm flexion. Reproduced with kind permission of Kinetic Control.

contraction of the local stability muscles in an attempt to specifically recruit their mechanical action independently of the global system. This approach uses nonfunctional movement but has the largest research base (Richardson et al 1999). Figure 12.5 illustrates a specific unloaded recruitment exercise for transversus abdominis. The second category (the B list) uses low-functional-load or non-neutral positions to retrain the integrative local and global stability muscle function (O'Sullivan et al 1997a). Stubbs et al (1998) demonstrated that mechanoreceptor stimulation in a joint ligament can produce reflex contraction of local joint muscles. Low functional loads and non-neutral positions may facilitate muscle recruitment via a mechanical pre-loading of the muscle through its fascial and connective tissue attachments. Figure 12.6 illustrates movement and load facilitation for lumbar multifidus. Clinically, this approach allows some co-activation recruitment of the global stability muscles along with the local

muscle system. However, it appears to be essential that the global stability muscles work within the range of tonic (low-threshold) recruitment.

The retraining of motor control dysfunction is a cognitive process requiring afferent feedback and different strategies are required for different problems. If specific facilitation (A list) is reasonably well performed then activation should be integrated into loaded activities and normal function. If specific facilitation is poorly performed then it is preferable to use other appropriate facilitation strategies (B list) until specific training is achieved. Integration into function can then be effected (Fig. 12.7) (Comerford & Mottram 2000).

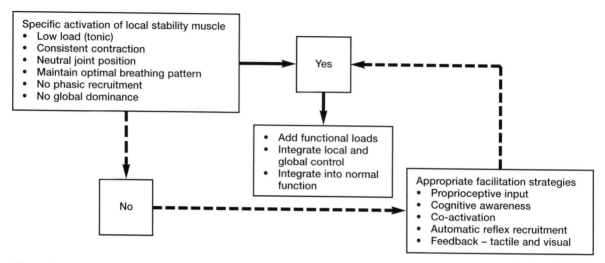

Figure 12.7 Facilitation strategies. Reproduced with kind permission of Kinetic Control.

GLOBAL STABILITY SYSTEM: CONTROL OF DIRECTION

II. RETRAIN DYNAMIC CONTROL OF THE DIRECTION OF STABILITY DYSFUNCTION

The strategy here is to control the give, and move the restriction. The priority is to retrain control of the stability dysfunction in the direction of symptom-producing movements. Low-load integration of local and global stabilizer recruitment is required to control and limit motion at the segment or region of give and then actively move the adjacent restriction. It is important to move only through as much range as the restriction allows or as far as the give is dynamically controlled. The ability to control directional stress and strain directly unloads mechanical provocation of pathology and is, therefore, the key strategy to symptom management. Motor control and coordination are the priorities.

Identify the direction of stability dysfunction

During the assessment of dynamic control of the direction of stability dysfunction, it is necessary to identify the give and restriction. It is important to note excessive range of movement or abnormal initiation of movement at the site about which the patient complains of symptoms. This is the 'give' (uncontrolled movement) or compensatory hypermobility used to keep function. During the movement test it is important to identify a loss of range of motion (the restriction) that presents either segmentally or multi-segmentally and to relate the symptoms that the patient complains of to the site and direction of 'give'.

Assessment of the patient's ability to actively control the give and move independently at the adjacent joint in the direction of provocation identifies stability dysfunction. A 'give' or compensation that: (i) cannot be actively controlled through appropriate range, or (ii) can only be controlled with difficulty (high perceived or actual effort) is a significant stability dysfunction. However, a 'give' or compensation that can be easily controlled actively under directional load is not a significant stability dysfunction, though this could be considered to be hypermobility with functional stability.

Although direction control or dissociation exercises are not normal functional movements, they are, however, movements and motor patterns that everyone should have the ability to perform. The dissociation or correction of the give is a test of motor control or recruitment. Using conscious activation of the stability muscles (both global and

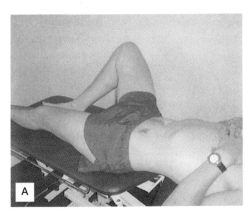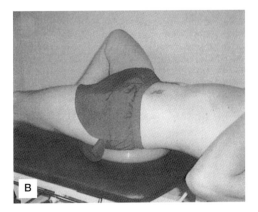

Figure 12.8 (A) Lumbopelvic rotation control. Slowly allow the bent leg to be lowered out to the side, keeping the foot supported beside the straight leg. The leg can be lowered out so far as no rotation of the pelvis occurs. The abdominal muscles, which stabilize the trunk, must coordinate with adductor muscles, which eccentrically lower the leg. (B) Lumbopelvic flexion control. A further progression would be to perform the exercise with a 'sit fit'under the pelvis creating an unstable base and increasing the proprioceptive challenge. Reproduced with kind permission of Kinetic Control.

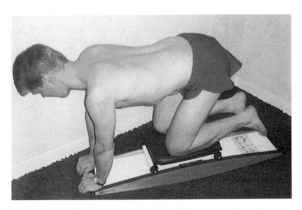

Figure 12.9 Lumbar flexion control. Backward rocking with independent hip flexion, but only as far as the neutral lumbopelvic position can be maintained. Progress until good control is achieved through half range (120° hip flexion) is easy. Performing this exercise on a 'fitter' provides an unstable base and increased proprioceptive challenge. Reproduced with kind permission of Kinetic Control.

local stabilizers) to hold the dysfunctional region or segment in a neutral position (± assisted or supported), the adjacent joint or motion segment is moved through its available range. Movement at the adjacent joint should only occur as far as isometric control (no movement) of the dysfunctional region can be maintained and the restriction at the adjacent joint allows. Slow, low-effort repetitions and movement only through the range that the dysfunction is controlled actively should be

performed. A general clinical guide is to perform 15–20 slow repetitions. This type of movement is performed until it starts to feel familiar and natural. It is important to remember that direction control movements can also be used to unload pathology, decrease mechanical provocation of pathology and assist in symptom management. This is important for early symptom control. Figure 12.8 illustrates control of lumbopelvic rotation and Figure 12.9 illustrates control of lumbar flexion.

GLOBAL STABILITY SYSTEM: CONTROL OF IMBALANCE

III. REHABILITATE GLOBAL STABILIZER CONTROL THROUGH RANGE

The global stability system is required to actively control the full available range of joint motion. These muscles are required to be able to control limb load whilst maintaining low-force, low-threshold recruitment and concentrically shorten through to the full passive inner range of joint motion. They must also be able to control limb load eccentrically against gravity and through any hypermobile outer range. The ability to control rotational forces is an especially important role of global stabilizers. Through range control is optimized by low-effort,

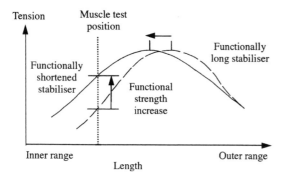

Figure 12.10 Regaining through range control. Shift the peak of the length–tension curve towards inner range and improve mechanical efficiency in inner range. Reproduced with kind permission of Kinetic Control.

sustained holds in the muscle's shortened position (Fig. 12.10) with controlled eccentric return especially of rotation. A useful clinical guide is to perform a 10-second, consistently sustained contraction repeated 10 times.

Figure 12.11 illustrates through range control for posterior gluteus medius and Figure 12.12 illustrates oblique abdominal loading.

IV. ACTIVE LENGTHENING OR INHIBITION OF THE GLOBAL MOBILIZERS

When the two joint global mobility muscles demonstrate a lack of extensibility due to overuse or adaptive shortening, compensatory overstrain or give may occur elsewhere in the kinetic chain in an attempt to maintain function. It then becomes necessary to lengthen or inhibit overactivity in the global mobilizers to eliminate the need for compensation. Figure 12.13 illustrates an active inhibitory restabilization lengthening technique for the hamstrings.

Active inhibitory restabilization

When short muscles are overactive and dominate their synergists an inhibitory lengthening technique called active inhibitory restabilization (AIR) is proposed. It involves the operator gently and slowly lengthening the muscle until the resistance causes a slight loss of proximal girdle or trunk stability. The operator then maintains

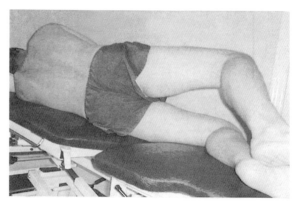

Figure 12.11 Through range control. Low-load inner range hold for posterior gluteus medius. Keeping the heels together (short lever and supported), the patient is instructed to lift the uppermost knee by turning out at the hip. The leg is turned out only as far as the neutral lumbopelvic position is maintained without substitution or fatigue. There must be no cramping or strain/pain in the buttocks or posterior thigh. Hold for 10 seconds at the position at which the hip can turn out comfortably with no loss of control or substitution, and repeat 10 times. Reproduced with kind permission of Kinetic Control.

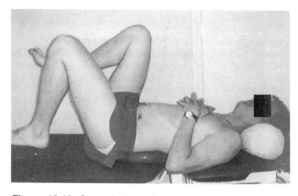

Figure 12.12 Control of rotational load. Oblique abdominal control of unilateral limb load. Slowly lift one foot off the floor and then lift the second foot off the floor and bring it up beside the first leg. Hold this position and, keeping the back stable (no pressure change), slowly lower one heel to the floor and lift it back to the start position. Repeat this movement, slowly alternating legs, for 10 seconds so long as stability is maintained (no pressure change), and then return both feet to the floor. This exercise may be progressed by placing a 'Sitfit' under the pelvis creating an unstable base and increasing the proprioceptive challenge. Reproduced with kind permission of Kinetic Control.

the muscle or limb in this position. Next, the subject is instructed to actively restabilize the proximal segment that had lost stability and sustain

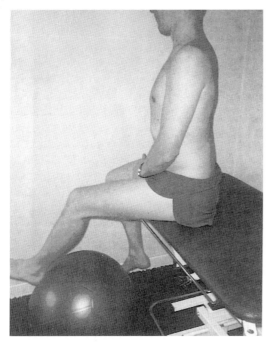

Figure 12.13 Active inhibitory restabilization for the hamstrings. The subject sits with the spine and pelvis in neutral alignment and the knee is extended to the point at which the lumbar spine starts to be pulled out of neutral into flexion or significant resistance is felt in the hamstrings. At this point the leg is passively supported and the patient is instructed to actively anterior tilt the pelvis (from the sacrum not the thoracic spine). The stretch should be held for 20–30 seconds and repeated 3–5 times. Reproduced with kind permission of Kinetic Control.

the correction. A clinical suggestion is to sustain the correction for 20–30 seconds and repeat 3–5 times. This active proximal restabilization pro-vides the force of the stretch, which the subject controls for safety. More importantly, it recipro-cally inhibits the overactive contractile elements of the tight muscle. A further bonus is that the sub-ject ideally uses a proximal stabilizer muscle (rather than a distal limb mobilizer) to provide the antagonistic inhibition and therefore facilitates and reinforces holding work for appropriate sta-bilizers. Home stretches should be left until the global stability system can control possible com-pensations during the stretch. However, manual mobilization of the articular restriction should commence as early as possible and techniques that regain myofascial extensibility without directly

Table 12.6 Integration of stability training into function.

- Specific exercise of the lateral abdominals and multifidus is effective in reducing pain and improving function in subjects with symptomatic spondylosis or spondylolisthesis.
- Specific exercise can alter the conscious and automatic patterns of recruitment ratios between internal oblique and rectus abdominis muscles in chronic low back pain (O'Sullivan et al 1995, 1997a, 1997b, 1998)

pulling on the muscle (e.g. myofascial trigger point release) can be commenced early as well.

INTEGRATION OF LOCAL AND GLOBAL STABILITY RETRAINING INTO NORMAL FUNCTION

O'Sullivan (1995, 1997a, 1997b, 1998) has demon-strated the clinical effectiveness and importance of the integration of the deep stability muscle sys-tem into functional movements, activities of daily living and even to high loads and provocative positions (Table 12.6). These exercises are per-formed initially as sustained contractions under low physiological load (low threshold, slow motor unit recruitment). This training is biased for the local stabilizers but functional control requires integration of local and global stabilizer muscle recruitment. In stability retraining motor control and recruitment are the priority, not strength and flexibility.

One of the greatest challenges facing therapists is the integration of specific training regimes into functional activities and making recruitment auto-matic. Because of individual behavioural traits and psychosocial factors there is no single strategy that is appropriate for every patient. Various approach-es have been categorized in order to identify a process that can accommodate individual differ-ences in motivation and compliance. Some patients benefit from a very structured process with very clear goals and progressions. Other patients, however, do not respond to this and do better with a non-structured, more flexible process with an end goal but without a rigid step-by-step pathway. Some patients respond to specific motor control retraining where they think about, try to feel or visualize a specific muscle activating. Other patients do not seem to be able to do this but appear to get the correct activation when they do not think about a specific muscle. Instead they seem to use nonspecific motor control strategies, such as correcting alignment or posture, achieving a certain position or moving in a certain way to get the activation required. By finding the right combination of structured or nonstructured and specific or nonspecific motor control retraining, there are many options (Fig. 12.14), so it should be possible to identify a combination that will maintain motivation and achieve compliance for most patients. Several options are presented below.

'Red dot' functional integration (nonstructured and specific)

Rothstein (1982) has suggested that to integrate an activity or skill into normal, automatic or unconscious function many repetitions must be performed under diverse functional situations. To do this, some form of 'reminder' is needed. Rothstein (1982) has proposed that small 'red dots' placed so that they are frequently seen will 'remind' the subject to perform a specific task each time they are observed. This process lends itself well to training of the local stability system. Frequent tonic activation of the key local stability muscle is suggested for dynamic postural re-education and integration into 'normal function'. Depending on the area of dysfunction, different

local stabilizer muscles may need to be facilitated (Comerford & Mottram 2000).

When the red dot is sighted, the subject is reminded to activate the key local stability muscle for their specific problem. The muscle is contracted at low effort (less than 25% of maximum voluntary contraction (MVC)), and is held for several seconds and repeated several times, without interrupting normal or functional activities. This process is repeated each time that a red dot is sighted. Red dots should be placed in appropriate positions (e.g. wristwatch, clock, telephone, coffee/tea making area, office drawer, bathroom mirror, under refrigerator door seal) as reminders to exercise.

Low-load spinal proprioception (structured and nonspecific)

The aim is to integrate stability muscle recruitment around neutral joint positions with automatic postural reflex responses. In the neutral joint position afferent information from the joint ligaments and capsules is minimized. Training is performed sitting or standing on a series of progressively unstable bases or supports. The eyes are open for initial training but as control improves they can be closed, the muscle system being thus relied on for proprioception. Figure 12.15 illustrates this process. The 'Pilates Reformer', the 'Fitter' (Fitter International Inc Calgary, Canada) and the 'Physio Ball' are also appropriate and useful tools.

Functional progressions for integration (structured and specific)

The integration of local stabilizer recruitment into normal function and occupational, recreational and sporting activities can be presented as a functional progression through a series of increasingly demanding tasks (Fig. 12.16). Recruitment of the local stability muscles must be integrated with the global stability muscles under low load for normal function. Activation must 'feel' easy (low perceived effort) and evoke confidence at each level before progression to the next level. There must be no substitution, fatigue or pain during the exercise programme.

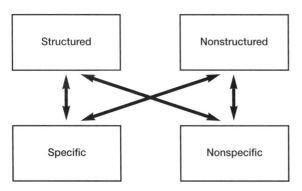

Figure 12.14 Processes of integration of stability training into function. Various combinations of structured or nonstructured with specific or nonspecific processes can be used to optimize motivation and compliance in the performance of therapeutic exercise.

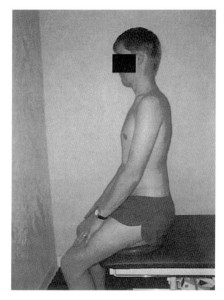

Figure 12.15 Proprioceptive challenge sit in neutral spinal alignment and balance (feet unsupported) on two Sitfits. As the unstable base causes alignment to move away from neutral the patient has to keep actively returning to the neutral position. Reproduced with kind permission of Kinetic Control.

PROGRESSION

a) Activation in neutral alignment with a variety of different postures or positions (progression: supported [arrow] unsupported)

b) Activation in neutral alignment without co-contraction rigidity (for the trunk: activation with normal relaxed breathing; for the limbs: activation without resistance to passive rotation)

c) Activation in neutral alignment on an unstable base (add a proprioceptive challenge) (Pilates is useful when startimg here with a low load)

d) Activation during directional control exercises (dissociation or recruitment reversals)

e) Activation during normal physiological movements (the trunk and girdles actively move away from neutral position)

f) Activation during functional activities (normal movements of the unloaded limbs and trunk – 'red dot' exercises)

g) Activation during stressful or provocative movements and positions (pathology and symptom specific)

h) Activation during occupational, recreational or sport specific skills

Figure 12.16 Structured sequential functional progression. Reproduced with kind permission of Kinetic Control.

Integrative dissociation (structured and nonspecific)

This process is based on the control of direction training discussed earlier in this article. Once the basic motor control skill of 'control the give and move the restriction' has been learnt, this strategy of controlling the region of dysfunction is incorporated with functionally orientated exercises where, so long as the problem region is controlled, any other movement is appropriate. This can be built into an exercise programme or just simply 'control the give while performing functional tasks'.

Control of the centre of gravity (non-structured and nonspecific)

The ability to move the centre of gravity of the body over its base of support at a global level and to maintain the centre of gravity of individual motion segments over their adjacent segment at a local level is essential for efficient movement. This is especially important during weight-transfer activities. The local stabilizer muscles are necessary to maintain correct alignment of the spine and girdle segments to provide a stable base for efficient limb and trunk movement (Crisco & Panjabi 1991; Cholewicki & McGill 1996). Cognitive retraining to develop self-awareness of body segments and develop position sense and voluntary control during weight-transfer activities can be used as part of integrative training.

The spine should be able to maintain a fairly neutral position during low-load weight-transfer activities and normal gait. The pelvis should not initiate or drag the trunk into weight transference. The shoulder girdle should not lead and produce large-range spinal movement. This should be performed while maintaining spinal neutral and maintaining the alignment of the centre of gravity of sequential segments: move forward to backward, side to side. This can be progressed to standing or sitting on an unstable base (balance board, Sitfit (Sissel UK, Ltd) Physio Ball, Pilates Reformer, Fitter, aerobic slide board etc.)

Table 12.7 Alternative approaches integration process.

Approach	Process
T'ai Chi	Structured and nonspecific
Alexander technique	Nonstructured and nonspecific
Pilates	Structured and nonspecific or specific
Yoga	Structured and nonspecific or specific
Physio Ball	Structured and nonspecific or specific

Other approaches

Many other approaches used in clinical practice have some potential to assist the integration of local and global stability retraining once the basic motor control correction has been learnt (Table 12.7).

CONCLUSION

Local and global retraining ideally should be retrained concurrently (Fig. 12.17). This appears to assist functional integration more efficiently that training one system in isolation or training one system initially and only progressing to the other system later. Priorities I and II are normally retrained concurrently and are started as early as possible. Priority I is progressed and integrated into function using whatever combination of process appear to achieve motivation and compliance. Priority III is an overlapping progression from Priority II. Priority IV is an overlapping progression from Priority III and is usually only commenced when the pathology is under control.

In clinical practice there is an increasing requirement to develop therapeutic strategies based on academic and clinical evidence and to integrate these strategies into our contemporary clinical frameworks. Our previous article in

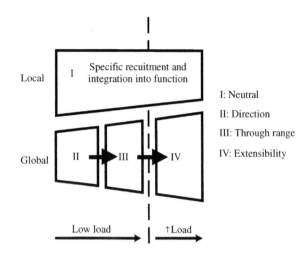

Figure 12.17 Local and global integration. Reproduced with kind permission of Kinetic Control.

Manual Therapy has attempted to draw together much of the evidence available in the literature to develop concepts and models of what constitutes good movement and what goes wrong in the presence of pain and pathology. In this article we have developed strategies of management for mechanical stability dysfunction. Our suggestions for the clinician are to look for give and restriction at an articular (segmental) and myofascial (multi-segmental) level and then to mobilize the 'restrictions', then stabilize the 'give' that relates to symptoms and pathology. Both the local and global stability systems should be retrained concurrently. Muscles may also become weak through disuse and they may require strength training as well as stability retraining. The therapist must also be aware of the influence of nonmechanical pain mechanisms on the patient's perception of symptoms. Finally, the specific training must be integrated into function.

REFERENCES

Bergmark A 1989 Stability of the lumbar spine. A study in mechanical engineering. Acta Orthopaedica Scandinavica 230(60): 20–24
Cholewicki J, McGill S 1996 Mechanical stability in the vivo lumbar spine: implications for injury and chronic low back pain. Clinical Biomechanics 11(1): 1–15
Comerford M, Mottram S 2000 Movement Dysfunction — Focus on Dynamic Stability and Muscle Balance:

Kinetic Control Movement Dysfunction Course. Kinetic Control, Southampton
Comerford M, Mottram S 2001 Movement and stability dysfunction — contemporary developments. Manual Therapy 6(1): 15–26
Crisco JJ, Panjabi MM 1991 The intersegmental and multisegmental muscles of the lumbar spine. Spine 16(7): 792–793

Hides JA, Richardson CA, Jull GA 1996 Multifidus recovery is not automatic after resolution of acute, first-episode low back pain. Spine 21(23): 2763–2769

Hodges PW, Richardson CA 1996 Inefficient muscular stabilization of the lumbar spine associated with low back pain: a motor control evaluation of transversus abdominis. Spine 21(22): 2640–2650

Janda V 1978 Muscles, central nervous motor regulation and back problems. In: Korr IM (ed) The Neurological Mechanisms in Manipulative Therapy. Plenum Press, New York, pp 27–41

Jull G, Barrett C, Magee R, Ho P 1999 Further clinical clarification of the muscle dysfunction in cervical headache. Cephalaegia 19(3): 179–185

O'Sullivan P, Twomey L, Allison G 1995 Evaluation of specific stabilizing exercises in the treatment of chronic low back pain with radiological diagnosis of spondylosis or spondylolisthesis. In: Proceedings of the 9th Biennial Conference of the Manipulative Physiotherapists Association of Australia. Gold Coast, 113–114

O'Sullivan PB, Twomey L, Allison G 1997a Evaluation of specific stabilizing exercises in the treatment of chronic low back pain with radiological diagnosis of spondylosis or spondylolisthesis. Spine 22(24): 2959–2967

O'Sullivan PB, Twomey L, Allison G, Sinclair J, Miller K, Knox J 1997b Altered patterns of abdominal muscle activation in patients with chronic low back pain. Australian Journal of Physiotherapy 43(2): 91–98

O'Sullivan P, Twomey L, Allison G 1998 Altered abdominal muscle recruitment in back pain patients following specific exercise intervention. Journal of Orthopaedics and Sports Physical Therapy 27(2): 114–124

Richardson C, Bullock MI 1986 Changes in muscle activity during fast, alternating flexion-extension movements of the knee. Scandanavian Journal of Rehabilitation Medicine 18: 51–58

Richardson C, Jull G, Hodges P, Hides J 1999 Therapeutic Exercise for Spinal Segmental Stabilization in Low Back Pain: Scientific Basis and Clinical Approach. Churchill Livingstone, Edinburgh

Rothstein JM 1982 Muscle biology. Clinical considerations. Physical Therapy 62(12): 1823–1830

Sahrmann SA 1992 Posture and muscle imbalance: faulty lumbar-pelvic alignment and associated musculoskeletal pain syndromes. Orthopaedic Division Review 13–20

Sahrmann SA 2001 Diagnosis & Treatment of Movement Impairment Syndromes. Mosby, USA

Stokes M, Young A 1984 Investigations of quadriceps inhibition: implications for clinical practice. Physiotherapy 70(11): 425–428

Stubbs M, Harris M, Solomonow M, Zhou B, Lu Y, Barrata RV 1998 Ligamento-muscular protective reflex in the lumbar spine of the feline. Journal of Electromyography and Kinesiology 8(4): 197–204

POSTSCRIPT

There are many variations in postures and patterns of movement used by individuals in their everyday functional activity. The majority are considered 'normal' and are not thought to be detrimental to the efficient pain-free functioning of the musculoskeletal system. However, some variations are considered to place abnormal stress and strain on the tissues and may contribute to musculoskeletal dysfunction, pain and pathology (Janda 1985, 1996; Comerford & Mottram 2001a; Adams et al 2002; Sahrmann 2002). As the pathology heals and the symptoms subside measurable dysfunction does not always automatically correct (Hides et al 1996; Hodges & Richardson 1996, 1999; Richardson et al 1999).

To date, measurement of motor control related to stability dysfunction has required complex measurement technology together with specialized training to analyse and interpret the results. There has therefore been a need to develop a 'clinic friendly' assessment system that is straightforward, functional and assists in clinical decision making, i.e. where to begin, when to progress and when to cease specific therapeutic exercises. A system of assessment, relating to motor control of low-load muscle function, has been developed to rate the performance efficiency of specific muscle tasks.

It appears that some inhibition of normal sensory-motor function is present in everyone experiencing pain (Grimby & Hannerz 1976; Stokes & Young 1984; Stokes et al 1992; Gandevia 1994; Hodges & Richardson 1996, 1999; Richardson et al 1999; Jull 2000). However, a number of these people recover and become painfree and do not experience recurrent or chronic pain episodes. Evidently they recover fully without the need for specific muscle retraining. All back pain patients who have been tested have demonstrated inhibition of transversus abdominis (Hodges & Richardson 1996, 1999). However, although the majority of these patients demonstrated recruitment inefficiency, there are many who can demonstrate efficient low-threshold recruitment of transversus abdominis in the presence of inhibition. Jull (2000) described an objective test of recruitment efficiency for the deep cervical flexor muscles. We have found that many neck pain patients can perform this test adequately during an episode of neck pain. We therefore believe that if low threshold voluntary recruitment of the muscles providing functional stability is efficient, then when the pathology heals and pain disappears, the muscle may automatically re-establish normal (ideal) function. The observation that some people get better and recover ideal function without any specific retraining supports this theory. However, if low-threshold voluntary recruitment in these muscles is inefficient, then when the pain or pathology disappears, the dysfunction in the muscle is likely to persist.

The assessment system, described below, does not measure muscle inhibition but has been developed to rate *low threshold voluntary recruitment efficiency*. Assessment is based on two elements:

1. Palpation of muscle activation with observation of the pattern of movement
2. Observation and subjective interpretation of the sense of effort or efficiency of performance

Table 12.8

Rating	Activation	Efficiency
✔✔	• correct muscle activation or • correct pattern of movement • without substitution	• efficient low-threshold muscle recruitment • sensation of low effort • without extra feedback
✔✗	• correct muscle activation or • correct pattern of movement • without substitution	• inefficient low-threshold muscle recruitment • sensation of high effort • requires tactile or visual feedback or unloading
✗✗	• incorrect muscle activation or • incorrect pattern of movement • due to substitution or excessive co-contraction	

Table 12.9 Local stabilizer control of neutral joint position.

	Requirements	✓ or ✗	Reason for ✗ (re-assess) (L) (R)
Dissociation pattern	• Correct dissociation pattern of normal functional load. (Instruction: [position] – prevent [site] give into [direction] and move [adjacent region] into [direction] by [description of movement])	❏	
	• Able to prevent give into the test direction	❏	
	• Dissociate through available range, or as far as benchmark standard (there is no requirement to dissociate excessive range) (Note any restriction or hypermobility below)	❏	
	• Prevent give during eccentric loading	❏	
	• Prevent give during concentric loading	❏	
	Final rating for dissociation pattern (✓ or ✗)		
Recruitment	• Looks easy and feels easy to prevent give into the test direction	❏	
	• No extra feedback needed (tactile or visual)	❏	
	• Available range at least meets the Benchmark Standard: ([range of dissociation])	❏	
	• No external support or unloading	❏	
	• Normal relaxed breathing	❏	
	• No fatigue	❏	
	Final rating for recruitment (✓ or ✗)		
	OVERALL RATING		

✓✓: If the muscle demonstrates **all** requirements for 'dissociation pattern' + **all** requirements for 'recruitment'
✓✗: If the muscle demonstrates **all** requirements for 'dissociation pattern' + fails **any** of the requirements for 'recruitment'
✗✗: If the muscle fails **any** of the requirements for 'dissociation pattern'

In order to keep the process 'clinician friendly', a '✔' or '✗' rating is given for each of these two elements. The ratings for both elements are combined to give one of three possible scores ranging from ✔✔ (correct muscle activation + efficient recruitment) through ✔✗ (correct muscle activation + inefficient recruitment) to ✗✗ (incorrect muscle activation due to substitution) (Table 12.8).

The test movements are not 'normal' movements but they are nevertheless movement patterns or skills that everybody has the ability to learn and perform easily (Comerford & Mottram 2001b). Even though the test manoeuvres may feel unfamiliar they are low load and should not be perceived as 'hard work'. As these test movements are not normal or habitual movements there is a requirement to teach the movement pattern so that the patient can practise the test movement or activation correctly. Verbal description, demonstration, hands-on facilitation and visual or tactile self-feed-

back should be used to ensure that the patient understands and has experienced the movement or activation required. Then this self-feedback is eliminated before rating and testing the efficacy of low-threshold voluntary recruitment.

This system has been developed around the requirements for stability function and the four principles of low-load stability rehabilitation suggested by Comerford and Mottram (2001a, 2001b). These principles are control of direction, control of neutral, control through range and control of extensibility.

CONTROL OF DIRECTION

Each direction is assessed separately. The ability to perform a direction specific dissociation manoeuvre is rated. To achieve a '✔✔' rating the patient must be able to demonstrate the direction specific recruitment pattern to control and prevent

Table 12.10 Global stabilizer control of direction specific give

	Requirements	✓ or ✗	Reason for ✗ (re-assess) (L)	(R)
Specific activation	• Correct activation pattern in unloaded posture (Instruction: [description of activation])	❏		
	• Sustained contraction for several seconds (even if not consistent or assymmetrical)	❏		
	• Maintain control of the neutral position	❏		
	• Without substitution or co-contraction rigidity	❏		
	• Without holding breath	❏		
	Final rating for activation (✓ or ✗)			
Recruitment	• Looks easy and feels easy	❏		
	• Consistent activation	❏		
	• Benchmark standard (Time: 15 seconds x 2 repetitions)	❏		
	• Normal relaxed breathing	❏		
	• No fatigue	❏		
	• No extra feedback (tactile or visual)	❏		
	• Good symmetry (compare left and right sides)	❏		
	• Able to recruit well in alternative postures (posture of provocation: [position])	❏		
	Final rating for recruitment (✓ or ✗)			
	OVERALL RATING			

✓✓ If the muscle demonstrates **all** requirements for 'specific activation' + **all** requirements for 'recruitment'
✓✗: If the muscle demonstrates **all** requirements for 'specific activation' + fails **any** of the requirements for 'recruitment'
✗✗: If the muscle fails **any** of the requirements for 'specific activation'

movement into that direction at one site while moving at another site and... it must look confident and feel easy (low sensation of effort with low threshold recruitment). If a loss of control into another direction is observed then this is a relative flexibility/relative stiffness issue related to another direction. The specific requirements for each section are detailed in Table 12.9.

CONTROL OF NEUTRAL

Each local stability muscle is assessed separately. The efficiency of specific muscle recruitment is rated in a neutral, midrange joint position. To achieve a '✔✔' rating the patient must be able to demonstrate the ability to specifically activate the local stability muscle correctly and... it must look confident and feel easy. The specific requirements for each section are detailed in Table 12.10.

CONTROL THROUGH RANGE

Each global stability muscle is assessed separately. The ability for global stability muscles to (i) shorten and move the joint through to its full inner range; (ii) isometrically hold that position (or any point in range) and (iii) eccentrically control lowering against gravity, is rated. To achieve a '✔✔' rating the patient must be able to demonstrate the ability to concentrically shorten the muscle sufficiently to move the joint through the full available range so that muscle active shortening is equal to joint passive inner range. If the available passive range is excessive or hypermobile then this range must be actively controlled and... actively shorten to at least the benchmark (ideal) minimum range, isometrically hold that position and control the eccentric return. The specific requirements for each section are detailed in Table 12.11.

Table 12.11 Global stabilizer through range control.

	Requirements	✓ or ✗	Reason for ✗ (re-assess) (L)	(R)
Muscle shortening	• The muscle can actively shorten through the available (including hypermobile) passive joint range in the position of the muscle's combined actions	❑		
	• Concentrically shorten against functional load and gravity	❑		
	• Can hold this position for at least 2–3 seconds	❑		
	• With passive fixation of the proximal girdle or trunk	❑		
	• Without substitution by other muscles	❑		
	Final rating for muscle shortening (✓ or ✗)			
Recruitment	• Available range at least meets the benchmark minimum range: (minimum range of active shortening])	❑		
	• Can hold position for the benchmark ideal (Time: 15 seconds x 2 repetitions)	❑		
	• Can smoothly control the eccentric return – including hypermobile outer range	❑		
	• Without fatigue	❑		
	• Without passive fixation of the proximal girdle or trunk (active unsupported control)	❑		
	• No external support or unloading	❑		
	• Relaxed breathing without breath-holding	❑		
	Final rating for recruitment (✓or ✗)			
	OVERALL RATING			

✓✓: If the muscle demonstrates **all** requirements for 'muscle shortening' + **all** requirements for 'recruitment'
✓✗: If the muscle demonstrates **all** requirements for 'muscle shortening' + fails **any** of the requirements for 'recruitment'
✗✗: If the muscle fails **any** of the requirements for 'muscle shortening'

CONTROL OF EXTENSIBILITY

Each global mobility muscle is assessed separately. The passive extensibility of the global mobility muscles and the ability for global stability muscles to control compensatory give during an active or active assisted stretch is rated. To achieve a '✓✓' rating the patient must be able to demonstrate passive extensibility to the benchmark (ideal) length and... demonstrate the ability to use this extensibility while actively maintaining proximal stability. The specific requirements for each section are detailed in Table 12.12.

CONCLUSION

The correction and rehabilitation of motor control stability dysfunction has been shown to decrease the incidence of recurrence of pain. Along with symptom management this is a primary short-term goal of therapeutic intervention. The patient frequently becomes symptom free before dysfunction is fully corrected. Treatment should not necessarily cease just because the symptoms have disappeared if dysfunction persists. A rating system (such as the one described) may be helpful for clinicians when assessing and treating their patients.

Table 12.12 Global mobilizer extensibility.

	Requirements	✓ or ✗	Reason for ✗ (re-assess) (L) (R)
Passive extensibility	• The muscle can passively lengthen to the benchmark standard (therapist controlled) ([minimum extensibility required for good function)	❏	
	Final rating for passive extensibility (✓ or ✗)		
Active control	• Active elongation (stretch) can reproduce the passive benchmark	❏	
	• With good active control of proximal stability	❏	
	• Without compensatory 'give' (relative flexibility)	❏	
	• No external support or assistance	❏	
	Final rating for active control (✓ or ✗)		

OVERALL RATING

✓✓: If the muscle demonstrates **all** requirements for 'passive extensibility' + **all** requirements for 'active control'
✓✗: If the muscle demonstrates **all** requirements for 'passive extensibility' + fails **any** of the requirements for 'active control'
✗✗: If the muscle fails **any** of the requirements for 'passive extensibility'

REFERENCES

Adams M, Bogduk N, Burton K, Dolan P 2002 The Biomechanics of Back Pain. Churchill Livingstone, Edinburgh

Comerford MJ, Mottram SL 2001a Movement and stability dysfunction – contemporary developments. Manual Therapy 6(1): 15–26

Comerford MJ, Mottram SL 2001b Functional stability retraining: Principles & strategies for managing mechanical dysfunction. Manual Therapy 6(1): 3–14

Gandevia SC 1994 The sensation of effort co-varies with reflex effects on the motorneurone pool: evidence and implications. International Journal of Industrial Ergonomics 13: 41–49

Grimby L, Hannerz J 1976 Disturbances in voluntary recruitment order of low and high frequency motor units on blockades of proprioceptive afferent activity. Acta Physiologica Scandinavica 96: 207–216

Hides JA, Richardson CA, Jull GA 1996 Multifidus recovery is not automatic after resolution of acute, first-episode low back pain. Spine 21(23): 2763–2769

Hodges PW, Richardson CA 1996 Inefficient muscular stabilisation of the lumbar spine associated with low back pain: a motor control evaluation of transversus abdominis. Spine 21(22): 2640–2650

Hodges PW, Richardson CA 1999 Altered trunk muscle recruitment in people with low back pain with upper limb movement at different speeds. Archives of Physical Medicine and Rehabilitation 80: 1005–1012

Janda V 1985 Pain in the locomotor system — A broad approach. In: Glasgow et al (ed) Aspects of Manipulative Therapy. Churchill Livingstone, Edinburgh pp148–151

Janda V 1996 Evaluation of muscle imbalance. In: Liebenson C (ed) Rehabilitation of the Spine. Williams & Wilkins, Baltimore

Jull GA 2000 Deep cervical flexor muscle dysfunction in whiplash. Journal of Musculoskeletal Pain 8(1/2): 143–154

Richardson C, Jull G, Hodges P, Hides J 1999 Therapeutic Exercise for Spinal Segmental Stabilization in Low Back Pain: Scientific Basis and Clinical Approach. Churchill Livingstone, Edinburgh

Sahrmann SA 2002 Diagnosis & Treatment of Movement Impairment Syndromes. Mosby, USA

Stokes MA, Cooper R, Morris G, Jayson MIV 1992 Selective changes in multifidus dimensions in patients with chronic low back pain. European Spine Journal 1: 38–42

Stokes M, Young A 1984 Investigations of quadriceps inhibition: implications for clinical practice. Physiotherapy 70(11): 425–428

13

The Mulligan Concept: its application in the management of spinal conditions

L. Exelby
Pinehill Hospital, Hitchen, North Herts, UK

The Mulligan Concept encompasses a number of mobilizing treatment techniques that can be applied to the spine; these include natural apophyseal glides (NAGs), sustained natural apophyseal glides (SNAGs) and spinal mobilizations with limb movements (SMWLMs). These techniques are described and the general principles of examination and treatment are outlined. Clinical examples are used to illustrate the Concept's application to the spine and how it has evolved and been integrated into constantly changing physiotherapy practice. New applications are considered which can assist in the correction of dysfunctional movement. This article reflects on the possible role that this Concept has to play within evidence-based practice. A future research direction is proposed in the light of presently available preliminary research results. *Manual Therapy* 2002 **7(2)**: 64–70.

INTRODUCTION

The Mulligan Concept is now an integral component of many manual physiotherapists' clinical practice. Brian Mulligan pioneered the techniques of this Concept in New Zealand in the 1970s. The Concept has its foundation built on Kaltenborn's (1989) principles of restoring the accessory component of physiological joint movement. Mulligan proposed that injuries or sprains might result in a minor positional fault to a joint thus causing restrictions in physiological movement. Unique to this Concept is the mobilization of the spine whilst the spine is in a weight-bearing position and directing the mobilization parallel to the spinal facet planes (Fig. 13.1) (Mulligan 1999). Passive oscillatory mobilizations called NAGs and sustained mobilizations with active movement called SNAGs are the mainstay of this Concept's spinal treatment (Mulligan 1999). Mulligan proposed that when an increase in pain-free range of movement occurs with a SNAG it primarily consists of the correction of a positional fault at the zygapophyseal joint, although a SNAG also influences the entire spinal functional unit (SFU). Recently, the evolution of this Concept has supported the use of a transverse glide applied to the spinous process with active spinal movement. A further development in the 1990s was spinal mobilizations with limb movements (SMWLMs). Here a sustained transverse glide to the spinous process of a vertebra is applied while the restricted peripheral joint movement is performed actively or passively (Mulligan 1999). The mobilization must result in a symptom-free movement. Mulligan (1999) proposed that the application of these techniques, was appropriate when peripheral joint limitation of movement could be spinal in origin. This has further evolved into simultaneous gliding of spinal and peripheral joints with movement. Mobilizations with movements (MWMs) is the terminology used when applying an accessory glide to an active peripheral joint movement and is described in other texts (Mulligan 1993, 1999; Exelby 1996).

Literature on the efficacy of Mulligan's techniques is lacking and dominated by descriptive or case report publications (Wilson 1994, 1997, 2001; Exelby 1995, 1996, 2001; Vicenzino & Wright 1995;

Hetherington 1996; O'Brien & Vicenzino 1998; Lincoln 2000; Miller 2000). Recently, however, research measuring the neurophysiological or mechanical effects has been conducted (Kavanagh 1999; Hall et al 2000; Vicenzino et al 2000; Abbot et al. 2001a, b). The bulk of this research is confined to peripheral MWMs. In this article, the principles of examination and treatment are outlined and clinical examples are used to illustrate the Concept's application to the spine and how it has evolved and been integrated into physiotherapy practice. New applications are described that can assist in the correction of dysfunctional movement. A future research direction is proposed in the light of preliminary research results.

EXAMINATION

By definition SNAGs involve manually facilitating restricted joint gliding to allow pain-free movement. This in itself can be a simple differential diagnostic tool. SNAGs and MWMs can be a powerful complementary assessment tool when differentiating between more complex clinical presentations, e.g. lumbar spine, sacroiliac joint and hip.

The Mulligan Concept of accessory gliding with active movement can be further expanded in our clinical practice to justify its place in the assessment of muscle dysfunction. When analysing a functional movement the cause of the symptoms can be established by integrating

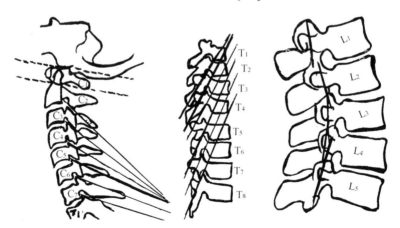

Figure 13.1 Orientation of zygapophyseal joints. (Reproduced by kind permission of Chartered Society of Physiotherapy from Physiotherapy 81(12): 724–729.)

this Concept with Sahrmann's theories (2002) namely 'the pathway of instantaneous centre of motion' and 'relative flexibility'. Clinically, a SNAG on a painful mobile level may not always achieve a full pain-free movement, whereas restricting the movement of a painful mobile segment or gliding a nearby stiff segment does achieve the desired result. For example, a patient with rightsided C5/6 cervical and upper arm symptoms of low irritability presented with a limitation of right cervical spine rotation. Full-range right rotation was achieved by applying a left unilateral SNAG on C1 in its horizontal treatment plane. Interventions at other levels had been unsuccessful. The possible explanation may be that the upper cervical spine segment was blocked causing lower cervical spine over-strain. Amevo et al (1992) demonstrated in cervical pain patients that abnormal instantaneous axes of rotation (IAR) in the upper cervical spine significantly correlated with pain found in the lower cervical spine segments.

This analysis of functional movement must be used in collaboration with other components of the assessment procedure and is valuable in helping to identify areas on which to focus more specific examination procedures. Intervertebral physiological and accessory active and passive motion testing (Maitland 1986) performed in weight bearing or lying is a necessity when the Concept is used in this way. While the Mulligan Concept is essentially an articular technique, the

principles can be applied to the myofascial system. Fascial tension can be altered or muscle trigger point pressure applied and the response to the movement restriction noted.

TREATMENT

The strength of this Concept also lies in its adaptability and ability to be integrated with most other commonly used musculoskeletal concepts (Wilson 1994, 1995; Exelby 1995). Some clinical examples will illustrate the diversity of this concept in multi-structural integrated treatments.

NAGS

Mulligan (1999) described NAGs for use in the cervical and upper thoracic spine. NAGs are passive oscillatory techniques performed parallel to the facet joint planes. The anatomical configuration of the upper two joints of the cervical spine necessitates a glide in a more horizontal plane. The NAGs are performed with the patient seated. A pillow supporting the arms will reduce tension in the neural tissue and myofascia around the neck and scapula. NAGs are invaluable when performed well and can be used on most spinal pathology. They are the treatment of choice for more acute inflammatory pathology (Exelby 1995; Mulligan 1999). In the author's experience they are less successful in the cervical spine if patients present with fixed forward neck postures with adaptive posterior soft tissue shortening. In this type of patient a NAG directed in a supero-anterior direction may be more difficult and compression of the facet joint surfaces instead could occur. NAGs are particularly useful in the cervical spine for mobilizing stiff joints that neighbour hypermobile segments. In this case they are modified, and applying the NAG with the thumb frees up the other fingers to fix the mobile segment anteriorly (Fig. 13.2). By positioning the patient in sidelying or supported, forward sitting NAGs can be performed on the rest of the thoracic spine and even the lumbar spine. In the thoracic spine they can be used for mobilizing segments that are

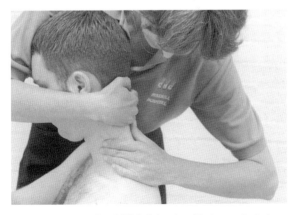

Figure 13.2 Localized NAG fixing level below anteriorly.

fixed in extension (Fig. 13.3). These patients often have an adverse response to postero-anteriorly directed mobilizations performed in the traditional prone position.

SNAGs

SNAGs as a treatment modality can be applied to all the spinal joints, the rib cage and the sacroiliac joint and are described in detail in Mulligan's book (1999). They provide a method to improve restricted joint range when symptoms are movement induced. The therapist facilitates the appropriate accessory zygapophyseal joint glide while the patient performs the symptomatic movement (Fig. 13.4). The facilitatory glide must result in full-range pain-free movement. Sustained end range holds or overpressure can be applied to the physiological movement. This previously symptomatic motion is repeated up to three times while the therapist continues to maintain the appropriate accessory glide. Further repetitions may be performed depending on the severity, irritability, and nature of the pathology (Maitland 1986). Failure to improve the comparable movement would indicate that the therapist has not found the correct contact point, spinal segment, amount of force or direction of mobilization, or that the technique is simply not indicated. SNAGs

are most successful when symptoms are provoked by a movement and are not multi-level (Mulligan 1999; Wilson 2001). They are not the treatment of choice in conditions that are highly irritable (Maitland 1986).

Although SNAGs are usually performed in functional weight-bearing positions they can be adapted for use in non-weight-bearing positions. For example they can be applied in lying to McKenzie lumbar spine extensions or to the lumbar spine joints in a four point kneel position (Exelby 2001).

FACILITATING FUNCTIONAL MOVEMENT PATTERNS WITH SNAGS

In problematic patients with mechanical stability dysfunction, treatment of the restriction may not result in long-lasting changes in symptoms. There is a need for these patients to change their posture and dysfunctional movement within their functional demands of daily living (O'Sullivan 2000). Various strategies used by physiotherapists may improve proprioception via joint and muscle receptor input to assist this functional adjustment. In the author's experience this concept can be modified so that an articular glide can be applied to an active corrected movement pattern, which can help to provide proprioceptive input to an

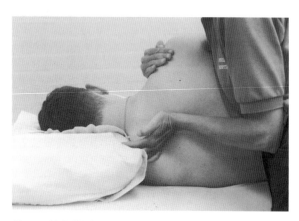

Figure 13.3 NAGs applied in sidelying position to promote flexion in an extended thoracic spine.

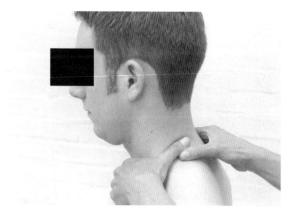

Figure 13.4 A unilateral SNAG applied to the left C5 zygapophyseal joint.

unfamiliar movement. The application can be progressed to more challenging positions and tasks.

An illustrative example may be a patient who presents with a loss of lower lumbar spine seg-

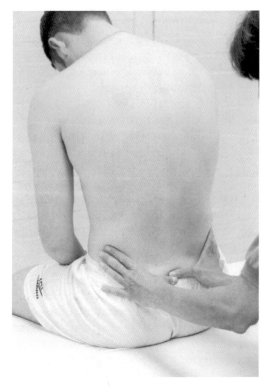

Figure 13.5 The upper lumbar spine is fixed in flexion; a SNAG is applied to the spinous process of L5 while the patient actively performs lower lumbar spine extension.

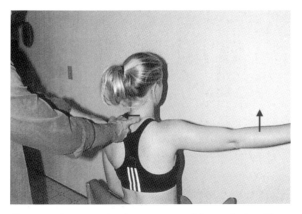

Figure 13.6 A sustained transverse glide applied to T1 while the patient performs active shoulder abduction.

mental lordosis and excessive upper lumbar spine extension. Passive intervertebral joint testing reveals a limitation of lower lumbar spine extension. A SNAG can be applied to these stiff joints in positions of sidelying, sitting or standing while the patient performs a localized anterior tilt with the upper lumbar spine fixed in some degree of flexion (Fig. 13.5).

SPINAL MOBILIZATION WITH LIMB MOVEMENTS

These techniques can be used for restricted upper or lower limb movements that could be as a result of a spinal joint dysfunction or abnormal neural dynamics (Mulligan 1994, 1995, 1999; Wilson 1994, 1995). A transverse glide is applied to a spinous process by the therapist. This transverse glide results in a rotation of the vertebra to which it is applied. The vertebra can be rotated either way and the neighbouring segment can also be fixed by applying an opposite glide to its spinous process (Mulligan 1999). The latter application is useful when stiff and mobile segments lie adjacent to each other. The direction and level of application is determined by a combination of examination findings such as the symptom referral pattern, palpation of the spine with the active limb movement, passive physiological intervertebral movements (PPIVMs), passive accessory intervertebral movements (PAIVMs) and alignment of the vertebrae. These examination procedures will help to provide a more comprehensive picture of the movement dysfunction and reduce experimental gliding with the restricted movement. The author has found in her clinical experience that a corrective glide on the implicated rotated segment achieves the best results.

SPINAL MOBILIZATIONS WITH ARM MOVEMENTS

Arm movements with cervical and upper thoracic glides can be applied in weight-bearing or non-weight-bearing positions (Mulligan 1994) (Fig. 13.6). They can be applied to a general functional movement, e.g. a back swing in golf or more specific neural testing positions. An example of the latter may be a limitation of the median nerve upper limb tension test (ULTT 1) (Butler 1991). The patient is positioned with the upper arm supported, the comparable movement being active elbow extension. The therapist applies a transverse glide on a spinous process that enables pain-free elbow extension. The glide is maintained and the pain-free elbow extension is repeated. Neural tissue must be given the respect it deserves: too much repetition of an aggravating movement when trying to identify a pain-easing glide may result in neural tissue irritation. Sound clinical decision making is necessary to decide if this technique is appropriate to the presenting clinical findings. In the above example C7 was restricted and rotated. Elbow extension was improved with a corrective transverse glide applied to the spinous process of C7 (Fig. 13.7).

SPINAL MOBILIZATIONS WITH LEG MOVEMENTS

In the lower limb the application of this technique is usually indicated when there is a restriction of the straight leg raise (SLR) (Mulligan 1995, 1999). Once the lumbar spine has been palpated, usually in prone, for intervertebral pain, restriction and alignment, the patient is placed in the sidelying position. Further spinal palpation can be carried out with limb movement to assess intervertebral mobility. A transverse glide is applied to a spinal segment while a second person performs a passive SLR. The neighbouring joint can be fixed with an opposing transverse glide. The spinal glide must result in a pain-free passive SLR. The technique can be successfully modified for use by a single therapist (Fig. 13.8). The thigh and hip are supported on a pillow; the transverse spinal glide must alleviate the symptoms provoked by active knee extension with or without ankle dorsiflexion. Applying ischaemic compression pressure to the piriformis trigger point (Travell & Simons 1992) while the patient performs active knee extension can also result in marked improvement in sciatic pain and SLR mobility when the spinal glides have been ineffectual. This has often proved more successful than releasing piriformis passively. The groups of patients that benefit particularly from this technique are those with a positive piriformis trigger point (Travell & Simons 1992) and more chronic symptoms, and post-spinal surgery patients. The latter are often left with residual moderate buttock and leg aching.

Other interfaces in the limbs (Wilson 1994, 1995; Exelby 1996) can be used in conjunction with passive joint or myofascial release work. It is important to remember that the full explanation for the changes in symptoms is probably far more complex than an alteration of local abnormal biomechanics alone.

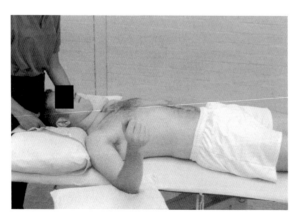

Figure 13.7 Active elbow extension performed in a modified ULLT 1 position. A transverse glide is applied to the C7 spinous process to correct its rotated position. This results in pain-free active elbow extension.

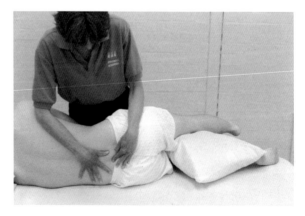

Figure 13.8 A SMWLM is performed in the sidelying position. The patient's hip is flexed and supported on a pillow. A corrective transverse glide is applied to L5 with L4 fixed while the patient performs active knee extension.

POSSIBLE MECHANISMS AND FUTURE RESEARCH

To date there is no published research establishing the efficacy of the treatment of the spine using this concept. An initial step may be to establish which subgroups of spinal conditions respond to particular techniques. Multi-centre collection of case study data could identify trends and form the framework on which to base larger studies. For instance, the case series on 'acute locked back' (Exelby 2001) could form the basis for further data collection and research.

A mobilization with an active movement (MWM) is only one component of the Mulligan Concept. Research can take many different pathways but one question in particular to be considered with MWMs is whether the application of a mobilization with an active movement can provide a greater modulatory affect on pain and the motor neurone pool than passive mobilization in isolation.

Two papers on the application of MWMs to a subgroup of patients with tennis elbow could provide some clues to these neurophysiological responses. A sustained lateral elbow glide with gripping resulted in immediate significant changes of pain-free grip strength (Abbot 2001a). The randomized, double blind controlled study of Vicenzino et al (2000) on tennis elbow patients evaluated the effects of the same elbow lateral glide technique on pain-free grip strength (PFGS) and pressure pain threshold (PPT). This study demonstrated an immediate 50% increase in PFGS, with only a 10% increase in PPT. Of particular interest in these studies is what can be interpreted as the significant modulatory affect on the motor neurone pool. Another study on a similar group of patients that received a cervical spine treatment resulted in a different response with a PPT increase in the order of 25–30% and a PFGS improvement of only 12–30% (Vicenzino et al 1996, 2000). Comparative studies on tennis elbow subjects will provide further information about the treatment responses of various therapeutic techniques. The use of electromyography (EMG) may give more insight into the interface between pain inhibition and motor response.

To establish the clinical efficacy of therapeutic approaches in the treatment of spinal conditions, methodology that more accurately reflects current clinical practice has been used with specific technique application left to the therapist's discretion. For example, to reflect present popular clinical practice 'manual therapy' has been compared to a 'spinal stabilization exercise programme' in a chronic low back pain subgroup (Goldby 2001) and a cervicogenic headache population (Jull 2000a). The Mulligan Concept in the light of its manual application to joints would not fit into the 'exercise category' and yet it is more than a passive mobilization especially in view of some of its applications to correct movement patterns as proposed by the author.

There is sufficient evidence to demonstrate that stimulation of joint receptors via passive mobilizations or manipulation will have an immediate reflex effect on segmental muscle activity (Thabe 1986; Taylor et al 1994; Murphy et al 1995). Colloca and Keller (2001), Herzog et al (1995), Katavich (1999) and Sabbahi et al (1990) have also considered the afferent input of manual therapy techniques on other tissues such as muscle. Despite this evidence, Jull's (2000a) RCT on the management of headaches revealed that manipulative therapy alone did not improve performance in the craniocervical test of deep flexor function and specific exercise alone did not improve cervical segmental motion as assessed by manual examination as effectively as manipulative therapy.

A number of investigative procedures are available to test muscle activity, e.g. EMG and ultrasound (Hides et al 1992, 1995; Hodges 1999; Jull 2000b; Moseley et al 2000), proprioceptive deficits (Revel et al 1991) and pain response (Vicenzino 1995). These could be used in comparative studies to determine whether there are advantages to the use of MWMs on segmental muscle activity, kinaesthetic sense and pain when compared to other passive manual therapy techniques or direct muscle facilitation. This direction for future research will establish what role these techniques have to play in the correction of movement patterns and the facilitation of local muscle activity.

CONCLUSION

The strength and enduring capabilities of this Concept lie in the founder's philosophy of encouraging integration of these techniques into the individual therapist's clinical practice. This has resulted in a constantly evolving concept that has stood the test of time. Clinical examples serve to illustrate the general use of this concept's principles and how it can also be incorporated with functional activity to assist in correcting joint positional faults within improved quality movement patterns. In the light of present physiotherapy evidence-based practice, a future research direction for this Concept is proposed.

Acknowledgements

The author would like to acknowledge R. Crowell and A. Lingwood for their guidance with the writing of this paper.

REFERENCES

Abbott JH, Patla CE, Jenson RH 2001a The initial effects of an elbow mobilisation with movement technique on grip strength in subjects with lateral epicondylalgia. Manual Therapy 6(3): 163–169

Abbott JH, Patla CE, Jenson RH 2001b Mobilisation with movement applied to the elbow affects shoulder range of motion in subjects with lateral epicondylalgia. Manual Therapy 6(3): 170–177

Amevo B, Aprill C, Bogduk N 1992 Abnormal instantaneous axes of rotation in patients with neck pain. Spine 17(7): 748–756

Butler DS 1991 Mobilisation of the Nervous System. Churchill Livingstone, Edinburgh, pp 147–152

Colloca CJ, Keller TS 2001 Electrom yographic reflex responses to mechanical force, manually assisted spinal manipulative therapy. Spine 26(10): 1117–1124

Exelby L 1995 Mobilisations with movement: a personal view. Physiotherapy 81(12): 724–729

Exelby L 1996 Peripheral mobilisations with movement. Manual Therapy 1(3): 118–126

Exelby L 2001 The locked facet joint: intervention using mobilisations with movement. Manual Therapy 6(2): 116–121

Goldby L, Moore A, Doust J, Trew M, Lewis J 2001 A randomized controlled trial investigating the efficacy of manual therapy, exercises to rehabilitate spinal stabilisation and an education booklet in the conservative treatment of chronic low back pain disorder. In: Proceedings of 1st International Conference on Movement Dysfunction 'Integrating Approaches. Edinburgh, Scotland, September, p. 19

Hall T, Cacho T, McNee C, Riches J, Walsh J 2000 Efficacy of the Mulligan SLR Technique. In: Singer KP (ed) Proceedings of the 7th Scientific Conference of the IFOMT in conjunction with the Biennial Conference of the MPAA. Perth, Australia, 9–10 November, pp 185–109

Herzog W, Conway PJ, Zhang YT, Gal J, Guimaraes ACS 1995 Reflex responses associated with manipulative treatments on the thoracic spine: a pilot study. Journal of Manipulative Physiological Therapeutics 18(4): 233–236

Hetherington B 1996 Case Study: Lateral Ligament strains of the ankle, do they exist? Manual Therapy 1(5): 274–275

Hides JA, Cooper DH, Stokes MJ 1992 Diagnostic ultrasound imaging for measurement of the lumbar multifidus in normal young adults. Physiotherapy Theory and Practice 8: 19–26

Hides J, Richardson C, Jull G, Davies S 1995 Ultrasound imaging in rehabilitation. Australian Journal of Physiotherapy 41(3): 187–193

Hodges PW 1999 Is there a role for transversus abdominis in lumbo-pelvic stability? Manual Therapy 4(2): 74–86

Jull GA 2000a The physiotherapy management of cervicogenic headache: A randomised controlled study. In: Singer KP (ed) Proceedings of the 7th Scientific Conference of the IFOMT in conjunction with the Biennial Conference of the MPAA. Perth, Australia, 9–10 November, p.100

Jull GA 2000b Deep cervical flexor muscle dysfunction in whiplash. Journal of Musculoskeletal Pain 8(1/2): 143–154

Kaltenborn FM 1989 Mobilisation of the Extremity Joints. 4th edn. Orthopaedic Physical Therapy Products, USA

Katavich L 1999 Neural mechanisms underlying manual cervical traction. The Journal of Manual and Manipulative Therapy 7(1): 20–25

Kavanagh J 1999 Is there a positional fault at the inferior tibiofibular joint in patients with acute or chronic sprains compared to normals? Manual Therapy 4(1): 19–24

Lincoln J 2000 Clinical instability of the upper cervical spine. Manual Therapy 5(1): 41–46

Maitland GD 1986 Vertebral Manipulation, 5th edn. Butterworths, London

Miller J 2000 Mulligan Concept — management of 'Tennis Elbow'. Orthopaedic Division Review, May/June: 45–46

Moseley GL, Hodges PW, Gandevia SC 2000 Deep and superficial fibres of multifidus are controlled independently during arm movements. In: Singer KP (ed) Proceedings of the 7th Scientific Conference of the IFOMT in conjunction with the Biennial Conference of the MPAA. Perth, Australia, 9–10 November, p. 127

Mulligan BR 1993 Mobilisations with movement. Journal of Manual & Manipulative Therapy 1(4): 154–156

Mulligan BR 1994 Spinal mobilisations with arm movement (further mobilisations with movement). The Journal of Manual and Manipulative Therapy 2(2): 75–77

Mulligan BR 1995 Spinal mobilisations with leg movement (further mobilisations with movement). The Journal of Manual and Manipulative Therapy 3(1): 25–27

Mulligan BR 1999 Manual therapy "Nags", "Snags", "MWMs" etc., 4th edn. Plane View Services, Wellington, New Zealand

Murphy BA, Dawson NJ, Slack JR 1995 Sacroiliac joint manipulation decreases the H-reflex. Electromyography and Clinical Neurophysiology 35: 87–94

O'Brien T, Vicenzino B 1998 A study of the effects of Mulligan's mobilisation with movement treatment of lateral ankle pain using a case study design. Manual Therapy 3(2): 78–84

O'Sullivan P 2000 Lumbar segmental instability: clinical presentation and specific stabilizing exercise management. Manual Therapy 5(1): 2–12

Revel M, Andre-Deshays C, Mineuet M 1991 Cervicocephalic kinesthetic sensibility in patients with cervical spine pain. Archives of Physical Medicine Rehabilitation 72: 288

Sabbahi MA, Fox AM, Druffle C 1990 Do joint receptors modulate the motoneuron excitability? Electromyography and Clinical Neurophysiology 30: 387–396

Sahrmann SA 2002 Diagnosis and Treatment of Movement Impairment Syndromes. Mosby, St Louis

Taylor M, Suvinen T, Rheade P 1994 The effect of Grade 4 distraction mobilisation on patients with temporomandibular pain-dysfunction disorder. Physiotherapy Theory and Practice 10: 129–136

Thabe H 1986 EMG as a tool to document diagnostic findings and therapeutic results associated with somatic dysfunctions in the upper cervical spinal joints and sacroiliac joints. Manual Medicine 2: 53–58

Travell JG, Simons DG 1992 Myofascial Pain and Dysfunction. The Trigger Point Manual. The Lower Extremities, Vol 2. Williams & Wilkins, Baltimore, pp 186–213

Vicenzino B 1995 An investigation of the effects of spinal manual therapy on the forequarter pressure and thermal pain thresholds and sympathetic nervous system activity in asymptomatic subjects: a preliminary report. In: Shacklock M (ed) Moving in on Pain. Butterworth–Heinnemann, Sydney, pp 185–193

Vicenzino B, Wright A 1995 Effects of a novel manipulative physiotherapy technique on tennis elbow: a single case study. Manual Therapy 1(1): 30–35

Vicenzino B, Collins D, Wright A 1996 The initial effects of a cervical spine manipulative physiotherapy treatment on the pain and dysfunction of lateral epicondylalgia. Pain 68: 69–74

Vicenzino B, Buratowski S, Wright A 2000 A preliminary study of the initial hypoalgesic effect of a mobilisation with movement treatment for lateral epicondylalgia. In: Singer KP (ed) Proceedings of the 7th Scientific Conference of the IFOMT in conjunction with the Biennial Conference of the MPAA. Perth, Australia, 9–10 November, pp 460–464

Wilson E 1994 Peripheral joint mobilisation with movement and its effects on adverse neural tension. Manipulative Therapist 26(2): 35–40

Wilson E 1995 Mobilisation with movement and adverse neural tension: an exploration of possible links. Manipulative Therapist 27(1): 40–46

Wilson E 1997 Central facilitation and remote effects: treating both ends of the system. Manual Therapy 2(2): 165–168

Wilson E 2001 The Mulligan Concept: NAGS, SNAGS, and mobilisations with movement. Journal of Bodywork and Movement Therapies 5(2): 81–89

14

The role of physiotherapy in the prevention and treatment of osteoporosis

Kim Bennell Karim Khan†
Heather McKay†*
*Centre for Sports Medicine Research and Education, School of Physiotherapy, The University of Melbourne, Melbourne, Australia
†Department of Family Medicine and Orthpaedics, University of British Columbia, Vancouver, Canada

Osteoporosis is an increasing public health problem that causes loss of life and reduced quality of life in sufferers. Strategies to improve bone density and reduce the likelihood of falls are important in the prevention of osteoporosis. Physiotherapists have a role to play in this condition through exercise prescription, therapeutic modalities, specific techniques and education. Appropriate treatment goals can be established following a thorough assessment of signs and symptoms, risk factors for osteoporosis and functional status. Levels of bone density measured from dual energy X-ray absorptiometry can help guide patient management. Since the aim is to maximize peak bone mass in children and adolescents, participation in a variety of high-impact activities should be encouraged. In the middle adult years, small increases in bone mass may be achieved by structured weight-training and weight-bearing exercise. In the older adult years, particularly if osteopenia or osteoporosis is present, the aim is to conserve bone mass, reduce the risk of falls, promote extended posture, reduce pain, and improve mobility and function. *Manual Therapy* (2000) **5(4)**: 198–213

INTRODUCTION

Osteoporosis is a metabolic bone disorder characterized by low bone mass and microarchitectural deterioration leading to skeletal fragility and increased fracture risk (Khan et al 2001). It is a major public health problem and one expected to increase with the significant ageing of the population (Kannus et al 1999). Osteoporosis consumes a large portion of the health-care budget, the greatest part of the cost being attributable to hip fractures (Randell et al 1995). However, far more importantly, osteoporosis causes loss of quality of life and loss of life in individuals, who otherwise may be in excellent health (Cooper & Melton 1992). Health practitioners have a role to play in this condition through exercise prescription, education and strategies to maximize function, reduce the risk of falls and manage pain. This article will provide an overview of physiotherapy management for bone health with an emphasis on the role of exercise during various stages of the lifespan.

FACTORS INFLUENCING THE RISK OF FRACTURE

Bone density and falls are two major determinants of the risk of fracture (Petersen et al 1996; Lespessailles et al 1998). An individual's peak bone mass is reached around the late teens and early 20s with up to 60% acquired during the pubertal years (Young et al 1995; Bailey 1997). A slow rate of bone loss starts at around age 40 years in both sexes and superimposed on this is an accelerated loss of bone in women at the menopause when oestrogen production ceases. Here rates of loss may be as great as 5–6% per year and are highest in the years immediately post-menopause (Riggs & Melton 1986; Fig. 14.1). It is now thought that one's peak bone mass is a better predictor of the risk of osteoporosis in later life than the amount of bone lost with age. Therefore, in addition to steps for minimizing bone loss, prevention strategies for osteoporosis are focusing on maximizing peak bone mass.

Approximately 60–80% of our peak bone mass is determined by our genes (Zmuda et al 1999). Other determinants include hormones, mechanical loading, nutrition, body composition and lifestyle factors, such as smoking and alcohol intake. Physiotherapists need to be aware of risk factors for osteoporosis as well as medical conditions and pharmacological agents that predispose to secondary osteoporosis (Table 14.1).

A greater propensity to fall will increase the risk of fracture (Parkkari et al 1999). Falls occur frequently in individuals over the age of 65 years (Hill et al 1999) and in residents in institutionalized care (Tinetti et al 1988; Campbell et al 1989). Many risk factors for fall initiation have been identified. These can be classified into intrinsic factors, for example, poor eyesight, reduced balance and reduced lower limb strength and extrinsic factors such as home hazards, multiple drug use and inappropriate footwear (Lord et al 1991; Lord et al 1994). Interestingly, those with osteoporosis appear to have different postural control strategies, specifically greater use of hip movement, than those without the disease (Lynn et al 1997).

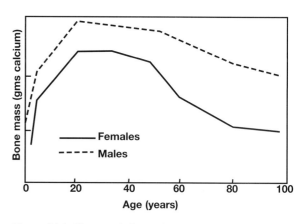

Figure 14.1 Changes in bone density with age in men and women.

MEASUREMENT OF BONE MINERAL DENSITY

Dual energy X-ray absorptiometry (DXA) is currently the technique of choice to measure bone density (Blake & Fogelman 1998). It has excellent measurement precision and accuracy, is relatively inexpensive and widely available. DXA uses a small amount of radiation (Lewis et al 1994) with the effective dose delivered being less than 1–3% of the annual natural background radiation one receives from living in a major city (Huda & Morin 1996).

DXA converts a three-dimensional body into a two-dimensional image, providing an integrated measure of both cortical and trabecular bone. The measurement of bone mineral density (BMD) is calculated by dividing the total bone mineral content (BMC) in grams by the projected area of the

Table 14.1 Risk factors for osteoporosis and medical conditions predisposing to secondary osteoporosis.

Risk factors for osteoporosis

- A family history of osteoporosis/hip fracture
- Post menopausal without hormone replacement therapy
- Late onset of menstrual periods
- A sedentary lifestyle
- Inadequate calcium and vitamin D intake
- Cigarette smoking
- Excessive alcohol
- High caffeine intake
- Amenorrhoea — loss of menstrual periods
- Thin body type
- Caucasian or Asian race

Medical conditions predisposing to secondary osteoporosis

- Anorexia nervosa
- Rheumatological conditions, e.g. rheumatoid arthritis, ankylosing spondylitis
- Endocrine disorders, e.g. Cushing's syndrome, primary hyperparathyroidism, thyrotoxicosis
- Malignancy
- Gastrointestinal disorders (malabsorption, liver disease, partial gastrectomy)
- Certain drugs (corticosteroids, heparin)
- Immobilization (paralysis, prolonged bed rest, functional impairment)
- Congenital disorders (Turner's syndrome, Klinefelter's syndrome)

specified region. It is therefore not a true volumetric density but an areal density expressed in g/cm^2. This has limitations particularly for paediatric populations where bone size rapidly changes during growth.

DXA scans are generally indicated if the individual is at risk for osteoporosis or if information is needed to help make a decision about pharmacological treatments or to monitor the success of treatment (Wark 1998). Repeated scans should be performed not less than 12 months apart as changes in bone density occur slowly. Furthermore, the same machine should be used as machines are calibrated differently. Bone density changes need to be more than 2–3% in order to represent true change and not simply measurement error.

INTERPRETATION OF DXA SCANS

Physiotherapists need to be able to interpret DXA scans as the results can guide patient management. There are three common methods of deriving a person's BMD from DXA (Fig. 14.2). The most direct method provides the unadjusted score in $g/cm2$ but this is less useful as it is influenced by the age of the subject. The two most useful BMD scores are the Z- and T-scores. The Z-score compares the person's BMD with that of an age-matched group (calculated as the deviation from the mean result for the age- and sex-matched group divided by the standard deviation of the group). This score indicates whether one is losing bone more rapidly than one's peers. The T-score is similarly defined but uses the deviation from the mean peak bone density of a young, healthy sex-matched group. The World Health Organization (1994) had defined bone mass clinically based on T-scores and has categorized it into normal, osteopenia, osteoporosis and established osteoporosis (Table 14.2). DXA-derived BMD scores have been shown clinically to predict fracture risk. There is a 1.9-fold increase in risk of vertebral fracture with each standard deviation decrease in lumbar spine BMD while there is a 2.6-fold increase in risk of hip fracture with each SD decrease in femoral neck BMD (Cummings et al 1993).

k = 1.235 d0 = 115.6 (1.000H)

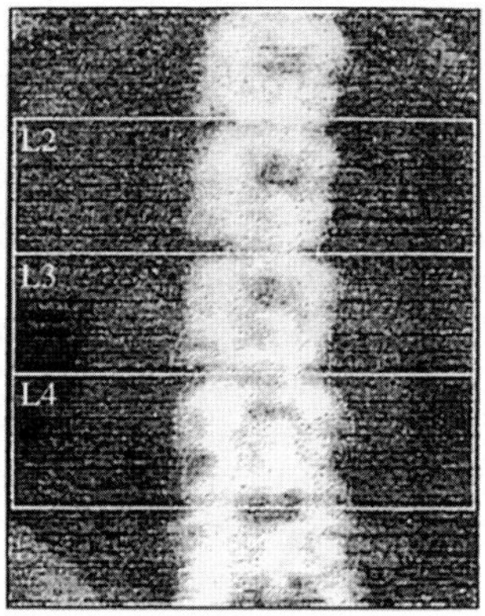

02-Jun-2000 14:37 [119 × 94]
Hologic QDR-1000/W (S/N 822)
Lumbar spine V4.76

Total BMD CV for L1–L4 1.0%

C.F.	0.999	1.063	1.000
Region	Area (cm²)	BMC (grams)	BMD (gms/cm²)
L2	10.00	6.42	0.642
L3	10.57	7.49	0.709
L4	13.05	10.59	0.811
Total	33.62	24.51	0.729

HOLOGIC

Lumbar spine
Reference database

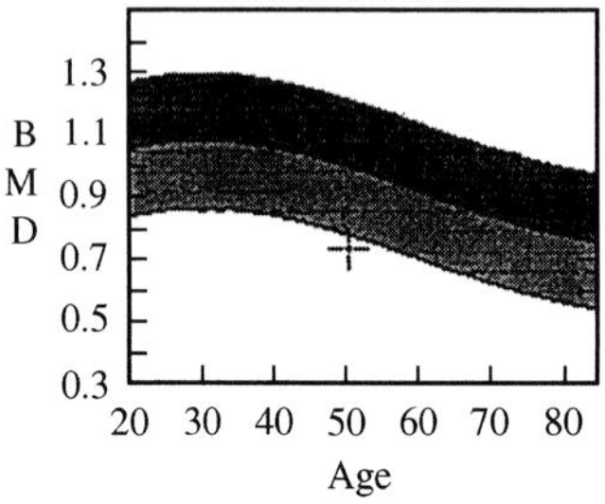

BMD (L2–L4) = 0.729 g/cm²

Region	BMD	T		Z	
N/A					
L2	0.642	−3.51	62%	−2.76	68%
L3	0.709	−3.41	65%	−2.62	71%
L4	0.811	−2.77	73%	−1.96	79%
L2 – L4	0.729	−3.18	68%	−2.40	73%

• Age and sex matched
T = peak bone mass
Z = age matched   TK   25 Oct 91

HOLOGIC

Figure 14.2 Results from a DXA scan of the lumbar spine of a 51-year-old woman showing the absolute bone density as well as T- and Z-scores. Since she has a T-score of –3.18 for the L2–4 she is considered to have osteoporosis at this site. A Z-score of –2.4 indicates that she also has lower bone density compared with her peers.

SIGNS AND SYMPTOMS OF OSTEOPOROSIS

Low bone density *per se* is asymptomatic and many individuals are unaware that they have osteopenia or osteoporosis until a fracture occurs. The common fracture sites are the hip, vertebrae and wrist and less commonly the ribs, pelvis and upper arm (Sanders et al 1999). Vertebral compression fractures can cause loss of height and this may occur suddenly or gradually over time.

Table 14.2 Diagnostic criteria for osteoporosis (World Health Organization 1994)

Classification	DXA result
Normal	Normal BMD greater than 1 standard deviation (SD) below the mean of young adults (T-score >−1)
Osteopenia	BMD between 1 and 2.5 SD below the mean of young adults (T-score −1 to −2.5)
Osteoporosis	BMD more than 2.5 SD below the mean of young adults (T-score ≤−2.5)
Severe or established osteoporosis	BMD more than 2.5 SD below the mean of young adults plus one or more fragility fractures

Height loss of more than 4 cm over 10 years has been found to be a clinical marker of reductions in bone density in postmenopausal women (Sanila et al 1994). A common clinical sign of advanced spinal osteoporosis is thoracic kyphosis or the 'dowager's hump'. This is due to anterior wedge fractures of the vertebral bodies (Ensrud et al 1997) but muscle weakness and pain may contribute (Cutler et al 1993). Postural changes may cause patients to complain of a 'pot belly' with a bulging stomach and concertina-like skin folds. These changes also result in less space within the thorax and abdominal region and increased intra-abdominal pressure. This can cause shortness of breath and reduced exercise tolerance, hiatus hernia, indigestion, heartburn and stress incontinence (Larsen 1998).

Some patients complain of spinal pain due to fractures, but not all fractures are symptomatic. Back pain may be due to nonskeletal causes such as facet joint and disc pathology. In established osteoporosis, the distance between the rib cage and the iliac crests decreases and, if severe, pain may be experienced due to the lower ribs pressing on the pelvis. This may be aggravated by sustained positions in flexion such as sitting.

PHYSIOTHERAPY ASSESSMENT

A complete subjective and physical assessment is needed but the choice of questions and procedures depends on several factors including the age of the patient, severity of the condition, DXA results, co-existing pathologies, functional status and reasons for consultation. Specific questioning for osteoporosis is shown in Table 14.3. There are a number of reliable and standardized measurement tools that can be used to gain a more accurate assessment of the patient's needs. The following section describes the key assessment procedures including those outlined in the excellent guidelines developed by Gisela Creed and Sarah Mitchell for the UK Chartered Society of Physiotherapy (1999).

POSTURE AND RANGE OF MOTION

Serial height measures should be recorded, especially in postmenopausal women and elderly men (Gordon et al 1991). The severity of cervical and thoracic deformity can be gauged, with the patient standing with their back against the wall, by measuring the distance of the tragus or the occiput to the wall (Laurent et al 1991; Fig. 14.3) as well as by measuring range of shoulder elevation (Crawford & Jull 1993), cervical rotation and lateral flexion, and hand behind back and head. A kyphometer or a flexicurve ruler is a simple, reliable and cost-effective alternative to X-rays for measuring spinal kyphosis (Lundon et al 1998). A digital camera may also provide a pictorial record of serial postural changes. Limitation of ankle dorsiflexion may increase the risk of falling and is best assessed in weight bearing (Bennell et al 1998).

MUSCLE STRENGTH AND ENDURANCE

The main muscles of interest include the quadriceps, ankle dorsiflexors, scapula retractors, trunk extensors, hip extensors and abdominals (especially transversus abdominis). Various isometric, isotonic or isokinetic methods can be used to assess strength. These may involve the measurement of one repetition maximum (1RM) or 3RM where the heaviest weight that the person can lift on one or three occasions is determined. However, this may be inappropriate for those with severe osteoporosis and certainly a short

Table 14.3 Relevant questions for subjective assessment in the area of bone health.

Category	Specific questions
DXA results	Date performed T- and Z-scores Amount of change with serial scans
Family history of osteoporosis	Which family member? Which sites?
Fracture	Site When? Related to minimal trauma?
Falls history	Number of falls in past year Mechanism of falls Associated injuries Risk factors, e.g. eyesight, home hazards
Medical history	Particularly with relation to risk factors including ovariectomy, eating disorder, endocrine disorder
Medication	Current or past especially long-term steroids, hormone replacement therapy, bisphosphonates
Menstrual history	Age of onset of periods Ever ≤8 periods per year and number of years? Menopausal status including age at menopause and number of years since menopause
Smoking habits	Number of cigarettes per day and number of years smoked currently or in past
Diet	Dietary restrictions such as vegetarianism, low fat Sources of daily calcium: yoghurt; cheese; milk Calcium supplementation: type and daily dose Amount of caffeine Number of glasses of alcohol per week
Exercise status	Amount and type of activity during youth Current exercise: type; intensity; duration; frequency Interests and motivational factors Exercise tolerance and shortness of breath
Posture	Noticed any loss of height? Difficulty lying flat in bed? Number of pillows needed Any activities encouraging bad posture?
Musculoskeletal problems and functional status	Pain, weakness, poor balance, incontinence Functional limitations
Social history	Occupation: full time/part time Hobbies Family

lever should be used. An inexpensive spring gauge purchased from a hardware shop can be used to assess isometric quadriceps strength with the patient seated (Lord et al 1994). Trunk extensors may be assessed using the trunk extension endurance measurement (Toshikazu et al 1996) although this is contraindicated in those with a severe thoracic kyphosis. The function of transversus abdominis can be assessed visually while the patient performs abdominal bracing in

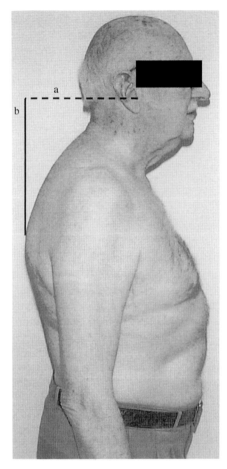

Figure 14.3 Assessing cervical and thoracic posture by measuring the distance of the tragus (A) to the wall (B) in standing. A more severe kyphosis will be reflected by a greater distance from the wall.

a variety of positions (Richardson & Jull 1995). Grip strength using a hand-held dynamometer provides a useful indicator of overall muscle strength while other functional tests such as sit-to-stand give an indication of lower limb strength.

AEROBIC CAPACITY

For relatively fit individuals without osteoporosis, a submaximal progressive exercise test using a treadmill or bike can provide an estimate of aerobic capacity. In older patients with moderate osteoporotic changes, simple tests which require minimal equipment, such as the 6-minute walk (Steele 1996) and the adapted shuttle walk test (Singh et al 1994), are suitable. Other walking tests may be more appropriate for the frail elderly and include the timed 6-minute walk and the 'timed up and go' test (Podsiadlo & Richardson 1991). If one is concerned about exercise tolerance, more sophisticated lung function tests such as forced vital capacity and forced expiratory volume in one second may be requested.

BALANCE

Depending on the person's functional level, reliable and valid measures include: (i) aspects of the clinical test of sensory interaction of balance (Shumway-Cook & Horak 1986; Cohen et al 1993) where the longest duration that the person can balance under different test conditions (eyes open/closed, standing on floor/foam) is timed; (ii) step test (Hill et al 1996) where the number of times the person can place the foot onto and off a step (7.5 or 15 cm high) in a 15-second period is counted; (iii) functional reach (Duncan et al 1990), which measures the maximal anterior–posterior distance that the person can reach in standing with the arm outstretched (Fig. 14.4).

PAIN AND FUNCTION

A history of osteoporotic fracture at any site is associated with a doubling of the risk of physical and functional limitation (Greendale et al 1995). Simple functional tests that can be administered in a clinical setting to establish the extent of disability and handicap include the 'timed up and go' (Podsiadlo & Richardson 1991) and the 'timed 6-minute walk' test (Hageman & Blanke 1986).

Self-administered questionnaires may provide useful additional information especially in those with more severe osteoporosis. The Osteoporosis Functional Disability Questionnaire and the Quality of Life Questionnaire of the European Foundation for Osteoporosis (QUAL-EFFO) are two valid and reliable disease-specific questionnaires developed for patients with back pain due to vertebral compression fractures

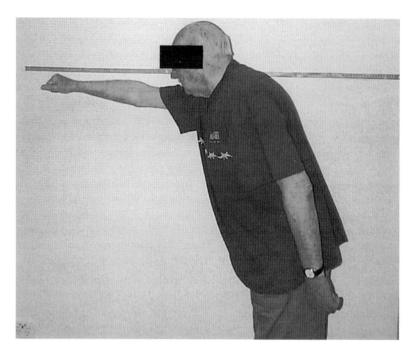

Figure 14.4 Functional reach, which measures the maximal anterior-posterior distance that the person can reach in standing with the arm outstretched, is a simple clinical measure of balance (Duncan et al 1990).

(Helmes et al 1995; Lips et al 1999). Use of other generic validated self-reported questionnaires that assess health-related qualify of life, such as the SF-36, allow comparison of the impact of disease and intervention across multiple studies and conditions.

Pain can also be assessed using visual analogue scales, the McGill pain questionnaire (Melzack 1975) and the monitoring of daily analgesic intake (Chartered Society of Physiotherapy 1999).

PHYSIOTHERAPY MANAGEMENT

Physiotherapy management will vary depending on assessment findings, particularly the patient's age, DXA results and functional status. The aims of treatment should be clearly established so that appropriate management can be instigated.

EXERCISE PRESCRIPTION FOR BONE LOADING

Loading of the skeleton occurs from the pull of contracting muscle and from ground reaction force during weight-bearing activity. Bone's ability to adapt to load is well recognized (Kerr et al 1996; Bennell et al 1997; Pettersson et al 1999a). Dramatic examples of the deleterious effect of unloading on bone can be seen with bed rest, space flight and immobilization (Arnaud et al 1992; Bauman et al 1999). While exercise influences bone material and structural properties, it is not known whether exercise reduces fracture rates, which is the ultimate goal. The fact that there are no randomized, controlled trials to answer this question reflects inherent methodological diffculties. However, large-scale epidemiological studies suggest that physical activity is associated with a lower risk of fracture in both men and women (Paganini-Hill et al 1991; Joakimsen et al 1999; Kujala et al 2000).

The mechanisms for bone adaptation are not entirely clear, but it is thought that mechanical strains sensed by bone are transduced into a cellular signal. This signal is then compared with 'optimal' strain for that particular bone site. If the bone strain is above or below the optimal range, then a skeletal remodelling or modelling response occurs. This concept proposed by Frost (1988) is known as the 'mechanostat theory'.

The skeletal effects of exercise at different ages

It is presently thought that exercise in childhood and adolescence produces much higher gains in bone mass than does exercise in adulthood. Unilateral loading studies involving adult female tennis and squash players showed that the beneficial effects on bone mineral acquisition and geometric adaptation were in the order of two to three times greater if the playing career was started before menarche (Kannus et al 1995; Haapasalo et al 1996). Retrospective studies in adult cohorts have reported that lifetime physical activity, especially during childhood, is associated with greater bone mass in adult females (McCulloch et al 1990; Cooper et al 1995; Khan et al 1998).

There are an increasing number of studies evaluating the effects of mechanical loading during growth. Cross-sectional and longitudinal cohort studies show greater bone mass in physically active children than in less-active controls (Slemenda et al 1991; McCulloch et al 1992; Grimston et al 1993; Bailey et al 1999; Lehtonen-Veromaa et al 2000). In intensely training elite athletes, such as gymnasts and weightlifters, the increases in bone mass can be as high as 30–80% (Conroy et al 1993; Bass et al 1998). Intervention studies in pre- and peri-pubertal girls (Morris et al 1997; McKay et al 2000; Heinonen et al 2000) and boys (Bradney et al 1998) show that even moderate levels of exercise have skeletal benefits. In one study, 30 minutes of weight-bearing and muscle-strengthening exercise performed three times per week led to 10% greater increases in bone density (Morris et al 1997). This would be sufficient to halve the risk of fracture if maintained

into the later years. In addition, it appears that childhood exercise stimulates the bone modelling process, expanding the bone size to produce a larger, possibly stronger bone (Haapasalo et al 1996; Bradney et al 1998). This phenomenon is generally not possible once growth has ceased. Skeletal exercise effects are not confined to healthy children. Exercise programmes in paediatric populations with disability, such as cerebral palsy, have led to improvements in bone density (Chad et al 1999).

There seems to be increasing evidence in favour of a fairly narrow critical period in childhood, probably determined by sexual maturation, where activity has a maximal positive effect on rapidly growing bone. This critical period appears to be in the peri-pubertal years (Tanner stage II and III) rather than the pre-pubertal years (Tanner stage I) but further research is required as current data conflict somewhat (Bass et al 1998; Haapasalo et al 1998). Certainly the skeleton is less responsive after menarche (Witzke & Snow 2000; Heinonen et al 2000). A supervised 9-month programme of step aerobics and jumps produced significant increases in bone mass in pre-menarcheal but not post-menarcheal girls (Heinonen et al 2000)

It is unknown whether skeletal gains can be maintained into the elderly years when fractures occur as no long-term exercise intervention study following children over this time has been carried out. Evidence to suggest that this is possible comes from the site-specific higher bone density related to unique loading patterns reported in retired athletes (Kirchner et al 1996; Bass et al 1998) and from exercise detraining studies (Kontulainen et al 1999). However, this issue is still unresolved as recent authors have suggested a gradual diminution of exercise effects over time (Karlsson et al 2000).

To emphasize the importance of exercise during growth is not to deny its importance later in life. The former is concerned mainly with acquisition and the latter mainly with conservation of bone. Exercise in adulthood is especially important considering that the adult skeleton is much more responsive to the adverse effects of unloading than to the beneficial effects of overloading.

Attention to lifestyle factors, such as diet, is also important during this time as the skeletal effects appear to be modulated by calcium intake (Specker 1996).

A recent meta-analysis evaluated the effect of exercise on bone mass in pre- and postmenopausal women (Wolff et al 1999). It concluded that randomized controlled trials consistently showed that exercise prevented or reversed about 1% of bone loss per year at both the lumbar spine and femoral neck. This was corroborated by other meta-analyses in post-menopausal women (Berard et al 1997; Kelley 1998) although Berard et al (1997) claimed this was confined to the lumbar spine. Much less attention has been paid to exercise in men. Results of the small number of trials ($n=8$) showed that targeted exercise can cause bone mass gains in the order of 2.6% at both the spine and hip in men over the age of 31 years (Kelley et al 2000).

Postmenopausal women do not seem to be as responsive to the same loading stimulus as pre-menopausal women. In a comparative study, 50 daily vertical jumps for 5 months produced a 2.8% increase in femoral neck BMD in premenopausal women but no change in postmenopausal women (Bassey et al 1998). Based on the mechanostat theory, it has been proposed that oestrogen deficiency increases the set points for the optimal strain range. Thus a greater loading stimulus is needed for bone adaptation than in an oestrogen-replete state (Dalsky 1990).

Since exercise *immediately* following menopause does not prevent the rapid bone loss that occurs at this time (Bassey & Ramsdale 1995; Maddalozzo & Snow 2000), it cannot be recommended as a substitute for hormone replacement therapy (HRT) (American College of Sports Medicine 1995). However, a combination of exercise and HRT appears to provide greater skeletal benefits than HRT alone (Kohrt et al 1995).

A small number of studies have evaluated the effect of exercise in women with diagnosed osteopenia (Bravo et al 1996; Hartard et al 1996) or osteoporosis (Preisinger et al 1996; Malmros et al 1998). While the emphasis in these groups is on preventing falls, improving function and reducing pain, exercise has been shown to conserve bone density.

In adulthood, exercise must be continued in order to maintain exercise-induced BMD levels (Dalsky et al 1988). Attrition rates from exercise are high even in supervised clinical trials (Bassey & Ramsdale 1994; Kerschan et al 1998). This reinforces the importance of developing strategies to improve compliance and encourage life-long participation in physical activity.

What types of exercise are best for improving bone strength?

Different activities will provide bone tissue with different strain environments and hence influence the overall adaptive response. Animal studies show that maximal skeletal effects are achieved with dynamic loads that are high in magnitude and rate, and unusual in distribution (Lanyon et al 1982; O'Connor et al 1982; Rubin & Lanyon 1984, 1985; Judex & Zernicke 2000). Relatively few loading cycles are necessary (Umemura et al 1997). It is also known that bone changes are localized to the areas directly loaded (Bennell et al 1997).

In humans, high-impact exercises, which generate ground reaction forces greater than two times body weight, are more osteogenic than low-impact exercises (Bassey & Ramsdale 1994; Heinonen et al 1996; Heinonen et al 1998). In a 8–12 month longitudinal study of well-trained females, gymnasts showed greater increases in spinal and femoral neck bone density than did runners, swimmers and controls (Taaffe et al 1997). In perimenopausal women, moderate intensity (70–80% V_{O_2} max) endurance exercise (cycling, jogging, treadmill walking) prevented bone loss at the femoral neck but not the lumbar spine while low-intensity callisthenics exercise was ineffective (Heinonen et al 1998). Exercise programmes reported in the literature have included various combinations of stair-climbing, aerobics, skipping, jumping, sprinting, dancing and jogging.

Since lean mass (Flicker et al 1995; Young et al 1995) and muscle strength (Madsen et al 1993) are positively correlated with bone density, weight training has been advocated for skeletal health. In premenopausal women, weight training has been shown to be of benefit at the lumbar spine

(Gleeson et al 1990; Snow-Harter et al 1992; Lohmann et al 1995), with a magnitude of effect similar to that gained with running (Snow-Harter et al 1992). Conversely, a study by Rockwell et al (1990) reported a 4% loss of vertebral bone mineral in 36-year-old women undertaking a mild weight-training intervention. This apparent detrimental effect could be due to the non-randomized design, small sample size, differences in baseline bone turnover levels and timing of measurements. The benefits of weight training for the hip region are unclear (Snow-Harter et al 1992; Lohmann et al 1995), although a significant improvement in bone density at the trochanter was seen following an 18-month programme (Lohmann et al 1995).

Loss of muscle mass and strength with age is well documented, especially after the sixth decade (Harries & Bassey 1990; Rutherford & Jones 1992). Maintenance of strength throughout the lifespan is associated with a reduced prevalence of functional limitations (Brill et al 2000). Progressive weight training even in the frail elderly can lead to large strength gains (Fiatarone et al 1990). Skeletal benefits of weight training in healthy postmenopausal women have been reported by some authors (Nelson et al 1994; Kerr et al 1996) but not others (Pruitt et al 1992; Nichols et al 1995), which may relate partly to the type of exercise regimen. In an elegant unilateral exercise study, Kerr et al (1996) compared two strength-training regimes that differed in the number of repetitions and the weight lifted. The strength programme (high loads, low repetitions) significantly increased bone density at the hip and forearm sites whereas the endurance programme (low loads, high repetitions) had no effect. Weight training has also been shown to increase bone density in men (Ryan et al 1994) and to conserve bone in women with osteoporosis and osteopenia (Hartard et al 1996).

Walking is frequently recommended in clinical practice to maintain skeletal integrity but controversy exists in the literature regarding its effcacy. Hatori et al (1993) found that 30 minutes of fast walking (7.2 km/h), performed three times a week at an intensity above the anaerobic threshold, increased spinal bone density. Slower walking (6.2 km/h) was ineffective. In general, however, the results of walking trials have not demonstrated significant effects at the spine or hip (Hatori et al 1993; Martin & Notelovitz 1993; Ebrahim et al 1997; Humphries et al 2000). This may relate to the fact that walking imparts relatively low magnitude, repetitive and customary strain to the skeleton. While walking has numerous health benefits, some of which may influence fracture risk, it should not be prescribed as the exercise of choice for skeletal loading in healthy ambulant individuals. Whether walking is effective in those with restricted mobility is yet to be researched.

Non-weight-bearing activities, such as cycling and swimming, do not stimulate bone adaptation despite increases in muscle strength (Orwoll et al 1989; Rico et al 1993; Taaffe et al 1995). This suggests that these activities do not generate sufficient strain to reach the threshold for bone adaptation.

Exercise dosage

The exact exercise dose required for maximal skeletal effects is not yet known. For an elderly or previously sedentary population, exercise should be gradually introduced to minimize fatigue and prevent soreness (Forwood & Larsen 2000). Exercise should be performed 2–3 times per week. Animal studies suggest that this is as effective for bone as daily loading (Raab-Cullen et al 1994).

For aerobic exercise, sessions should last between 15 and 60 min. The average conditioning intensity recommended for adults without fragility fractures is between 70% and 80% of their functional capacity. Individuals with a low functional capacity may initiate a programme at 40–60% (Forwood & Larsen 2000).

Adults commencing a weight-training programme may perform a few weeks of familiarization (Kerr et al 1996) followed by a single set of 8–10 repetitions at an intensity of 40–60% of 1RM. This can be progressed to 80%, even in the very elderly (Fiatorone et al 1994; American College of Sports Medicine 1998). In a study of postmenopausal women with diagnosed osteopenia, strength training at 70% 1RM was safe and effective for maintaining hip and spine bone mass (Hartard et al 1996). Programmes should include 8–10 exercises involving the major muscle groups.

Supervision, particularly in the beginning, with attention to safe lifting technique is paramount.

Periodic progression of exercise dosage is needed otherwise bone adaptation will cease. Increasing the intensity or weight bearing is more effective than increasing the duration of the exercise. A periodic increase in a step-like fashion may be better than progression in a linear fashion (Forwood & Larsen 2000). Nevertheless, there comes a point where gains in bone mass will slow and eventually plateau. This is because each person has an individual biological ceiling that determines the extent of a possible training effect (American College of Sports Medicine 1995).

In women, the intensity and volume of exercise should not compromise menstrual function. The incidence of menstrual disturbances in athletes is greater than that in the general female population (Malina et al 1978; Skierska 1998). Amenorrhoea (loss of menstrual cycles) and oligomenorrhoea (3–8 cycles per year) are associated with bone loss, particularly at the lumbar spine (Drinkwater et al 1984; Rutherford 1993; Pettersson et al 1999b). Endurance athletes are more susceptible to bone loss than athletes involved in high-impact sports (Robinson et al 1995). Of concern is evidence that even long-term resumption of regular menses fails to restore the bone deficits (Keen & Drinkwater 1997; Micklesfield et al 1998). Patients with menstrual disturbances should be referred to an appropriate medical practitioner for further investigation.

CLINICAL RECOMMENDATIONS FOR EXERCISE PRESCRIPTION

In children and adolescents, the goal is to maximize peak bone mass. A variety of weight-bearing, high-impact activities should be encouraged as part of the physical education curriculum in schools and during extra-curricular sport and play. In the premenopausal adult years, the emphasis is on structured exercise to load bone. This could involve high-impact activities and weight-training. A healthy lifestyle should be promoted and in females, attention paid to regular menstrual cycles. In the older adult years, a variety of exercise modes are needed to target clin-

Table 14.4 Exercises which may be included in a weight-training programme for healthy adults.

Weight-training exercises

- Biceps curl
- Overhead press
- Wrist curl
- Reverse wrist curl
- Triceps extension
- Forearm pronation/supination
- Bench press
- Leg press
- Half squats
- Hip abduction/adduction
- Hamstring curl
- Hip flexion
- Hip extension

ically relevant hip, spine and forearm sites. Progressive weight training (Table 14.4) and low-impact exercise are appropriate given that high-impact loading may be injurious. Other activities for balance, posture and aerobic fitness could include a fast walking programme, cycling, swimming and specific exercises.

While exercise should be directed at improving or maintaining bone density, in osteoporotic and older patients the exercise focus shifts from specifically loading bone to preventing falls and improving function. Figure 14.5 shows how a patient's bone density may influence the aims of treatment and the types of exercise chosen (Forwood & Larsen 2000). However, it must be remembered that the divisions are relatively arbitrary and should only be used as a guide. Other factors that will influence the choice of exercise programme include the patient's age, previous fractures, co-morbid musculoskeletal or medical conditions, lifestyle, interests and current fitness level. Exercises to avoid in osteoporotic patients include high-impact loading, abrupt or explosive movements, trunk flexion, twisting movements and dynamic abdominal exercises.

POSTURE AND FLEXIBILITY

In patients with osteopenia or osteoporosis, treatment should aim to minimize the flexion load on the spine, promote extended posture and improve chest expansion. Increased physical activity is

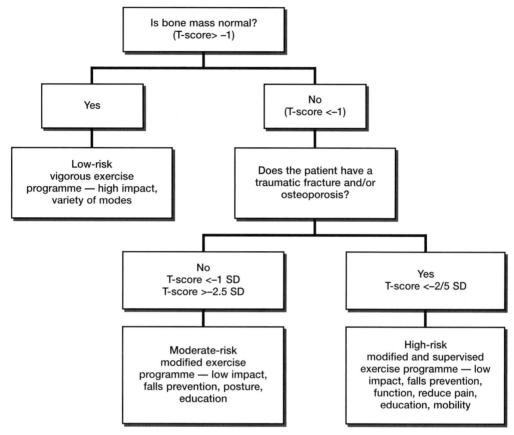

Figure 14.5 Devising an exercise programme based on DXA determined fracture risk. Adapted from Forwood and Larsen (2000).

associated with a reduced risk of vertebral deformity (Chow & Harrison 1987; Silman et al 1997). Land or water exercises can be designed to encourage diaphragmatic breathing, strengthen the hip, back and neck extensors and scapula retractors, and stretch the major upper and lower limb muscles (Bravo et al 1997; Chartered Society of Physiotherapy 1999). Postural re-education and dynamic stabilization for the trunk and limb girdles are particularly important to normalize mechanical forces (Figs 14.6 & 14.7). Stronger back extensors have been shown to be related to smaller thoracic kyphosis (Sinaki et al 1996). Patients can be advised to spend time lying in prone or prone on elbows to stimulate thoracic extension. Postural taping (Fig. 14.8) or bracing may be required to assist with maintenance of correct posture and for pain relief. Advice can be given about correct ways to lift as well as correct posture during standing, lying, sitting and bending.

FALLS REDUCTION

In elderly individuals or where falls risk factors have been identified, treatment should be directed towards reducing falls and their consequences. Patients who report multiple falls may benefit from referral to a falls clinic or to medical specialists for further evaluation and multi-faceted interventions. Such interventions may be effective in reducing fall frequency (Tinetti et al 1994) depending upon the programme and setting (McMurdo

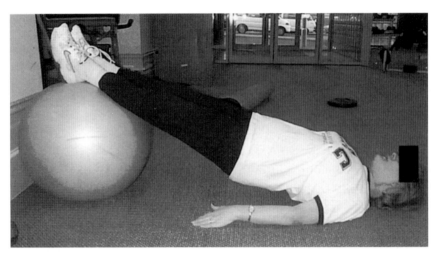

Figure 14.6 Hip extension exercises using a ball assist with trunk and pelvic stability.

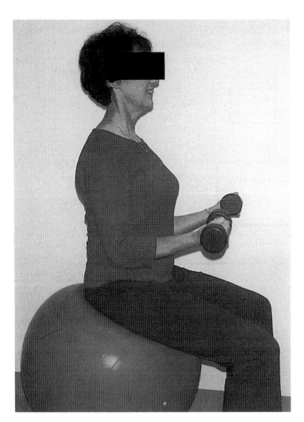

Figure 14.7 Upper limb exercises can be performed while sitting on a ball to increase dynamic stability and trunk control.

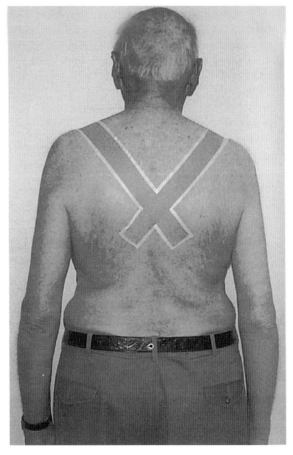

Figure 14.8 Taping may be used to facilitate thoracic extension and improve posture.

et al 2000). Home hazard modification may be required often in consultation with an occupational therapist. Consideration should be given to prescription of gait aids and external hip protectors in appropriate patients. Hip protectors have been shown to attenuate fall impact (Parkkari et al 1995, 1997) and to halve the incidence of hip fractures in institutionalized older persons (Lauritzen et al 1993). Specific deficits, such as restrictions in range of ankle dorsiflexion, can be improved through therapist techniques or self-stretches.

There are numerous studies demonstrating the positive effect of various forms of land and water-based exercise on balance and strength deficits in elderly individuals (McMurdo & Rennie 1993; Nelson et al 1994; Morganti et al 1995; Lord 1996; Simmons & Hansen 1996; Bravo et al 1997; Kronhed & Moller 1998). However, of the randomized, controlled trials of exercise in older persons using falls as an outcome measure (Reinsch et al 1992; MacRae et al 1994; Mulrow et al 1994; Lord et al 1995; Wolf et al 1996; Buchner et al 1997; Campbell et al 1997; McMurdo et al 1997; Campbell et al 1999), only a few report beneficial exercise effects. The effective exercise programmes included T'ai Chi (Wolf et al 1996) and physiotherapy-prescribed combined lower limb strengthening and balance training (Buchner et al 1997; Campbell et al 1997, 1999). The fact that other studies have failed to show significant results may be partly due to differences in exercise dimensions (type, duration, frequency and intensity), populations studied and falls definition.

At this stage, no definitive exercise prescription guidelines to prevent falls can be made on the basis of published studies. However, there is sufficient evidence to recommend a broad-based exercise programme comprising balance training, resistive exercise, walking and weight-transfer as part of a multi-faceted intervention to address all falls risk factors (Khan et al 2001).

PAIN-RELIEVING TECHNIQUES

Exercise has been shown to reduce back pain and improve psychological well-being in post-menopausal women with osteopenia (Bravo et al 1996; Preisinger et al 1996) and with established osteoporosis (Malmros et al 1998). In a randomized, controlled trial of 53 women with spinal crush fracture and back pain, a 10-week physiotherapy programme consisting of balance training, muscle strengthening and lumbar stabilization exercises, was effective in decreasing analgesic use and back pain and increasing quality of life and level of daily function (Malmros et al 1998).

Hydrotherapy may be beneficial due to the heat and unloading effects (Bravo et al 1997) and is particularly useful for building patient confidence prior to commencing a land-based exercise programme. Other pain-relieving techniques include ice, hot packs, soft tissue massage, TENS, interferential therapy and shortwave diathermy. Gentle spinal mobilization can be performed even in patients with osteoporosis and osteopenia, provided care is taken and techniques well short of end range are used. However, forceful joint manipulation is contraindicated. To deal more positively with chronic pain, cognitive and behavioural strategies or relaxation techniques may be employed by the physiotherapist.

EDUCATION

A large part of the physiotherapist's role is to provide osteoporosis education and to empower the individual to take control of the condition. In many cases, patients may be anxious and require reassurance and advice about safe activities. Information about lifestyle behaviours such as diet and smoking should be provided and there is an abundance of printed literature and web sites available for this purpose. The provision of educational material has been shown to change such behaviours in premenopausal women (Jamal et al 1999). Physiotherapists should continually update their knowledge about self-help groups, community programmes, and reputable gymnasiums and exercise classes in the local area. Osteoporosis organizations are found in many countries and states and provide a range of useful services and resources. The physiotherapist may need to liaise with other medical and health professionals for overall patient care.

CONCLUSION

Physiotherapists have a role to play in both the prevention and management of osteoporosis. Appropriate treatment goals can be established following a thorough assessment. Since the aim is to maximize peak bone mass in children and adolescents, participation in a variety of high-impact activities should be encouraged. In the middle adult years, small increases in bone mass may be achieved by structured weight-training and weight-bearing exercise. In the older adult years, particularly if osteopenia or osteoporosis is present, the aim is to conserve bone mass, reduce the risk of falls, promote extended posture, reduce pain, and improve mobility and function. Management consists of various physiotherapy techniques and specific exercise prescription. Education is an essential part of the physiotherapist's role in promoting skeletal health throughout the lifespan.

REFERENCES

American College of Sports Medicine 1995 Position stand on osteoporosis and exercise. Medicine and Science in Sports and Exercise 27: i–vii

Arnaud SB, Sherrard DJ, Maloney N, Whalen RT, Fung P 1992 Effects of 1–week head-down tilt bed rest on bone formation and the calcium endocrine system. Aviation, Space, and Environmental Medicine 63: 14–20

Bailey DA 1997 The Saskatchewan paediatric bone mineral accrual study-bone mineral acquisition during the growing years. International Journal of Sports Medicine 18: S191–194

Bailey DA, McKay HA, Mirwald RL, Crocker PRE, Faulkner RA 1999 A six-year longitudinal study of the relationship of physical activity to bone mineral accrual in growing children: The University of Saskatchewan bone mineral accrual study. Journal of Bone and Mineral Research 14: 1672–1679

Bass S, Pearce G, Bradney M, Hendrich E, Delmas PD, Harding A, Seeman E 1998 Exercise before puberty may confer residual benefits in bone density in adulthood: studies in active prepubertal and retired female gymnasts. Journal of Bone and Mineral Research 13: 500–507

Bassey EJ, Ramsdale SJ 1994 Increase in femoral bone density in young women following high impact exercise. Osteoporosis International 4: 72–75

Bassey EJ, Ramsdale SJ 1995 Weight-bearing exercise and ground reaction forces — a 12-month randomized controlled trial of effects on bone mineral density in healthy postmenopausal women. Bone 16: 469–476

Bassey EJ, Rothwell MC, Littlewood JJ, Pye DW 1998 Pre- and postmenopausal women have different bone mineral density responses to the same high-impact exercise. Journal of Bone and Mineral Research 13: 1805–1813

Bauman WA, Spungen AM, Wang J, Pierson RN Jr, Schwartz E 1999 Continuous loss of bone during chronic immobilization: a monozygotic twin study. Osteoporosis International 10: 123–127

Bennell KL, Malcolm SA, Khan KM et al 1997 Bone mass and bone turnover in power athletes, endurance athletes and controls: a 12-month longitudinal study. Bone 20: 477–484

Bennell K, Talbot R, Wajswelner H, Techovanich W, Kelly D 1998 Intra-rater and inter-rater reliability of a weight-bearing lunge measure of ankle dorsiflexion. Australian Journal of Physiotherapy 44: 175–180

Berard A, Bravo G, Gauthier P 1997 Meta-analysis of the effectiveness of physical activity for the prevention of bone loss in postmenopausal women. Osteoporosis International 7: 331–337

Blake GM, Fogelman I 1998 Applications of bone densitometry for osteoporosis. Endocrinology and Metabolism Clinics of North America 27: 267–288

Bradney M, Pearce G, Naughton G et al 1998 Moderate exercise during growth in prepubertal boys — changes in bone mass, size, volumetric density, and bone strength — a controlled prospective study. Journal of Bone and Mineral Research 13: 1814–1821

Bravo G, Gauthier P, Roy PM et al 1996 Impact of a 12-month exercise programme on the physical and psychological health of osteopenic women. Journal of the American Geriatrics Society 44: 756–762

Bravo G, Gauthier P, Roy P, Payetter H, Gaulin P 1997 A weight-bearing, water-based exercise programme for osteopenic women: its impact on bone, functional fitness, and well-being. Archives of Physical Medicine and Rehabilitation 78: 1375–1380

Brill PA, Macera CA, Davis DR, Blair SN, Gordon N 2000 Muscular strength and physical function. Medicine and Science in Sports and Exercise 32: 412–416

Buchner DM, Cress ME, de Lateur BJ et al 1997 The effect of strength and endurance training on gait, balance, fall risk, and health services use in community-living older adults. Journal of Gerontology 52: M218–M224

Campbell AJ, Borrie MJ, Spears GF 1989 Risk factors for falls in a community-based prospective study of people 70 years and older. Journal of Gerontology 44: M112–117

Campbell AJ, Robertson MC, Gardner MM, Norton RN, Buchner DM 1999 Falls prevention over 2 years: a randomized controlled trial in women 80 years and older. Age and Ageing 28: 513–518

Campbell AJ, Robertson MC, Gardner MM, Norton RN, Tilyard MW, Buchner DM 1997 Randomised controlled trial of a general practice programme of home based exercise to prevent falls in elderly women. British Medical Journal 315: 1065–1069

Chad KE, Bailey DA, McKay HA, Zello GA, Snyder RE 1999 The effect of a weight-bearing physical activity programme on bone mineral content and estimated volumetric density in children with spastic cerebral palsy. Journal of Pediatrics 135: 115–117

Chartered Society of Physiotherapy 1999 Physiotherapy Guidelines for the Management of Osteoporosis. Chartered Society of Physiotherapy, London

Chow RK, Harrison JE 1987 Relationship of kyphosis to physical fitness and bone mass on post-menopausal women. American Journal of Physical Medicine 66: 219–227

Cohen H, Blatchly C, Gombash L 1993 A study of the clinical test of sensory interaction and balance. Physical Therapy 73: 346–351

Conroy BP, Kraemer WJ, Maresh CM et al 1993 Bone mineral density in elite junior Olympic weight lifters. Medicine and Science in Sports and Exercise 25: 1103–1109

Consensus Development Conference 1993 Diagnosis, prophylaxis and treatment of osteoporosis. American Journal of Medicine 94: 646–650

Cooper C, Cawley M, Bhalla A, Egger P, Ring F, Morton L, Barker D 1995 Childhood growth, physical activity and peak bone mass in women. Journal of Bone and Mineral Research 10: 940–947

Cooper C, Melton L 1992 Epidemiology of osteoporosis. Trends in Endocrinology and Metabolism 3: 224–229

Crawford HJ, Jull GA 1993 The influence of thoracic posture and movement on range of arm elevation. Physiotherapy Theory and Practice 9: 143–148

Cummings SR, Black DM, Nevitt MC et al 1993 Bone density at various sites for prediction of hip fractures. Lancet 341: 72–75

Cutler WB, Friedmann E, Genovese-Stone E 1993 Prevalence of kyphosis in a healthy sample of pre- and postmenopausal women. American Journal of Physical Medicine & Rehabilitation 72: 219–225

Dalsky GP 1990 Effect of exercise on bone: permissive influence oestrogen and calcium. Medicine and Science in Sports and Exercise 22: 281–285

Dalsky GP, Stocke KS, Ehansi AA, Slatopolsky E, Lee WC, Birge SJ 1988 Weight-bearing exercise training and lumbar bone mineral content in postmenopausal women. Annals of Internal Medicine 108: 824–828

Drinkwater BL, Nilson K, Chesnut lll CH, Bremner WJ, Shainholtz S, Southworth MB 1984 Bone mineral content of amenorrheic and eumenorrheic athletes. The New England Journal of Medicine 311 5: 277–281

Duncan P, Weiner K, Chandler J, Studenski S 1990 Functional reach: a new clinical measure of balance. Journal of Gerontology 45: M192–197

Ebrahim S, Thompson P, Baskaran V, Evans K 1997 Randomized placebo-controlled trial of brisk walking in the prevention of postmenopausal osteoporosis. Age and Ageing 26: 253–260

Ensrud KE, Black DM, Harris F, Ettinger B, Cummings SR 1997 Correlates of kyphosis in older women. Journal of the American Geriatrics Society 45: 682–687

Fiatarone M, Marks E, Ryan N, Meredith C, Lipstitz L, Evans W 1990 High-intensity training in nonagenarians. Journal of the American Medical Association 263: 3029–3034

Fiatarone MA, O'Neill EF, Ryan ND et al 1994 Exercise training and nutritional supplementation for physical frailty in very elderly people. New England Journal of Medicine 330: 1769–1775

Flicker L, Hopper JL, Rodgers L, Kaymakci B, Green RM, Wark JD 1995 Bone density determinants in elderly women: a twin study. Journal of Bone and Mineral Research 10: 1607–1613

Forwood M, Larsen J 2000 Exercise recommendations for osteoporosis: a position statement for the Australian and New Zealand Bone and Mineral Society. Australian Family Physician 29: 761–764

Frost HM 1988 Vital biomechanics: proposed general concepts for skeletal adaptations to mechanical usage. Calcified Tissue International 42: 145–156

Gleeson P, Protas E, LeBlanc A, Schneider V, Evans H 1990 Effects of weight lifting on bone mineral density in premenopausal women. Journal of Bone and Mineral Research 5: 153–158

Gordon CC, Cameron Chumlea WC, Roche AF 1991 Stature, recumbent length, and weight. In: Lohman TG, Roche AF, Martorell R (eds) Anthropometric Standardization Reference Manual, Abridged Edition. Human Kinetics, Champaign, pp 3–8

Greendale GA, Barrettconnor E, Ingles S, Haile R 1995 Late physical and functional effects of osteoporotic fracture in women the Rancho Bernado study. Journal of the American Geriatrics Society 43: 955–961

Grimston SK, Willows ND, Hanley DA 1993 Mechanical loading regime and its relationship to bone mineral density in children. Medicine and Science in Sports and Exercise 25: 1203–1210

Haapasalo H, Kannus P, Sievanen H, et al 1998 Effect of long-term unilateral activity on bone mineral density of female junior tennis players. Journal of Bone and Mineral Research 13: 310–319

Haapasalo H, Sievanen H, Kannus P, Heinonen A, Oja P, Vuori I 1996 Dimensions and estimated mechanical characteristics of the humerus after long-term tennis loading. Journal of Bone and Mineral Research 11: 864–872

Hageman P, Blanke 1986 Comparison of gait of young women and elderly women. Physical Therapy 66: 1382–1387

Harries UJ, Bassey EJ 1990 Torque-velocity relationships for the knee extensors in women in their 3rd and 7th decades. European Journal of Applied Physiology 60: 187–190

Hartard M, Haber P, Ilieva D, Preisinger E, Seidl G, Huber J 1996 Systematic strength training as a model of therapeutic intervention. American Journal of Physical Medicine and Rehabilitation 75: 21–28

Hatori M, Hasegawa A, Adachi H et al 1993 The effects of walking at the anaerobic threshold level on vertebral bone loss in postmenopausal women. Calcified Tissue International 52: 411–414

Heinonen A, Kannus P, Sievanen H et al 1996 Randomised, controlled trial of effect of high-impact exercise on selected risk factors for osteoporotic fractures. Lancet 348: 1343–1347

Heinonen A, Oja P, Sievanen H, Pasanen M, Vuori I 1998 Effect of two training regimens on bone mineral density in healthy perimenopausal women: a randomised, controlled trial. Journal of Bone and Mineral Research 13: 483–490

Heinonen A, Sievanen H, Kannus P, Oja P, Pasanen M, Vuori I 2000 High-impact exercise and bones of growing girls. A 9-month controlled trial. Calcified Tissue International Osteoporosis Int 11(12): 1010–17

Helmes E, Hodsman A, Lazowski D et al 1995 A questionnaire to evaluate disability in osteoporotic patients with vertebral compression fractures. Journals of Gerontology Series A — Biological Sciences and Medical Sciences 50: M91–M98

Hill K, Bernhardt J, McGann A, Maltese D, Berkovits D 1996 A new test of dynamic standing balance for stroke patients: reliability, validity, and comparison with healthy elderly. Physiotherapy Canada 48: 257–262

Hill K, Schwarz J, Flicker L, Carroll S 1999 Falls among healthy, community-dwelling, older women: a prospective study of frequency, circumstances, consequences and prediction accuracy. Australian and New Zealand Journal of Public Health 23: 41–48

Huda W, Morin RL 1996 Patient doses in bone mineral dosimetry. British Journal of Radiology 69: 422–425

Humphries B, Newton RU, Bronks R et al 2000 Effect of exercise intensity on bone density, strength, and calcium turnover in older women. Medicine and Science in Sports and Exercise 32: 1043–1050

Jamal SA, Ridout R, Chase C, Fielding L, Rubin LA, Hawker GA 1999 Bone mineral density testing and osteoporosis education improve lifestyle behaviors in premenopausal women: a prospective study. Journal of Bone and Mineral Research 14: 2143–2149

Joakimsen RM, Fonnebo V, Magnus JH, Stormer J, Tollan A, Sogaard AJ 1999 The Truomso study — physical activity and the incidence of fractures in a middle-aged population. Journal of Bone and Mineral Research 13: 1149–1157

Judex S, Zernicke RF 2000 High-impact exercise and growing bone: relation between high strain rates and enhanced bone formation. Journal of Applied Physiology 88: 2183–2191

Kannus P, Haapasalo H, Sankelo M et al 1995 Effect of starting age of physical activity on bone mass in the dominant arm of tennis and squash players. Annals of Internal Medicine 123: 27–31

Kannus P, Niemi S, Parkkari J, Palvanen M, Vuori I, Jarvinen M 1999 Hip fractures in Finland between 1970 and 1997 and predictions for the future. Lancet 353: 802–805

Karlsson MK, Linden C, Karlsson C, Johnell O, Obrant K, Seeman E 2000 Exercise during growth and bone mineral density and fractures in old age. Lancet 355: 469–470

Keen AD, Drinkwater BL 1997 Irreversible bone loss in former amenorrheic athletes. Osteoporosis International 7: 311–315

Kelley GA 1998 Exercise and regional bone mineral density in postmenopausal women — a meta-analytic review of randomized trials. American Journal of Physical Medicine and Rehabilitation 77: 76–87

Kelley GA, Kelley KS, Tran ZV 2000 Exercise and bone mineral density in men: a meta-analysis. Journal of Applied Physiology 88: 1730–1736

Kerr D, Morton A, Dick I, Prince R 1996 Exercise effects on bone mass in postmenopausal women are site-specific and load-dependent. Journal of Bone and Mineral Research 11: 218–225

Kerschan K, Alacamlioglu Y, Kollmitzer J et al 1998 Functional impact of unvarying exercise programme in women after menopause. American Journal of Physical Medicine and Rehabilitation 77: 326–332

Khan KM, Bennell KL, Hopper JL et al 1998 Self-reported ballet classes undertaken at age 10 to 12 years are associated with augmented hip bone mineral density in later life. Osteoporosis International 8: 165–173

Khan K, McKay H, Kannus P, Bailey D, Wark J, Bennell K 2001 Physical Activity and Bone Health. Human Kinetics, Champaign, Ill, USA, pp181–198

Kirchner EM, Lewis RD, O'Connor PJ 1996 Effect of past gymnastics participation on adult bone mass. Journal of Applied Physiology 80: 226–232

Kohrt W, Snead D, Slatopolsky E, Birge SJ 1995 Additive effects of weight-bearing exercise and estrogen on bone mineral density in older women. Journal of Bone and Mineral Research 10: 1302–1311

Kontulainen S, Kannus P, Haapasalo H et al 1999 Changes in bone mineral content with decreased training in competitive young adult tennis players and controls: a prospective 4-yr follow-up. Medicine and Science in Sports and Exercise 31: 646–652

Kronhed A, Moller M 1998 Effects of physical exercise on bone mass, balance skill and aerobic capacity in women and men with low bone mineral density, after one year of training — a prospective study. Scandinavian Journal of Medicine and Science in Sports 8: 290–298

Kujala UM, Kaprio J, Kannus P, Sarna S, Koskenvuo M 2000 Physical activity and osteoporotic hip fracture risk in men. Archives of Internal Medicine 160: 705–708

Lanyon LE, Goodship AE, Pye CJ, MacFie JH 1982 Mechanically adaptive bone remodelling. Journal of Biomechanics 15: 141–154

Larsen J 1998 Osteoporosis. In: Sapsford R, Bullock-Saxton J, Markwell S (eds) Women's Health. A Textbook for Physiotherapists. WB Saunders, London, pp 412–453

Laurent MR, Buchanon WW, Bellamy N 1991 Methods of assessment used in ankylosing spondylitis clinical trials. A review. British Journal of Rheumatology 30: 326–329

Lauritzen JB, Petersen MM, Lund B 1993 Effect of external hip protectors on hip fractures. Lancet 341: 11–13

Lehtonen-Veromaa M, Mottonen T, Nuotio I, Heinonen OJ, Viikari J 2000 Influence of physical activity on ultrasound and dual-energy X-ray absorptiometry bone measurements in peripubertal girls: a cross-sectional study. Calcified Tissue International 66: 248–254

Lespessailles E, Jullien A, Eynard E et al 1998 Biomechanical properties of human os calcanei: relationships with bone density and fractal evaluation of bone microarchitecture. Journal of Biomechanics 31: 817–824

Lewis MK, Blake GM, Fogelman I 1994 Patient dose in dual X-ray absorptiometry. Osteoporosis International 4: 11–15

Lips P, Cooper C, Agnusdei D et al 1999 Quality of life in patients with vertebral fractures: validation of the Quality of Life questionnaire of the European Foundation for Osteoporosis (QUALEFFO). Osteoporosis International 10: 150–160

Lohmann T, Going S, Pamenter R et al 1995 Effects of resistance training on regional and total bone mineral density in premenopausal women: a randomized prospective study. Journal of Bone and Mineral Research 10: 1015–1024

Lord S 1996 The effects of a community exercise programme on fracture risk factors in older women. Osteoporosis International 6: 361–367

Lord SR, Clark RD, Webster IW 1991 Physiological factors associated with falls in an elderly population. Journal of the Geriatrics Society 39: 1194–1200

Lord SR, Sambrook PN, Gilbert C et al 1994 Postural stability, falls and fractures in the elderly: results from the Dubbo Osteoporosis Epidemiology Study. Medical Journal of Australia 160: 684–691

Lord SR, Ward JA, Williams P, Strudwick M 1995 The effect of a 12-month exercise trial on balance, strength, and falls in older women: a randomized controlled trial. Journal of the American Geriatrics Society 43: 1198–1206

Lundon KMA, Li AMW, Bibershtein S 1998 Interrater and intrarater reliability in the measurement of kyphosis in postmenopausal women with osteoporosis. Spine 23: 1978–1985

Lynn SG, Sinaki M, Westerlind KC 1997 Balance characteristics of persons with osteoporosis. Archives of Physical Medicine and Rehabilitation 78: 273–277

MacRae PG, Feltner ME, Reinsch S 1994 A 1-year exercise programme for older women: effects on falls, injuries and physical performance. Journal of Ageing and Physical Activity 2: 127–142

Maddalozzo GF, Snow CM 2000 High intensity resistance training: effects on bone in older men and women. Calcified Tissue International 66: 399–404

Madsen OR, Schaadt O, Bliddal H, Egsmose C, Sylvest J 1993 Relationship between quadriceps strength and bone mineral density of the proximal tibia and distal forearm in women. Journal of Bone and Mineral Research 8: 1439–1444

Malina RM, Spriduso WW, Tate C, Baylor AM 1978 Age at menarche and selected menstrual characteristics in athletes at different competitive levels and in different sports. Medicine and Science in Sports and Exercise 10: 218–222

Malmros B, Mortenson L, Jensen MB, Charles P 1998 Positive effects of physiotherapy on chronic pain and performance in osteoporosis. Osteoporosis International 8: 215–221

Martin D, Notelovitz M 1993 Effects of aerobic training on bone mineral density of postmenopausal women. Journal of Bone and Mineral Research 8: 931–936

McCulloch RG, Bailey DA, Houston CS, Dodd BL 1990 Effects of physical activity, dietary calcium and selected lifestyle factors on bone density in young women. Canadian Medical Association Journal 142: 221–227

McCulloch RG, Bailey DA, Whalen RL, Houston CS, Faulkner RA, Craven BR 1992 Bone density and bone mineral content of adolescent soccer athletes and competitive swimmers. Pediatric Exercise Science 4: 319–330

McKay HA, Petit MA, Schutz RW, Prior JC, Barr SI, Khan KM 2000 Augmented trochanteric bone mineral density after modified physical education classes: a randomized school-based exercise intervention study in prepubescent and early pubescent children. Journal of Pediatrics 136: 156–162

McMurdo M, Rennie L 1993 A controlled trial of exercise by residents of old peoples' homes. Age and Ageing 22: 11–15

McMurdo ME, Mole PA, Paterson CR 1997 Controlled trial of weight bearing exercise in older women in relation to bone density and falls. British Medical Journal 314: 22

McMurdo MET, Millar AM, Daly F 2000 A randomized controlled trial of fall prevention strategies in old peoples' homes. Gerontology 46: 83–87

Melzack R 1975 The McGill pain questionnaire: major properties and scoring methods. Pain 1: 277–299

Micklesfield LK, Reyneke L, Fataar A, Myburgh KH 1998 Long-term restoration of deficits in bone mineral density is inadequate in premenopausal women with prior menstrual irregularity. Clinical Journal of Sport Medicine 8: 155–163

Morganti CM, Nelson ME, Fiatorone MA, Dallal GE, Economos CD, Crawford BM, Evans WJ 1995 Strength improvements with 1 yr of progressive resistance training in older women. Medicine and Science in Sports and Exercise 27: 906–912

Morris FL, Naughton GA, Gibbs JL, Carlson JS, Wark JD 1997 Prospective ten-month exercise intervention in premenarcheal girls: positive effects on bone and lean mass. Journal of Bone and Mineral Research 12: 1453–1462

Mulrow CD, Gerety MB, Kanten D et al 1994 A randomized trial of physical rehabilitation for very frail nursing home residents [see comments]. Journal of the American Medical Association 271: 519–524

Nelson M, Fiatarone M, Morganti C, Trice I, Greenberg R, Evans W 1994 Effects of high-intensity strength training on multiple risk factors for osteoporotic fractures: a randomized controlled trial. Journal of the American Medical Association 272: 1909–1914

Nichols JF, Nelson KP, Sartoris DJ 1995 Bone mineral responses to high-intensity strength training in active older women. Journal of Ageing and Physical Activity 3: 26–38

O'Connor JA, Lanyon LE, MacFie H 1982 The influence of strain rate on adaptive bone remodelling. Journal of Biomechanics 15: 767–781

Orwoll ES, Ferar J, Oviatt SK, McClung M, Huntington K 1989 The relationship of swimming exercise to bone mass in men and women. Archives of Internal Medicine 149: 2197–2220

Paganini-Hill A, Chao A, Ross RK, Henerson B 1991 Exercise and other factors in the prevention of hip fracture: The Leisure World study. Epidemiology 2: 16–25

Parkkari J, Kannus P, Heikkila J, Poutala J, Heinonen A, Sievanen H, Vuori I 1997 Impact experiments of an external hip protector in young volunteers. Calcified Tissue International 60: 354–357

Parkkari J, Kannus P, Heikkila J, Poutala J, Sievanen H, Vuori I 1995 Energy-shunting external hip protector attenuates the peak femoral impact force below the theoretical fracture threshold — an in vitro biomechanical study under falling conditions of the elderly. Journal of Bone and Mineral Research 10: 1437–1442

Parkkari J, Kannus P, Palvanen M et al 1999 Majority of hip fractures occur as a result of a fall and impact on the greater trochanter of the femur: a prospective controlled hip fracture study with 206 consecutive patients. Calcified Tissue International 65: 183–187

Petersen MM, Jensen NC, Gehrchen PM, Nielsen PK, Nielsen PT 1996 The relation between trabecular bone strength and bone mineral density assessed by dual photon and dual energy X-ray absorptiometry in the proximal tibia. Calcified Tissue International 59: 311–314

Pettersson U, Nordstrom P, Lorentzon R 1999a A comparison of bone mineral density and muscle strength in young male adults with different exercise levels. Calcified Tissue International 64: 490–498

Pettersson U, Stalnacke BM, Ahlenius GM, Henriksson-Larsen K, Lorentzon R 1999b Low bone mass density at multiple skeletal sites, including the appendicular skeleton in amenorrheic runners. Calcified Tissue International 64: 117–125

Podsiadlo D, Richardson S 1991 The timed 'up and go': a test of basic functional mobility for frail elderly persons. Journal of the American Geriatric Society 39: 142–148

Preisinger E, Alacamlioglu Y, Pils K et al 1996 Exercise therapy for osteoporosis: results of a randomised, controlled trial. British Journal of Sports Medicine 30: 209–212

Pruitt LA, Jackson RD, Bartels RL, Lehnhard HJ 1992 Weight-training effects on bone mineral density in early post-menopausal women. Journal of Bone and Mineral Research 7: 179–185

Raab-Cullen DM, Akhter MP, Kimmel DB, Recker RR 1994 Bone response to alternate-day mechanical loading of the rat tibia. Journal of Bone and Mineral Research 9: 203–211

Randell A, Sambrook PN, Nguyen TV 1995 Direct clinical and welfare costs of osteoporotic fracture in elderly men and women. Osteoporosis International 5: 427–432

Reinsch S, Macrae P, Lachenbruch PA, Tobis JS 1992 Attempts to prevent falls and injury: a prospective community study. Gerontologist 32: 450–456

Richardson CA, Jull GA 1995 Muscle control – pain control. What exercises would you prescribe? Manual Therapy 1: 2–10

Rico H, Revilla M, Hernandez ER, Gomez-Castresana F, Villa LF 1993 Bone mineral content and body composition in postpubertal cyclist boys. Bone 14: 93–95

Riggs BL, Melton LJI 1986 Involutional osteoporosis. New England Journal of Medicine 314: 1676–1686

Robinson TL, Snow-Harter C, Taaffe DR, Gillis D, Shaw J, Marcus R 1995 Gymnasts exhibit higher bone mass than runners despite similar prevalence of amenorrhea and oligomenorrhea. Journal of Bone and Mineral Research 10: 26–35

Rockwell JC, Sorensen AM, Baker S, Leahey D, Stock JL, Michaels J, Baran DT 1990 Weight training decreases vertebral bone density in premenopausal women: a prospective study. Journal of Clinical Endocrinology and Metabolism 71: 988–993

Rubin CT, Lanyon LE 1984 Regulation of bone formation by applied dynamic loads. The Journal of Bone and Joint Surgery 66-A: 397–402

Rubin CT, Lanyon LE 1985 Regulation of bone mass by mechanical strain magnitude. Calcified Tissue International 37: 411–417

Rutherford OM 1993 Spine and total body bone mineral density in amenorrheic endurance athletes. Journal of Applied Physiology 74: 2904–2908

Rutherford OM, Jones DA 1992 The relationship of muscle and bone loss and activity levels with age in women. Age and Ageing 21: 286–293

Ryan AS, Trueth MS, Rubin MA et al 1994 Effects of strength training on bone mineral density: hormonal and bone turnover relationships. Journal of Applied Physiology 77: 1678–1684

Sanders KM, Nicholson GC, Ugoni AM, Pasco JA, Seeman E, Kotowicz MA 1999 Health burden of hip and other fractures in Australia beyond 2000 — Projections based on the Geelong Osteoporosis Study. Medical Journal of Australia 170: 467–470

Sanila M, Kotaniemi A, Viikare J, Isomake H 1994 Height loss rate as a marker of osteoporosis in post-menopausal women with rheumatoid arthritis. Clinical Rheumatology 13: 256–260

Shumway-Cook A, Horak F 1986 Assessing the influence of sensory interaction on balance: suggestions from the field. Physical Therapy 66: 1548–1550

Silman AJ, O'Neill TW, Cooper C, Kanis J, Felsenberg D, The European Vertebral Osteoporosis Study Group 1997 Influence of physical activity on vertebral deformity in men and women: results from the European Vertebral Osteoporosis Study. Journal of Bone and Mineral Research 12: 813–819

Simmons V, Hansen PD 1996 Effectiveness of water exercise on postural mobility in the well elderly: an experimental study on balance enhancement. Journal of Gerontology 51A: M233–M238

Sinaki M, Ito E, Rogers JW, Bergstralh EJ, Wahner HW 1996 Correlation of back extensor strength with thoracic kyphosis and lumbar lordosis in estrogen-deficient women. American Journal of Physical Medicine and Rehabilitation 75: 370–374

Singh SJ, Morgan SJ, Hardman AE, Rowe AE, Bardsley PA 1994 Comparison of oxygen uptake during a conventional treadmill test and the shuttle walking test in chronic airflow limitation. European Respiratory Journal 11: 2016–2020

Skierska E 1998 Age at menarche and prevalance of oligoamenorrhea in top Polish athletes. American Journal of Human Biology 10: 511–517

Slemenda CW, Miller JZ, Hui SL, Reister TK, Johnston CC Jr 1991 Role of physical activity in the development of skeletal mass in children. Journal of Bone and Mineral Research 6: 1227–1233

Snow-Harter C, Bouxsein ML, Lewis BT, Carter DR, Marcus R 1992 Effects of resistance and endurance exercise on bone mineral status of young women: a randomized exercise intervention trial. Journal of Bone and Mineral Research 7: 761–769

Specker BL 1996 Evidence for an interaction between calcium intake and physical activity on changes in bone mineral density. Journal of Bone and Mineral Research 11: 1539–1544

Steele B 1996 Timed walking tests of exercise capacity in chronic cardiopulmonary illness. Journal of Cardiopulmonary Rehabilitation 16: 25–33

Taaffe DR, Robinson TL, Snow CM, Marcus R 1997 High-impact exercise promotes bone gain in well-trained female athletes. Journal of Bone and Mineral Research 12: 255–260

Taaffe DR, Snow-Harter C, Connolly DA, Robinson TL, Brown MD, Marcus R 1995 Differential effects of swimming versus weight-bearing activity on bone mineral status of eumenorrheic athletes. Journal of Bone and Mineral Research 10: 586–593

Tinetti M, Baker D, McAvay G et al 1994 A multifactorial intervention to reduce the risk of falling among elderly people living in the community. New England Journal of Medicine 331: 822–827

Tinetti ME, Speechley M, Ginter SF 1988 Risk factors for falls among elderly persons living in the community. New England Journal of Medicine 319: 1701–1707

Toshikazu I, Shirado O, Suzuki H, Takahashi M, Kanedo K, Strax TE 1996 Lumbar trunk muscle endurance testing: an inexpensive alternative to a machine for evaluation. Archives of Physical Medicine and Rehabilitation 77: 75–79

Umemura Y, Ishiko T, Yamauchi T, Kurono M, Mashiko S 1997 Five jumps per day increase bone mass and breaking force in rats. Journal of Bone and Mineral Research 12: 1480–1485

Wark JD 1998 How to prevent and treat osteoporosis. Australian Doctor July: I–VII

Witzke KA, Snow CM 2000 Effects of plyometric jump training on bone mass in adolescent girls. Medicine and Science in Sports and Exercise 32: 1051–1057

Wolf SL, Barnhart HX, Kutner NG, McNeely E, Coogler C, Xu T 1996 Reducing frailty and falls in older persons: an investigation of Tai Chi and computerized balance training. Journal of the American Geriatrics Society 44: 489–497

Wolff I, van Croonenborg JJ, Kemper HCG, Kostense PJ, Twisk JWR 1999 The eÄect of exercise training programmes on bone mass: a meta-analysis of published controlled trials in pre- and postmenopausal women. Osteoporosis International 9: 1–12

World Health Organization 1994 Assessment of fracture risk and its application to screening for osteoporosis. Report of WHO Study Group. World Health Organization, Geneva, p. 129

Young D, Hopper JL, Nowson CA, et al 1995 Determinants of bone mass in 10- to 26-year-old females: a twin study. Journal of Bone and Mineral Research 10: 558–567

Zmuda JM, Cauley JA, Ferrell RE 1999 Recent progress in understanding the genetic susceptibility to osteoporosis. Genetic Epidemiology 16: 356–367

POSTSCRIPT

EXERCISE FOR BONE LOADING

Although it has been recognized that strain parameters such as magnitude, rate, frequency and distribution play a role in the bone's response to loading, the critical importance of strain rate has recently been highlighted (Burr et al 2002). Strain produces fluid flow within the bone fluid compartment that generates shear stresses on bone cells. These shear stresses will be proportional to the rate of fluid flow. As bone is loaded more quickly at a higher strain rate, fluid velocity and thus shear stresses increase. This proportional relationship between fluid shear stresses on cells and strain rate predicts that the net bone response to loading should be proportional to strain rate. Thus, exercises incorporating faster movements may be more effective for stimulating bone even if the strain magnitude is lower.

Animal loading studies have demonstrated that bone cells desensitize soon after a loading session is initiated. It seems that the bone cells reach a saturation point whereby they are unresponsive to further stimuli. This point may be reached after as little as 50–100 repetitions of loading. It is evident that bone cells then require a recovery period before they can respond again to their mechanical environment. In a series of short- and long-term rat forearm loading experiments, Robling and colleagues (2000, 2001, 2002) demonstrated that the anabolic effect of loading was greater when the stimulus was broken down into smaller bouts separated by recovery periods than when the loading stimulus was delivered in a single uninterrupted bout. In previously stimulated bone cells, mechanosensitivity was restored after approximately 4–8 hours of load-free recovery. Even modest periods of rest restored some degree of mechanical sensitivity with bone formation rates proportional to the recovery time. Furthermore, a 30-second rest between loading cycles appears to be more effective than 3 seconds of rest within the one loading session (Umemura et al 2002). Taken together, these data suggest that lengthy exercise sessions are less beneficial to bone than shorter sessions and that greater success might be achieved if exercise is broken down into smaller sessions with recovery in between (Burr et al 2002). Short rest periods between each repetition may also increase the osteogenic response.

REFERENCES

Burr DB, Robling AG, Turner CH 2002 Effects of biomechanical stress on bones in animals. Bone 30: 781–786

Robling AG, Burr DB, Turner CH 2000 Partitioning a daily mechanical stimulus into discrete loading bouts improves the osteogenic response to loading. Journal of Bone and Mineral Research 15: 1596–1602

Robling AG, Burr DB, Turner CH 2001 Recovery periods restore mechanosensitivity to dynamically loaded bone. Journal Experimental Biology 204: 3389–3399

Robling AG, Hinant FM, Burr DB, Turner CH 2002 Shorter, more frequent mechanical loading sessions enhance bone mass. Medicine and Science in Sports and Exercise 34: 196–202

Umemura Y, Sogo N, Honda A 2002 Effects of intervals between jumps or bouts on osteogenic response to loading. Journal of Applied Physiology 93: 1345–1348

15

Fear of movement/(re)injury, avoidance and pain disability in chronic low back pain patients

J. W. S. Vlaeyen   *G. Crombez[†]*
*Department of Medical, Clinical and Experimental Psychology, Maastricht University and Pain Management and Research Centre, University Hospital Maastricht, The Netherlands
[†]Department of Experimental Clinical and Health Psychology, University of Ghent, Belgium

Chronic pain syndromes such as chronic low back pain are responsible for enormous costs for healthcare and society. For these conditions a pure biomedical approach often proves insufficient. Numerous studies have shown that there is little direct relationship between pain and disability and suggest that the biopsychosocial approach offers the foundations for a better insight into how pain can become a persistent problem. The main assumption is that pain and pain disability are not only influenced by organic pathology, if found, but by psychological and social factors. In this contribution, a behavioural analysis of chronic musculoskeletal pain will be discussed, with special attention to the role of pain-related fear in the development and maintenance of chronic pain disability, and the behavioural rehabilitation perspective of chronic pain management. *Manual Therapy* (1999) **4(4)**: 187–195.

INTRODUCTION

Pain is a universal experience. There is, however, very little known about its mechanisms and influencing factors. From a biomedical perspective, pain has been considered as almost synonymous with tissue damage. The French philosopher René Descartes was one of the first to present a biomedical model of pain. In his model there are direct and unique pain pathways from the peripheral nervous system to the brain, in the same way a bell in the church tower rings when the rope attached to it is being pulled. For Descartes, pain was a reflex of the mind upon nociceptive stimulation of the body. It is considered as a symptom that is isomorphically related to the extent of bodily damage in the organism. According to this perspective, pain treatment consists of two acts: (i) localization of the underlying pathology; and (ii) removal of the pathology with appropriate remedy or cure. In the absence of bodily damage, the mind was assumed to be at fault, and psychic pathology was inferred. This model has been extremely influential. Even today, most medical pain treatments are based on its assumptions. The limitations of the biomedical model became apparent during the late seventies. It became clear that no absolute relationship exists between the amount of tissue damage and the severity of the pain experience (e.g. Jensen et al 1994).

In a nice example of a Kuhnian shift of paradigm, the gate-control theory of Melzack and Wall (1965) adequately dealt with some of the shortcomings of the biomedical model. The gate-control theory has also figuratively opened the gate for research on the role of psychological variables moderating and mediating pain. This theory clearly stated that cortical processing was involved in the integration of both sensory–discriminative and affective–motivational aspects of pain. A revolutionary idea was that pain was not only the result of nociceptive information ascending from the periphery, but was profoundly moderated by descending pathways that amplify or inhibit nociceptive input in the spinal cord. According to the gate-control theory, the balance between sensory and central inputs determines the presence or absence of pain.

About a decade after the publication of the gate-control theory, Fordyce (1976) introduced his influential book *Behavioural Methods for Chronic Pain and Illness*. His work stemmed from the obvious shortcomings of the attempts of traditional health care to resolve chronic pain problems. Fordyce was the first to apply the principles of operant conditioning (Skinner 1953) to problems of chronic pain. Central was the idea that 'pain

behaviour', which refers to observable signs of pain and suffering, should be the focus of treatment. There are at least two assumptions to this approach. First, the factors that maintain the pain problem can be different from those that have initiated it. Pain behaviours may be subject to a graded shift from structural/mechanical to environmental control. Secondly, biomedical findings do not eliminate the possibility that psychological or social factors contribute to the level of pain disability.

After the so-called cognitive revolution in behavioural science, Turk et al (1983) emphasized the role of attributions, efficacy expectations, personal control and problem-solving within a cognitive–behavioural perspective on chronic pain. The additional assumptions of this approach are as follows. First, individuals actively process information regarding internal stimuli and external events. Secondly, thoughts and beliefs may alter behaviour by their direct influence on emotional and physiological responses. Thirdly, individuals can become active participants in their treatment if they learn skills to deal with their problems (Gatchel & Turk 1996). This has now become the prevailing approach in current chronic pain management.

TRIPLE RESPONSE MODE IN CHRONIC PAIN

It is clear that a strict biomedical model of pain is insufficient in explaining the complexity of the pain experience. The International Association for the Study of Pain (1986) has adopted this perspective and defined pain therefore as 'a sensory and emotional experience associated with actual or potential tissue damage, or described in terms of such damage'. This definition radically breaks with the biomedical model in which pain and tissue damage are almost synonymous. Tissue damage is not even a necessary condition for pain. Pain is also considered an emotional experience. In line with this idea, we will further elaborate the view that pain, just like an emotion, is a multidimensional experience. In particular, the three-systems model of emotions will be applied to the

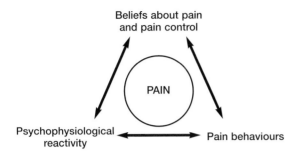

Figure 15.1 Pain as a hypothetical construct which can only be inferred by observable psychophysiological reactivity, pain cognitions and pain behaviours (based on Öhman 1987 and Vlaeyen 1991).

experience of pain (Fig. 15.1). According to this model, emotions are always subjective and never observable in themselves. They can only be inferred by their effects at an observable level. Likewise, (chronic) pain can best be approached as a hypothetical construct that can be inferred by at least three partially independent response systems: (i) psychophysiological reactivity; (ii) overt pain behaviours; and (iii) attention, attributions and expectations (Vlaeyen et al 1989).

PSYCHOPHYSIOLOGICAL REACTIVITY

Like any emotional experience, pain may variably affect several bodily systems including the muscular (Fig. 15.2), cardiovascular, respiratory and electrodermal systems (see Flor et al 1992 for an extensive review). Although some of the psychophysiological responses during pain may be biologically hardwired and relatively specific to pain, psychophysiological reactivity to pain is also specific for particular groups of subjects (response stereotypy) and is also extremely sensitive to the environment in which pain emerges. In particular, the issue of response stereotypy has attracted much research attention. The idea is that stress causes an overreactivity in particular physiological systems, which may initiate and maintain pain problems. In a well-controlled laboratory study with chronic low back pain patients, Flor et al (1985) measured electromyography (EMG) activity of various muscle sites while patients were

exposed to a neutral situation (reciting the alphabet) and to two different stressors: a mental arithmetic task (general stress) and talking about a life event or pain episode (personally relevant stress). Of interest was that, as compared to healthy controls and patients with medical complaints other than back pain, the chronic low back pain patients responded with elevated EMG activity only in the lower left paraspinal muscles, but this muscular reactivity was only observed in the personally relevant stress situation. Likewise, patients with chronic pain in the temporomandibular (cheek) region responded to personal stress with high EMG activity in the masseter muscle (involved in chewing). In similar situations, patients with headache responded with an overreactivity in the frontalis muscle (Flor et al 1992). In other words, psychophysiological reactivity to personal stressors appears to be symptom-specific. This increased muscular reactivity to pain or psychosocial stressors may contribute to a reduced ability to tolerate pain, and subsequently to functional limitations and pain disability (Feuerstein 1991). Despite the existing evidence, the function of response stereotypy in the initiation or maintenance of chronic pain is still unclear and poorly researched.

OVERT PAIN BEHAVIOURS

The overt–motoric responses cover a wide range of gross motor behaviours, referred to in the pain literature as pain behaviours. Fordyce (1986) demonstrated the clinical and theoretical relevance of observable pain behaviours. The importance of assessing pain behaviours lies in the fact that they elicit reinforcing responses from the social environment, which can maintain these behavioural expressions. For example, Lousberg et al (1990) reported that chronic low back pain patients with solicitous spouses reported more pain during a treadmill test than patients with nonsolicitous spouses. In addition, pain behaviours are always incompatible with physical activity. The longer these pain behaviours exist, the lower activity levels will be which, in turn, may worsen the pain problem, as long-standing inactivity may lead to the so-called disuse or deconditioning syndrome (Fig. 15.3).

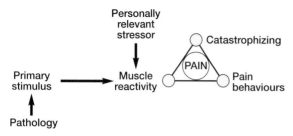

Figure 15.2 Factors that influence muscular reactivity in chronic musculoskeletal pain.

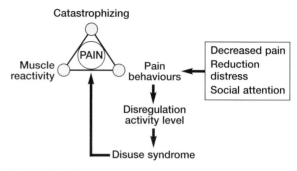

Figure 15.3 Factors that influence pain behaviours in chronic musculoskeletal pain.

ATTENTION, ATTRIBUTIONS AND EXPECTATIONS

Pain seems to be designed to capture attention. Among many other competing demands in the environment, pain is quickly selected as the focus of attention. Once selected it is often diffcult to disengage from. When pain demands the attention of the individual, three kinds of appraisal processes are hypothesized to occur (Lazarus et al 1970): primary, secondary and tertiary reappraisals. Primary appraisals concern the immediate meaning of the invading stimulus: 'Am I okay or in trouble?' Beecher (1959) was one of the first to point to the effects of the meaning attached to pain. In one of his classic studies he investigated the differences in pain responses between a group of male civilian patients undergoing major surgery and a group of soldiers with comparable wounds. He found that four-fifths of the civilians requested analgesics whereas only one-third of the soldiers wanted medication. His explanation for this discrepancy was that for the soldiers, the painful wound meant an escape from the battlefield. In contrast, the major surgery was a calamitous event for the civilian. A typical example of an extreme negative appraisal of pain in clinical practice is catastrophizing about pain. Pain is then appraised as extremely threatening and as having catastrophic consequences, such as the patient reporting 'I can't seem to keep it out of my mind', 'I feel I can't stand it anymore' or 'I think that fate hit me'. It is well documented that pain catastrophizing is related to high pain reports and diffi-

culties in directing attention away from pain (Crombez et al 1998a). Catastrophic thinking about pain is also known to increase distress (Sullivan et al 1995). Distress symptoms can, in turn, increase pain by reducing pain tolerance levels and by triggering unnecessary sympathetic arousal (Ciccone & Grzesiak 1984). Additional evidence for the importance of catastrophizing is provided in a study comparing chronic pain patients seeking help (consumers) with people with chronic pain who were not receiving treatment, and who were recruited via advertisements in local newspapers (non-consumers). The results revealed that the consumers reported much higher levels of pain catastrophizing than the non-consumers (Reitsma & Meijler 1997). A prospective study by Burton et al (1995) concerning predictors of back pain chronicity at 1 year after the acute onset is also worth mentioning in this context. These researchers found that catastrophizing, as measured by the Coping Strategies Questionnaire (Rosenstiel & Keefe 1983), was the most powerful predictor: almost seven times more important than the best of the clinical and historical variables for the acute back pain patient. One possible explanation comes from cognitive psychology. There is some evidence that individuals who catastrophize demonstrate a lack of confidence in their problem-solving abilities (Davey et al 1996), and therefore are more likely to avoid daily hassles rather than actively approach them in a problem-solving manner. This lack of initiative to change undesirable events may add to the disablement process.

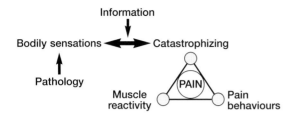

Figure 15.4 Factors that influence catastrophizing beliefs in chronic musculoskeletal pain.

AVOIDANCE LEARNING AND PAIN-RELATED FEAR

In an attempt to explain how and why some individuals with musculoskeletal pain develop a chronic pain syndrome, several models have been developed including the 'fear-avoidance model of exaggerated pain perception' (Lethem et al 1983), and, more recently, a 'cognitive model of fear of movement/(re)injury' (Vlaeyen et al 1995a). The central concept of these models is fear of pain, or the more specific fear that physical activity will cause (re)injury. Two opposing behavioural responses to these fears are postulated: confrontation and avoidance. In the absence of a serious somatic pathology in the majority of patients with musculoskeletal pain, confrontation with daily activities, despite pain, is conceptualized as an adaptive response which may lead to the reduction of fear and the promotion of recovery. In contrast, avoidance leads to the maintenance or exacerbation of fear, possibly resulting in a phobic state.

Avoidance refers to 'the performance of a behaviour which postpones or averts the presentation of an aversive event' (Kazdin 1980). In the case of pain, a patient may no longer perform certain activities because he/she anticipates that these activities increase pain and suffering. In the acute phase, avoidance behaviours such as resting, limping or the use of supportive equipment are effective in reducing suffering from nociception. Later on, these protective pain and illness behaviours may persist in anticipation of pain, instead of as a response to it. Longlasting avoid-ance of motoric activities can have detrimental consequences, both physically (loss of mobility, muscle strength and fitness, possibly resulting in the 'disuse syndrome') (Bortz 1984; Verbunt et al 2003) and psychologically (loss of self-esteem, deprivation of reinforcers, depression, somatic preoccupation). All these consequences may augment disability (Vlaeyen & Linton 2000).

In 1990, Kori et al introduced the term 'kinesio-phobia' (kinesis = movement) for the condition in which a patient has an 'excessive, irrational, and debilitating fear of physical movement and activity resulting from a feeling of vulnerability to painful injury or reinjury'. These authors also developed the Tampa Scale for Kinesiophobia (TSK) as a measure for fear of movement/(re)injury. When a fearful subject is exposed to the feared situation, a behavioural response (escape and avoidance) and a cognitive response (catastrophic thinking), as well as a psychophysiological response (increased physiological arousal), can typically be observed (Lang 1968). Does this triple response mode model also hold for pain-related fear?

PAIN-RELATED FEAR AND AVOIDANCE/ESCAPE

It has been repeatedly shown that pain-related fear is associated with escape/avoidance behaviours. That is, poor behavioural performance (Vlaeyen et al 1995a; Crombez et al 1998b, 1999) and self-reported disability (McCracken et al 1992; Vlaeyen et al 1995b; Asmundson et al 1997; Crombez et al 1999) are more strongly associated with pain-related fear than with pain severity or biomedical findings. For example, using the Fear Avoidance Beliefs Questionnaire, Waddell et al (1993) demonstrated that fear-avoidance beliefs about work are strongly related to disability in daily living and work lost in the past year, and more so than pain variables such as anatomical pattern of pain, time pattern and pain severity. McCracken et al (1992) showed that, in a group of chronic low back pain (CLBP) patients, greater pain-related anxiety was associated with higher predictions of pain and less range of motion during a procedure involving a passive but painful straight leg raising test. Using the TSK, Vlaeyen et al (1995a) found that fear of movement/(re)injury was the most powerful predictor in the performance of a simple weight-lifting task, and similar findings were reported by Crombez et al (1999) with a knee flexion and extension unit of the Cybex System. These effects of fear also appear to generalize towards other activities of daily life. Asmundson et al (1997) found that patients classified as 'dysfunctional' with the Multidimensional Pain Inventory (Kerns et al 1985) reported more pain-related fear than those classified as 'interpersonally distressed' or as 'adaptive copers'. In the studies by Vlaeyen et al (1995b) and Crombez et al (1999), pain-related fear was was strongly associated with self-reported disability levels, while current pain intensity, biomedical findings and general distress were not predictive of pain disability.

PAIN-RELATED FEAR AND CATASTROPHIZING

There is also evidence that pain-related fear is associated with catastrophic thinking about pain. McCracken and Gross (1993) found a strong association between fear of pain and pain catastrophizing in chronic pain patients. Similarly, Vlaeyen et al (1995a; b) found that in CLBP patients, fear of movement/(re)injury was strongly related to catastrophizing, and the authors suggested that catastrophizing is likely to be a precursor of pain-related fear. In line with this idea, Crombez et al (1998a) found that pain-free volunteers with a high frequency of catastrophic thinking about pain became more fearful when threatened with the possibility of occurrence of intense pain than students with a low frequency of catastrophic thinking.

FEAR-INDUCED MUSCULAR REACTIVITY

One study has dealt with the question of whether pain-related fear is associated with muscular reactivity. Vlaeyen et al (1999a) asked 31 CLBP patients to watch a neutral nature documentary, followed by a fear-eliciting video-presentation (a dummy patient vigorously engaging in heavy physical exercise), while surface EMG recordings were made from the muscles of the lower back and lower legs. Unexpectedly, paraspinal EMG-activity decreased during video-exposure, rather than increased. The decrement, however, tended to be substantially less in fearful patients than in the non-fearful patients. The findings extend the symptom-specificity model of psychophysiological reactivity to the area of pain-related fear, and support the idea that pain-related fear perpetuates pain and pain disability through muscular reactivity.

SUMMARY

These studies, as well as the studies by Rose et al (1992) and Waddell et al (1993), provide support for the validity of the pain-related fear concept. It should be noted, however, that these are cross-sectional in nature, leaving the question of whether fear of movement/(re)injury is secondary to the experience of LBP, or if it is one of the determinants of becoming a chronic pain patient. The recent prospective study by Klenerman et al (1995) provides support for the latter. They collected both psychological and biomedical measures from a sample of 300 acute LBP patients within 1 week of presentation, and at 2 months, so as to predict the 12 month outcome. The data showed that subjects who had not recovered by 2 months (7.3%) became CLBP patients. Moreover, fear of pain early on turned out to be one of the most powerful predictors of chronicity. Linton et al (1999) included a large sample from the general population in their prospective cohort study with the aim to examine whether pain catastrophizing and fear-avoidance in pain-free individuals predict subsequent episodes of musculoskeletal pain. They found that individuals who scored above the median score of a modified version of the Fear Avoidance Beliefs Questionnaire (FABQ) (Waddell et al 1993) had twice as much chance of having a pain episode in the following year.

Based on the findings of recent studies, a biopsychosocial model is proposed (Fig. 15.5) that represents the mechanisms of how fear of movement/(re)injury contributes to the maintenance of chronic pain disability in CLBP. It begins with the injury occurring during the acute phase.

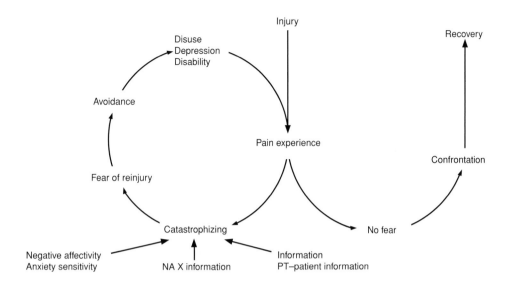

Figure 15.5 Theoretical model of pain-related fear as a determinant of CLBP disability. If pain, possibly caused by an injury, is interpreted as threatening (pain catastrophizing), pain-related fear evolves. This leads to avoidance behaviours, followed by disability, disuse and depression. The latter will maintain the pain experiences, thereby fuelling the vicious circle of increasing fear and avoidance. In noncatastrophizing patients, no pain-related fear and rapid confrontation with daily activities is likely to occur, leading to fast recovery. Pain catastrophizing is hypothesized as the result of the interaction between negative affectivity (as a personality characteristic) and (threatening) information provided by others, such as the health-care provider. (Based on Vlaeyen and Linton, 2000, with permission from the International Association for the Study of Pain, (IASP).

Painful experiences that are intensified during movement, will elicit catastrophizing cognitions in some individuals and more adaptive cognitions in others. Patients who catastrophize are more likely to become fearful. Fear of movement/(re)injury subsequently leads to increased avoidance and, in the long run, to disuse, depression and increased disability (Philips 1987; Council et al 1988). Both depression and disuse are known to be associated with decreasing pain tolerance levels (Romano & Turner 1985; McQuade et al 1988), and hence promote the painful experiences. In addition to the avoidance of threatening physical activities, pain disability may also persist because of increased attention from others, as well as the avoidance of social conflicts or responsibilities. In patients with more adaptive cognitions, confrontation rather than avoidance is likely to occur, promoting health behaviours and early recovery.

In the proposed model, pain catastrophizing is considered a main precursor of pain-related fear. What do we know about the origins of catastrophizing? On the one hand, there is evidence that catastrophizing is associated with relatively stable personality traits such as negative affectivity (NA). NA reflects a general tendency to experience subjective distress and dissatisfaction (Watson & Clark 1984). High NA subjects are hypervigilant, consistently scan their environment for signs of trouble, and interpret ambiguous stimuli in a negative and threatening manner (Watson & Pennebaker 1989). Catastrophizing may, however, also be influenced by external factors such as the characteristics of the therapist–patient interaction. People in the direct environment, including health-care providers, may verbally and nonverbally convey the message that there might be something dangerously wrong with the back. It is likely that this threatening information will be incorporated into the individual's personal beliefs and convictions. More generally, studies have demonstrated that patient–therapist interaction patterns have an impact on patients' health outcomes (Kaplan et al 1989). More likely, however, is that information provided by therapists, and how this information is perceived by the patient, moderates the influence of NA on catastrophizing. Future studies testing the causality assumed in this model need to be carried out.

CONSEQUENCES FOR CLINICAL MANAGEMENT

What can be the implications of the current findings for the treatment of musculoskeletal pain? First, clinicians are often requested to make judgements about the present and future functional capacity of patients on the basis of dynamometry. The assumption made is that lumbar (isokinetic) dynamometry provides objective and unbiased measures and that it can quantify maximal functional capacity. Menard et al (1994), for example, found a difference in the pattern of dynamometry in two groups of LBP patients who differed only in the propensity of abnormal illness behaviour (as indicated by the Waddell score), and proposed that fear of pain of movement might be one of the possible explanations. The plausibility of this explanation is corroborated by other studies (Vlaeyen et al 1995a; Crombez et al 1996) in which a relation between fear of movement/(re)injury and behavioural performance is demonstrated. This means that a valid assessment of functional capacity cannot be carried out without controlling for pain-related fear.

Second, keeping in mind that the relatively small percentage of chronic back pain patients are responsible for 75–90% of the societal costs (Van Tulder et al 1995), the early identification of patients at risk of becoming disabled might lead to more specific and preventive interventions, the reduction of disability and associated costs (Linton 1998). Catastrophizing, pain-related fear and fear of movement/(re) injury, in particular, must be considered such a risk factor. Pain-related fear may be an essential aspect of a broader early assessment of psychosocial 'yellow flags' (Kendall et al 1997). For this subgroup, an early cognitive–behavioural intervention might be war-

ranted. According to the suggestions made by Turner (1996) and Von Korff (1996) for behavioural interventions in primary care, such an intervention could be designed in three steps: screening, education and exposure.

In terms of screening, a number of relatively short questionnaries are now available, which have the potential to identify back pain patients whose level of disability may be mainly determined by pain-related fear, and not by pain intensity or biomedical status. Examples are the Acute Low Back Pain Screening Questionnaire (Linton & Halldèn 1996), the Tampa Scale for Kinesiophobia (TSK) (Kori et al 1990; Vlaeyen et al 1995a, b) or the Fear Avoidance Beliefs Questionnaire (FABQ) (Waddell et al 1993; Crombez et al 1999). These appear appropriate for use in a primary care setting as well. In the case of elevated scores, it is worth enquiring about the essential stimuli: What is the patient actually afraid of? So far, there is a lack of standardized tools for identifying these stimuli. In addition to checklists of daily activities, the presentation of visual materials, such as pictures of back-stressing activities and movements, might be worthwhile (Kugler et al 1999). They can be helpful in the development of graded hierarchies. Such a hierarchy of back-stressing activities reflects the full range of situations that a patient avoids, beginning with those that provoke only mild discomfort, and ending with activities or situations that are well beyond the patient's present abilities. Each situation is then rated by the patient on a 0–100 scale according to the amount of fear it causes (Fig. 15.6). In our experience, abrupt changes in movements (e.g. suddenly being hit) or activities consisting of repetitive spinal compressions (e.g. lifting, jumping) are frequently mentioned stimuli that chronic back pain patients fear. These situations are feared because of beliefs about the causes of pain, such as ruptured or severely damaged nerves ('If I lift heavy weights, the nerves in my back might be damaged'). Such a screening may also be supplemented by information about the precipitants (situational or internal) of the pain-related fear, and about the direct and indirect consequences. This screening might also include other areas of life stresses, as they might increase arousal levels and indirectly fuel pain-related fear.

The second step consists of unambiguously educating the patient in such a way that the patient views his pain as a common condition that can be self-managed, rather than as a serious disease or a condition that needs careful protection. Although cognitive–perceptual factors, such as catastrophizing in particular, are associated with pain-related fear, didactic lectures and rational argument may facilitate behaviour change, but are not as effective as direct experiences.

Therefore, the third, and probably most essential, step consists of graded exposure to the situations the patients has identified as 'dangerous' or 'threatening'. Such a cognitive–behavioural approach is always introduced with a careful explanation of the fear-avoidance model (Fig. 15.5), using the patient's individual symptoms, beliefs and behaviours to illustrate how vicious

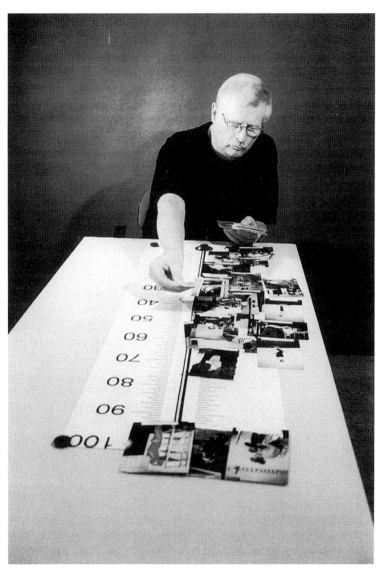

Figure 15.6 Application of PHODA in a patient with chronic low back pain.

circles maintain the pain problem. Subsequently, the most common approach would be to devise individually tailored practice tasks based on a graded hierarchy of fear-eliciting situations. Such a graded exposure is quite similar to the graded activity programmes in that it gradually increases activity levels despite pain (Fordyce et al 198,; 1986; Lindström et al 1992), but is dissimilar in that it pays special attention to the idiosyncratic aspects of the pain-related fear stimuli. For example, if the patient fears the repetitive spinal compression produced by riding a bicycle on a bumpy road, then the graded exposure should include an activity that mimics that specific activity, and not just a stationary bicycle. Such an approach gives the individual an opportunity to correct the inaccurate predictions about the relationship between activities and harm. The vast literature on behavioural treatments learns that graded exposure has proven to be the most effective treatment ingredient for individuals suffering from excessive fears and phobias (Davey 1997). Preliminary results of a controlled study examining the effectiveness of such an approach in 'kinesiophobic' back pain patients are very promising indeed (Vlaeyen et al 1999b).

CONCLUSION

In this article, we have reviewed current views on psychophysiologic, behavioural and cognitive factors capable of modulating painful experiences and associated pain behaviours in patients with CLBP. In particular, we have highlighted the mediating role of pain-related fear in the maintenance of chronic pain disability. The empirical evidence promises to provide a new foundation for the early identification of risk patients, prevention, assessment and treatment. Yet, we have only scratched the surface of this area so we need to remain careful regarding the conclusions drawn. Given the compelling evidence reached to date, however, pain-related fear needs to be considered in clinical practice and given priority in research.

Acknowledgements

We are grateful to Roeland Lysens, Peter Heuts, Madelon Peters, Anja van den Hout, Jeanine Verbunt, Piet Portegijs, Mario Geilen, Albére Köke, Jeroen de Jong and the staff of the Department of Pain Rehabilitation of the Hoensbroeck Rehabilitation Center for ongoing, inspiring discussions.

REFERENCES

Asmundson GJG, Norton GR, Allerdings MD 1997 Fear and avoidance in dysfunctional chronic back pain patients. Pain 69: 231–236

Beecher HK 1959 Measurement of Subjective Responses. Oxford University Press, Oxford

Bortz WM 1984 The disuse syndrome. Western Journal of Medicine 141: 691–694

Burton AK, Tillotson KM, Main CJ, Hollis S 1995 Psychosocial predictors of outcome in acute and subchronic low back trouble. Spine 20: 722–728

Ciccone DS, Grzesiak RC 1984 Cognitive dimensions of chronic pain. Social Sciences in Medicine 12: 1339–1345

Council JR, Ahern DK, Follick MJ, Kline CL 1988 Expectancies and functional impairment in chronic low back pain. Pain 33: 323–331

Crombez G, Vervaet L, Lysens R, Eelen P, Baeyens F 1996 Do pain expectancies cause pain in chronic low back patients? A clinical investigation. Behaviour Research and Therapy 34: 919–925

Crombez G, Eccleston C, Baeyens F, Eelen P 1998a When somatic information threatens, catastrophic thinking enhances attentional interference. Pain 75: 187–198

Crombez G, Vervaet L, Lysens R, Baeyens F, Eelen P 1998b Avoidance and confrontation of painful, back straining movements in chronic back pain patients. Behaviour Modification 22: 62–77

Crombez G, Vlaeyen JWS, Heuts PHTG, Lysens R 1999 Fear of pain is more disabling than pain itself. Evidence on the role of pain-related fear in chronic back pain disability. Pain 80: 329–340

Davey GCL 1997 Phobias. A Handbook of Theory, Research and Treatment. Wiley, Chichester

Davey GCL, Jubb M, Cameron C 1996 Catastrophic worrying as a function of changes in problem-solving confidence. Cognitive Therapy and Research 20: 333–344

Feuerstein M 1991 A multidisciplinary approach to the prevention, evaluation, and management of work disability. Journal of Occupational Rehabilitation 1: 5–12

Flor H, Turk DC, Birbaumer N 1985 Assessment of stress-related psychophysiological reactions in chronic back pain patients. Journal of Consulting and Clinical Psychology 53: 354–364

Flor H, Birbaumer N, Schugens MM, Lutzenberger W 1992 Symptom-specific psychophysiological responses in chronic pain patients. Psychophysiology 29: 452–460

Fordyce WE 1976 Behavioural Methods for Chronic Pain and Illness. Mosby, St Louis

Fordyce WE, Shelton JL, Dundore DE 1982 The modification of avoidance learning in pain behaviours. Journal of Behavioural Medicine 5: 405–414

Fordyce WE, Brockway J, Bergman J, Spengler D 1986 A control group comparison of behavioural versus traditional management methods in acute low back pain. Journal of Behavioural Medicine 2: 127–140

Gatchel RJ Turk DC 1996 Psychological Approaches to Pain Management. A Practitioner's Handbook. Guilford Press, New York

International Association for the Study of Pain 1986 Classification of chronic pain, descriptions, descriptions of pain syndromes and definitions of pain terms. Pain Supplement 3: 1–225

Jensen MC, Brant-Zawadzki M, Obuchowski N, Modic MT, Malkasian D, Ross JS 1994 Magnetic resonance imaging of the lumbar spine in people without back pain. New England Journal of Medicine 331: 69–73

Kaplan SH, Greenfeld S, Ware JE 1989 Assessing the effects of physician-patient interactions on the outcomes of chronic disease. Medical Care 27: 110–127

Kazdin AE 1980 Behaviour Modification in Applied Settings (revised edn). Dorsey Press, Homewood

Kendall NAS, Linton SJ, Main CJ 1997 Guide to assessing psychosocial yellow flags in acute low back pain: Risk factors for long-term disability and work loss. Accident Rehabilitation & Compensation Insurance Corporation of New Zealand and the National Health Committee, New Zealand

Kerns RD, Turk DC, Rudy TE 1985 The West Haven-Yale Multidimensional Pain Inventory (WHYMPI). Pain 23: 345–356

Klenerman L, Slade PD, Stanley IM et al 1995 The prediction of chronicity in patients with an acute attack of low back pain in a general practice setting. Spine 4: 478–484

Kori SH, Miller RP, Todd DD 1990 Kinisophobia: a new view of chronic pain behaviour. Pain Management Jan/Feb: 35–43

Kugler K, Wijn J, Geilen M, de Jong J, Vlaeyen JWS 1999 The photograph series of daily activities (PHODA) (CD-rom version). Institute for Rehabilitation Research and School for Physiotherapy, Heerlen, the Netherlands

Lang P 1968 Fear reduction and fear behaviour: problems in treating a construct. Research in Psychotherapy 3: 90–102

Lazarus RS, Averill JR, Opton EM 1970 Towards a cognitive theory of emotion. In: Arnold MB (ed) Feelings and Emotions. Academic Press, New York

Lethem J, Slade PD, Troup JDG, Bentley G 1983 Outline of a fear-avoidance model of exaggerated pain perceptions. Behaviour Research and Therapy 21: 401–408

Lindström I, Öhlund C, Eek C, Wallin L, Peterson L, Fordyce WE, Nachemson AL 1992 The effect of graded activity on patients with sub-acute low back pain: a randomized prospective clinical study with an operant conditioning behavioural approach. Physical Therapy 72: 279–290

Linton SJ 1998 The socioeconomic impact of chronic back pain: is anyone benefiting? Pain 75: 163–168

Linton SJ, Halldén K 1996 Risk factors and the natural course of acute and recurrent musculoskeletal pain: developing a screening instrument. Proceedings of the 8th World Congress on Pain. IASP Press, Seattle

Linton SJ, Buer N, Vlaeyen JWS, Hellsing A-L 1999 Are fear-avoidance beliefs related to the inception of an episode of back pain? A prospective study. Psychology and Health (in press)

Lousberg R, Schmidt AJM, Groenman NH 1990 The relationship between spouse solicitousness and pain behaviour. Searching for more experimental evidence. Pain 51: 75–80

McCracken LM, Gross RT 1993 Does anxiety affect coping with pain? Clinical Journal of Pain 9: 253–259

McCracken LM, Zayfert C, Gross RT 1992 The Pain Anxiety Symptoms Scale: development and validation of a scale to measure fear of pain. Pain 50: 63–67

McQuade KJ, Turner JA, Buchner DM 1988 Physical fitness and chronic low back pain. Clinical Orthopaedics and Related Research 233: 198–204

Melzack R, Wall PD 1965 Pain mechanisms: a new theory. Science 150: 978

Menard MR, Cooke C, Locke SR, Beach GN, Butler TB 1994 Pattern of performance in workers with low back pain during a comprehensive motor performance evaluation. Spine 2: 1359–1366

Öhman A 1987 The psychophysiology of emotion: an evolutionary-cognitive perspective. Advances in Psychophysiology 2: 79–127

Philips HC 1987 Avoidance behaviour and its role in sustaining chronic pain. Behaviour Research and Therapy 25: 273–279

Reitsma B, Meijler WJ 1997 Pain and patienthood. Clinical Journal of Pain 13: 9–21

Romano JM, Turner JA 1985 Chronic pain and depression. Does the evidence support a relationship? Psychological Bulletin 97: 311–318

Rose M, Klenerman L, Atchinson L, Slade PD 1992 An application of the fear-avoidance model to three chronic pain problems. Behaviour Research and Therapy 30: 359–365

Rosenstiel AK, Keefe FJ 1983 The use of coping strategies in chronic low back pain patients: relationship to patient characteristics and current adjustment. Pain 17: 33–44

Skinner BF 1953 Science and Human Behaviour. Macmillan, New York

Sullivan MJL, Bishop SR, Pivik J 1995 The pain catastrophizing scale: development and validation. Psychological Assessment 7: 524–532

Turk DC, Meichenbaum D, Genest M 1983 Pain and Behavioural Medicine. A Cognitive-behavioural Perspective. Guilford Press, New York

Turner JA 1996 Educational and behavioural interventions for back pain in primary care. Spine 21: 1851–1858

Van Tulder MW, Koes BW, Bouter LM 1995 A cost-of-illness study of back pain in the Netherlands. Pain 62: 233–240

Verbunt J, Van der Heijden G, Vlaeyen JWS, Heuts PHGT, Pons C, Knottnerus A 2003 The disuse syndrome: facts and fiction in chronic musculoskeletal pain. Eur J Pain 7:9–21

Vlaeyen JWS 1991 Chronic Low Back Pain: Assessment and Treatment from Behavioural Rehabilitation perspective. Swets & Zeitlinger, Amsterdam

Vlaeyen JWS, Linton SJ 2000 Fear-avoidance and its consequences in chronic musculoskeletal pain: a state of the art Pain 85:317–332

Vlaeyen JWS, Snijders AMJ, Schuerman JA, van Eek H, Groenman NH, Bremer JJCB 1989 Chronic pain and the three-systems model of emotions. A critical examination. Critical Reviews in Physical and Rehabilitation Medicine 2: 67–76

Vlaeyen JWS, Kole-Snijders AMJ, Boeren RGB, van Eek H 1995a Fear of movement/(re)injury in chronic low back pain and its relation to behavioural performance. Pain 62: 363–372

Vlaeyen JWS, Kole-Snijders AMJ, Rotteveel A, Ruesink R, Heuts PHTG 1995b The role of fear of movement/(re)injury in pain disability. Journal of Occupational Rehabilitation 5: 235–252

Vlaeyen JWS, Seelen HAM, Peters M, De Jong P, Aretz E, Beisiegel E, Weber, W 1999a Fear of movement/(re)injury and muscular reactivity in chronic low back pain patients: an experimental investigation. Pain 82: 297–304

Vlaeyen JWS, de Jong J, Geilen M, Heuts PGHT, Van Breukelen G 2001 Graded exposure in the treatment of pain-related fear: a replicated single case experimental design in patients with chronic low back pain. Beh Res Ther 39: 151–66

Von Korff M 1996 A research program for primary care pain management: back pain. In: Campbell JN (ed) Pain — an Updated Review. IASP Press, Seattle 457–465

Waddell G, Newton M, Henderson I, Somerville D, Main C 1993 A Fear-Avoidance Beliefs Questionnaire (FABQ) and the role of fear-avoidance beliefs in chronic low back pain and disability. Pain 52: 157–168

Watson D, Clark LA 1984 Negative affectivity: the disposition to experience aversive emotional states. Psychological Bulletin 96: 465–490

Watson D, Pennebaker JW 1989 Health complaints, stress, and distress: exploring the central role of negative affect. Psychology Review 96: 234–254

POSTSCRIPT

The fear-avoidance model presented in our article has been further elaborated by empirical research. The conclusions can be summarized as follows: first that studies support the idea that the relationship between pain-related fear and self-reported pain is mediated by attentional processes; secondly, that more empirical evidence supports the efficiency of graded-exposure *in vivo* treatment in the treatment of CLBP patients who report substantial fear of movement/(re)injury; and thirdly, there is growing evidence that some health-care providers may be fearful of engaging their CLBP patients in physical activity, and that this may have an impact on the treatment process.

1. ATTENTION MEDIATES BETWEEN PAIN-RELATED FEAR AND SELF-REPORTED PAIN

Probably the most important function of anxiety is to facilitate the early detection of potentially threatening situations. In line with this reasoning, highly anxious individuals demonstrate hypervigilance. Hypervigilance for threatening information is the inclination to attend selectively to threat-related rather than neutral stimuli. In laboratory studies with healthy subjects and experimentally induced pain stimuli, there is evidence that the role of anxiety on pain perception is mediated by attentional processes (Arntz et al 1994; Eccleston and Crombez 1999; Keogh et al 2001). There is very little research that has directly examined hypervigilance in pain patients who report pain-related fear (Asmundson et al 1997). Crombez et al (1996) and Eccleston et al (1997) used a primary task paradigm, in which subjects were requested to direct the attentional focus towards a mental task while receiving painful stimuli. Degradation in task performance in a mental task was also taken as an index of attentional interference due to body hypervigilance. These researchers found that disruption of attentional performance was most pronounced in chronic pain patients who reported pain-related

fear, somatic awareness and high pain intensity. Using a more direct body scanning reaction time paradigm in our laboratory, we found that the latency in detecting non-noxious electrical stimuli to various body sites was predicted by pain-related fear in both fibromyalgia (Peters et al 2000) and chronic low back pain (Peters et al 2002).

2. GRADED EXPOSURE *IN VIVO* WITH BEHAVIOURAL EXPERIMENTS FOR PAIN-RELATED FEAR

In an analogy with the treatment of phobias, the efficacy of graded exposure to back-stressing movements has been tested for back pain patients reporting substantial fear of movement/(re)injury. A detailed description of the exposure *in vivo* protocol can be found in Vlaeyen et al 2002a. In the first experiment, four consecutive patients with high fear of movement/(re)injury (Tampa Scale for Kinesiophobia score > 40), were randomly assigned to one of two interventions (Vlaeyen et al 2001). In intervention A, patients received the exposure first, followed by operant graded activity. In intervention B, the sequence of treatment modules was reversed. Daily measures of pain-related cognitions and fears were recorded with visual analogue scales. Using time series analysis, we found that improvements occurred during the exposure *in vivo*, and not during the graded activity. Further analysis of the pre–post treatment differences also revealed that decreases in pain-related fear concurred with decreases in pain catastrophizing and pain disability. In a similar subsequent study (Vlaeyen et al 2002b), patients also carried an ambulatory activity monitor at home for 1 week after each treatment module. Results were identical to those of the previous study. In addition, this study revealed that improvements concurred with decreases in pain vigilance, and an increase in physical activity as measured with an ambulatory activity monitor. As the exposure in the two previous studies was embedded within a multidisciplinary treatment programme, the results may be confounded. However, this is unlikely as two other recent studies have supported the efficacy of exposure *in vivo* as a single treatment (Vlaeyen et al 2002c; Linton et al 2002a). Finally, studies have started to disentangle the underlying processes of exposure in order to optimize treatment effects. Crombez et al (2002), and Goubert et al (2002) have shown that during exposure, patients are reluctant to change their general belief that back stressing movements hurt and are harmful. Patients rather accept exceptions ('This particular movement does not cause any harm, but all the others do.'). In order to maximize generalization of extinction, it is recommended that exposure treatment is conducted in several different contexts, varying the specific movements, and that exposure sessions are distributed widely over time.

3. ARE HEALTH-CARE PROVIDERS FEARFUL?

What are the origins of catastrophic beliefs about pain and pain-related fear in patients with chronic musculoskeletal pain? Fears can originate from traumatic experience. CLBP patients who retrospectively reported a sudden traumatic pain onset, scored higher on the TSK than patients who reported that the pain complaints started gradually (Vlaeyen et al 1995a). Additionally, there is evidence that a large percentage of people with chronic musculoskeletal pain meet DSM-IV criteria for post-traumatic stress disorder(Asmundson et al 1998). Fearful appraisals about pain may be fuelled by intense, unexpected and novel bodily sensations. There are other sources as well. Pain-related fear may also be influenced by external information from the social environment. Significant others, including health-care providers, may verbally and nonverbally convey the message that there might be something dangerously wrong with the back. It is likely that this threatening information will be incorporated into the individual's personal beliefs and convictions. Rainville (1995) conjectured that 'Patients' attitudes and beliefs [and thereby patients' disability levels] may be derived from the projected attitudes and beliefs of health care providers'. Empirical studies seem to support this idea. A recent study showed that therapists with a biomechanical view on back pain scored daily physical activities as more harmful, and were less likely to recommend return to daily life activities compared with the more behaviourally oriented therapists. This suggests that some health-care providers are also fearful about their patients being vulnerable to re-injuring themselves (Houben et al in press). Health-care providers with higher levels of such fears also have an increased risk for believing sick leave to be a good treatment, not providing good information about activities, and being uncertain about identifying patients at risk for developing persistent pain problems(Linton et al 2002b).

REFERENCES

Arntz A, Dreessen L, De Jong P 1994 The influence of anxiety on pain: attentional and attributional mediators. Pain 56(3): 307–14.

Asmundson GJ, Kuperos JL, Norton GR 1997 Do patients with chronic pain selectively attend to pain-related information?: preliminary evidence for the mediating role of fear. Pain 72(1–2): 27–32

Asmundson GJ, Norton GR, Allerdings MD, Norton PJ, Larsen DK 1998 Posttraumatic stress disorder and work-related injury. Journal of Anxiety Disorders 12(1): 57–69.

Crombez G, Eccleston C, Baeyens F, Eelen P 1996 The disruptive nature of pain: an experimental investigation. Behaviour Research Therapy 34(11–12): 911–918.

Crombez G, Eccleston C, Vansteenwegen D, Vlaeyen JWS, Lysens R, Eelen P 2002Exposure to movement in low back pain patients: restricted effects of generalisation. Health Psychology 2002 21: 573–8

Eccleston C, Crombez G 1999 Pain demands attention: a cognitive-affective model of the interruptive function of pain. Psychological Bulletin 125(3): 356–366.

Eccleston C, Crombez G, Aldrich S, Stannard C 1997 Attention and somatic awareness in chronic pain. Pain 72(1–2): 209–215

Goubert L, Francken G, Crombez G, Vansteenwegen D, Lysens R 2002 Exposure to physical movement in chronic back pain patients: no evidence for generalization across different movements. Behaviour Research Therapy 40(4) :415–29

Houben RMA, Ostelo RWJG, Vlaeyen JWS, Wolters PMJC, Peters ML, Stomp-van den Berg SGM. Health care providers' orientations towards common low back pain predict perceived harmfulness of physical activities and recommendations regarding return to normal activity. The Clinical Journal of Pain (in press)

Keogh E, Ellery D, Hunt C, Hannent I 2001 Selective attentional bias for pain-related stimuli amongst pain fearful individuals. Pain 91(1–2): 91–100

Linton SJ, Overmeer T, Janson M, Vlaeyen JWS, de Jong JR 2002a Graded in vivo exposure treatment for fear-avoidant pain patients with functional disability: a case study. Cognitive Behaviour Therapy 31(2): 49–58

Linton SJ, Vlaeyen J, Ostelo R 2002b The back pain beliefs of health care providers: Are we fear-avoidant? Journal of Occupational Rehabilitation 12(4): 223–232

Peters ML, Vlaeyen JW, van Drunen C 2000 Do fibromyalgia patients display hypervigilance for innocuous somatosensory stimuli? Application of a body scanning reaction time paradigm. Pain 86(3): 283–292

Peters ML, Vlaeyen JW, Kunnen AM 2002 Is pain-related fear a predictor of somatosensory hypervigilance in chronic low back pain patients? Behaviour Research Therapy 40(1): 85–103

Rainville J, Bagnall D, Phalen L 1995 Health care providers' attitudes and beliefs about functional impairments and chronic back pain. Clinical Journal of Pain 11(4): 287–295

Vlaeyen JWS, de Jong JR, Sieben JM, Crombez G 2002a Graded exposure in vivo for pain-related fear. In: Turk DC, Gatchel RJ (eds) Psychological Approaches to Pain Management. A Practitioner's Handbook. 2nd ed. New York, Guilford, pp210–233

Vlaeyen JW, de Jong J, Geilen M, Heuts PH, van Breukelen G 2001 Graded exposure in vivo in the treatment of pain-related fear: a replicated single-case experimental design in four patients with chronic low back pain. Behaviour Research Therapy 39(2): 151–166

Vlaeyen JW, De Jong J, Geilen M, Heuts PH, Van Breukelen G 2002b The treatment of fear of movement/(re)injury in chronic low back pain: further evidence on the effectiveness of exposure in vivo. Clinical Journal of Pain 18(4): 251–261

Vlaeyen JWS, de Jong JR, Onghena P, Kerckhoffs-Hanssen M, Kole–Snijders AMJ 2002c Can pain-related fear be reduced? The application of cognitive-behavioral exposure in vivo. Pain Res Manag 7: 144–153

Vlaeyen JW, Kole-Snijders AM, Boeren RG, van Eek H 1995a Fear of movement/(re)injury in chronic low back pain and its relation to behavioral performance. Pain 62(3): 363–72

Index